Practical Nursing

Introduction to Practical Nursing, Pharmacology Math, and Drug Dosage and Therapy

Subcourses MD0905 & MD0906

Edition 100

Practical Nursing

Introduction to Practical Nursing, Pharmacology Math, and Drug Dosage and Therapy

Subcourses MD0905 & MD0906

Edition 100

Practical Nursing: Introduction to Practical Nursing, Pharmacology Math, and Drug Dosage and Therapy

PharmaLogika

PharmaLogika, Inc.
PO Box 461
Willow Springs, NC 27592

www.pharmalogika.com

PharmaLogika Books is an imprint of PharmaLogika, Inc.

Author / Editor: Mindy J. Allport-Settle

Published by PharmaLogika, Inc.

Printed in the United States of America.

ISBN 1-9372580-2-5
ISBN-13 978-1-937258-02-3

Contents

Pharmacology Math

Introduction to Practical Nursing

Drug Dosage and Therapy

Overview

About this Book

The United States Army is recognized internationally as the standard for complete, efficient and effective adult education. The Army has a tradition of pioneering training systems (including computer-based training) that then transition into the corporate sector.

This manual has been continuously tested and updated to successfully educate every member of the modern United States Army. The needs of the instructor, the student, and the Army are perfectly balanced. This is the model all educators strive to follow when developing and delivering training programs.

Included Documents and Features

Pharmacology Math

1. Basic Math
    - Section I. Basic Arithmetic
    - Section II. Fractions
    - Section III. Decimals
    - Section IV. Percentages
    - Section V. Ratio and Proportion
2. Pharmacology
    - Section I. Ratio and Proportion Operations
    - Section II. Systems of Measurement
    - Section III. Computing Medication Dosages
    - Section IV. Computing Intravenous Infusion Rates
    - Section V. Basic Dose Calculations

Introduction to Practical Nursing

1. The Practical Nurse in the AMEDD
   - Section I. Review of the AMEDD
   - Section II. The Role of the M6
2. The M6 Practical Nurse Course
   - Section I. The Resident Course
   - Section II. The Practical Nurse Preparatory Correspondence Course
3. Duties and Responsibilities of the M6 Practical Nurse
   - Section I. Clinical Duties and Responsibilities of the Practical Nurse
   - Section II. Managerial Duties and Responsibilities of the M6 Practical Nurse

Drug Dosage and Therapy

1. Dosage Calculations
   - Section I. Interpreting Medical Orders
   - Section II. Ratio and Proportion
   - Section III. The Metric System
   - Section IV. The Apothecary System
   - Section V. Conversions
   - Section VI. Percentage Solutions
   - Section VII. Injection Dose Calculations
   - Section VIII. Pediatric Dose Calculations
2. Basic Pharmacology; Antiseptics and Disinfectants; Other Topical Drugs; Gastrointestinal Agents; Respiratory Drugs; Local Anesthetics
   - Section I. Introduction to Pharmacology
   - Section II. Antiseptics and Disinfectants
   - Section III. Other Topical Drugs
   - Section IV. Antacids
   - Section V. Cathartics
   - Section VI. Antidiarrheals
   - Section VII. Respiratory Drugs
   - Section VIII. Local Anesthetics

3. Central Nervous System Drugs
   - Section I. The Central Nervous System
   - Section II. Sedative-Hypnotics
   - Section III. Antipsychotic Tranquilizers and Related Antidepressants
   - Section IV. Narcotic Analgesics
   - Section V. Nonaddictive Analgesics and Antipyretics
   - Section VI. CNS Stimulants
4. Autonomic and Cardiovascular Drugs
   - Section I. The Autonomic Nervous System
   - Section II. Anticholinergic (Parasympatholytic) Drugs
   - Section III. Adrenergic (Sympathomimetic) Drugs
   - Section IV. Vasodilator Drugs
   - Section V. Fluid and Electrolyte Therapy
   - Section VI. Antihistamines
   - Section VII. Other Agents
5. Drugs Used to Prevent and Treat Infection I
   - Section I. Microbiology
   - Section II. Biologicals (Immunizing Agents)
   - Section III. Penicillins and Cephalosporins; Erythromycin
   - Section IV. Tetracyclines
6. Drugs Used to Prevent and Treat Infection II
   - Section I. Aminoglycosides
   - Section II. Sulfonamides
   - Section III. Antifungal Agents
   - Section IV. Antimalarial Drugs
   - Section V. Anthelmintic Drugs
   - Section VI. Other Agents

Exercises to Support Each Section

Introduction

As a member of the Army Nurse Corps, your role as an Army Officer will afford you the chance to care for your patients in a variety of settings. Army Nurses have autonomy to practice nursing in a way that is unmatched by civilian health care facilities. Your professional judgment will be the driving force behind leading your nursing team to provide full spectrum patient care.

The Army Nurse Corps believes in a holistic nursing philosophy. You'll identify and organize multi-disciplinary resources for patients and their families to help them with inpatient, outpatient and home care. You'll be able to understand the special concerns and needs of your Soldier patients because you're also a Soldier, which allows you to better serve them. Identifying with your fellow Soldiers is essential to providing effective health care. Explore your options in the Army Nurse Corps below.

History of the Army Nurse Corps

The United States Army Nurse Corps (NC) was formally established by the U.S. Congress in 1901. It is one of the six medical Special Branches (or "Corps") of officers which – along with medical enlisted soldiers – comprise the Army Medical Department (AMEDD).

The NC is the nursing service for the U.S. Army and provides qualified nursing staff in support of the Department of Defense medical plans. This NC is composed entirely of registered nurses (RNs).

Ready, Caring, Proud

Since 1901, Army nurses have demonstrated again and again their total commitment to the highest standards of military nursing excellence. Both men and women have served as Army nurses since 1775, but the Army Nurse Corps did not become a part of the Army Medical Department until 1901. The distinguished contributions of female contract nurses during and following the

1898 Spanish-American War became the justification and demonstrated the need for a permanent female nurse corps.[1]

When the United States entered World War I in 1917, there were only 4,093 nurses on active duty. By November 1918, there were 21,460 Army nurses, with 10,000 serving overseas. During the war, nurses served primarily in base, evacuation, and mobile surgical hospitals in the United States, France, Hawaii, Puerto Rico, and the Philippines. They also provided care on hospital trains in France and transport ships carrying wounded home across the Atlantic. Approximately 270 nurses lost their lives in the conflict.

When the United States entered World War II, fewer than 7,000 nurses were on active duty. By 1945, more than 57,000 Army Nurses were assigned to hospital ships and trains, flying ambulances, field hospitals, evacuation stations, and general hospitals at home and overseas. In Europe, Army nurses assisted in developing the concept of recovery wards for immediate postoperative nursing care. Military nursing gained a greater understanding of the process of shock, blood replacement, and resuscitation. Air evacuation from the combat zone by fixed wing aircraft brought patients to definitive treatment quickly. Army flight nurses helped to establish the incredible record of only five deaths in flight per 100,000 patients.

Nurses endured hardships caring for their patients. In May 1942, with the fall of Corregidor in the Philippines, 67 Army nurses became Japanese prisoners of war. During the thirty-seven month captivity, the women endured primitive conditions and starvation rations, yet they continued to care for the ill and injured in the internment hospital. On Anzio, nurses dug their foxholes outside their tents and cared for patients under German shellfire. Their example bolstered the spirits of the soldiers who shared the same tough experience. By war's end, 215 brave nurses died for their country.

Army nurses once again played a major role in support of combat troops when President Truman ordered United States forces into Korea in June, 1950. Army nurses cared for combat troops during the landing on Inchon; the advance across the 38th parallel into North Korea; the amphibious landing on the east coast of Korea; the drive toward the Yalu River; and the retreat to the 38th parallel. Throughout the Korean War, 540 Army nurses served on the embattled peninsula.

Mobility and increased patient acuity characterized service in Vietnam. Evacuation by helicopter brought wounded to medical units located within

---

[1] Army Nurse Corps Historical Collection documents summarized by MAJ Debora Cox, Past ANC Historian (1 August 2001). Available on the U.S. Army website at: http://history.amedd.army.mil/ANCWebsite/about.html

minutes flying time of the battlefield. The UH-1H helicopter ambulance, nicknamed the "Dustoff," not only transported patient from battle locations fifty percent faster than in Korea, but also provided triage and resuscitative services for casualties. Trauma care specialization, as well as shock/trauma units, developed from this experience. The "chain of evacuation" from Vietnam was extraordinary. A soldier could be wounded on the battlefield one day and two days later be in an Army hospital in the continental United States. In Vietnam, of the nearly 5,000 Army Nurses who served in forty-four hospitals, eight women made the ultimate sacrifice for their nation.

During Operation Desert Storm, approximately 2,200 nurses served in forty-four hospitals. Two of every three nurses in the Arabian Gulf were from the Army National Guard or Army Reserves. This was the first major conflict that DEPMEDS, Deployable Medical Systems, were used. Another unique feature was that Army hospital staff coexisted with host nation personnel in fixed facilities forming joint national professional organizations. Before, during, and after the 100-hour ground war, U.S. forces sustained a disease and non-battle injury rate that was the lowest ever recorded in a conflict.

Recent years have seen Army nurses active throughout the world both in armed conflicts and humanitarian endeavors. In 1983, they supported combat troops in Grenada; in 1989 in Panama; and in 1991 in the Middle East. Since December 1995, Army nurses have been deployed with medical units in support of NATO alliance troops in Haiti, Bosnia, Herzegovina and Kosovo. Nurses have continued to serve proudly during relief efforts following natural disasters such as Hurricane Mitch in 1998. Today, the legacy of these military nurses lives on. Currently, Army nurses serve throughout the world in support of multiple military and humanitarian actions in support of the Global War On Terrorism.

The Corps' recent professional evolution reflects not only the requirement of a transformational Army, but also its expanded roles in support of the health care needs of the nation. Army nurses compete with other members of the Army Medical Department for command positions. For example, our current Chief, Major General Gale S. Pollock, is the first Army Nurse Corps Chief to be appointed a 2-star general. She is also the Commanding General of Tripler Amy Medical Center, Pacific Regional Medical Command, United States Army Pacific Surgeon and Lead Agent-TRICARE Pacific Honolulu, Hawaii.

Throughout its history, the Army Nurse Corps has earned the deep respect and gratitude of the American people because of its dedication to providing the best possible care to our soldiers and their families while serving our country in war and peace. Army nurses have unselfishly come to the aid of victims of disaster and disease throughout the world. Over time, the mission has grown broader, yet there has been one constant - the devotion of the individual nurse in providing excellent nursing care.

Today, as our soldiers stand on point for our nation, defending freedom across the globe, they can rest assured, should they get wounded or ill, an Army nurse will be by their side during their hour of need. Because any time our nation calls: "Ready, Caring, and Proud," Army nurses always respond.

Army Nurse Corps Campaign Plan

Situation

The nation's nursing shortage continues to have the potential to negatively impact the quality and safety of patient care both in civilian and military medical treatment facilities (MTF). Insufficient Army nursing capacity and in some cases low density specialties can threaten the viability of current and future AMEDD missions.[2]

The use of different nursing care delivery models in MTFs increases practice variance, limits the capability to codify evidence-based nursing practice and causes imbalanced nursing workload to workforce ratios across the AMEDD. An inability to offer innovative, flexible career programs that promote nurse retention further decrements the steadystate workforce that is needed for workforce optimization. An irrelevant long-range leader succession plan and appropriate force structure precludes optimization of key leader knowledge and skills required for organizational traction and momentum. No corporate, cohesive nurse training blueprint exists that leverages human capital asymmetric advantages such as junior nurses' capabilities to innovate in complex, uncertain environments that can mitigate gaps in technology and nursing capacity. The sustained increased demand for Army nurses is beginning to exceed the sustainable supply. As a result, Army nursing's ability to respond proactively to new and different contingencies is decreasing. Twenty-first century persistent conflicts demand fullspectrum Army nurses who are versatile in their ability to accomplish a broad range of tasks and agile thinkers who can exploit opportunities in complex environments.

Hospital-based Army Nurse Corps' medical occupational specialties and additional skill identifiers were developed for a hospital-based environment in an era where the Army was downsizing. New MOS/ASI's are required to provide the right expeditionary and interoperable capability in support of the strength of our Nation: America's Army. Emerging global trends impacting the

[2] Available for download from the U.S. Army website ar: http://armynursecorps.amedd.army.mil/campaign/campaignplanonwebpagemarch09.pdf

Army demand an analysis and optimization of the Army Nurse Corps force horizon.

Key Assumptions

- The nursing shortage is a looming public health crisis that has the potential to erode access to and quality of military health care.
- Nurses are critical to meeting the increasing healthcare needs of vulnerable populations.
- Competitive-edge strategies will attract and retain qualified nurses and nurse candidates from an increasingly diverse population.
- Nurses have a responsibility to impact needed changes in healthcare delivery systems and models of care.
- Nurses function as partners in an interdisciplinary healthcare delivery system.
- Current and future military healthcare delivery systems demand predictive models that delineate required nursing capacities and capabilities.
- Current and future changes in nursing workload texture demand measurement systems that capture workload quality and quantity; promote nurse staffing models and improve nursing care performance improvement.

Purpose

This Army Nurse Corps Campaign Plan establishes priorities for the Corps and codifies campaign planning as the systematic process for blueprinting the future.

Major improvements in agility often require new work systems, simplification of work processes, or an ability to rapidly change direction towards improvement. Subsequently, a major long-term investment associated with nursing care excellence is the investment in creating and sustaining an assessment system focused on outcomes.

The priorities drive strategic planning and are conducted to nest with the AMEDD's and Army's mission and vision. These priorities include measures of effectiveness ("are we doing the right things") and measures of performance ("are we doing things right") that indicate when the priority has been accomplished and becomes sustainable. On receipt of this Plan, all Action

Officers will form a process action team to develop their strategy and way ahead. The strategy must include resources required, designated benchmarks (date or condition), priority or enabling tasks identified, and a timeline for execution.

The plan is evaluated yearly by the ANC Executive Board and approved by the Chief, AN. The Deputy Chief, AN evaluates progress on the plan monthly and reports accordingly to the Chief, AN. Transparency is optimum and the Chief AN will provide updates to DSG, TSG and Congress as often as requested.

An effective Army Nurse Corps depends on the continuous measurement and analysis of performance. Subsequently, campaign planning occurs yearly to evaluate performance, codify and internalize best practices and transform key work processes and systems to achieve performance excellence.

Army Nurse Corps Campaign Plan Mission and End State

A. Mission

Task

Re-posture the Army Nurse Corps to deliver patient driven, familycentric evidence-based nursing care; provide full-spectrum leadership for professional nursing and in support of the Army Medical Department.

Purpose

Optimize Army Nursing as a key enabler for the Military Health System.

Corps Chief Intent

I intend to provide continuous, responsive and essential nurse advocacy for the AMEDD's strategic imperatives. All actions and tasks must lead and work toward promoting the wellness of Warriors, their families, and all entrusted to our care; supporting the delivery of patient and family healthcare and ultimately, positioning the Army Nurse Corps as a key enabler for the future of military medicine.

B. End State

In the near term, the Army Nurse Corps executed effective strategies that provided evidence-based nursing care and developed full spectrum leaders: optimized their footprint through aggressive validation of priorities; repostured the force structure to create current and future capacity and capability and maximized performance excellence. Leveraged Strategic Communication that engaged key audiences and created, strengthened, and preserved conditions favorable for the advancement of Army Nurse Corps' interests and objectives. Codified a robust clinical delivery system nested with competencies, capabilities, and evidence-based ideology. Transformed Army Nurses into Full Spectrum Leaders, agile and responsive to all conditionsbased missions.

In the far term, the Army Nurse Corps codified and internalized best organizational strategies that provided a relentless focus on organizational improvement, agility and responsiveness.

In the long term, the Army Nurse Corps consistently achieved performance excellence, fostered innovation, built knowledge and capabilities, and insured organizational credibility and sustainability.

Campaign Plan Objectives

Leader Development: "Build our bench"

A persistent, sustainable nurse leader succession plan created full-spectrum leaders who were adaptive to any conditions-based mission; provided a persuasive voice at key echelons of influence in the AMEDD, and innovated doctrine to blueprint the future of the Army Nurse Corps.

Warrior Care: "Back to basics"

Optimized nursing care delivery systems that wrapped nursing capability around AMEDD strategic goals and mission; Warrior/patient driven/family-centric care models embraced evidence-based practice to achieve best patient outcomes.

Evidence-based Management: "Optimize performance"

Evidence-based methodology optimized business practices and cost-capabilities by blending analysis, measuring, and re-designing into daily performance.

Human Capital: "Portfolio of Expertise"

The Army Nurse Corps footprint is optimized through validation of priorities and the force structure is repostured for conditions-based capability and capacity.

Army Nursing Team Creed

I am a member of the Army Nursing Team[3]

- My patients depend on me and trust me to provide compassionate and proficient care always.
- I nurture the most helpless and vulnerable and offer courage and hope to those in despair.
- I protect the dignity of every individual put in my charge.
- I tend to the physical and psychological wounds of our Warriors and support the health, safety, and welfare of every retired Veteran.
- I am an advocate for family members who support and sustain their Soldier during times of War.
- It is a privilege to care for each of these individuals and I will always strive to be attentive and respectful of their needs and honor their uniquely divine human spirit.

We are the Army Nursing Team

- We honor our professional practice standards and live the Soldier values.
- We believe strength and resiliency in difficult times is the cornerstone of Army Nursing.
- We embrace the diversity of our team and implicitly understand that we must maintain a unified, authentically positive culture and support each other's physical, social, and environmental well-being.
- We have a collective responsibility to mentor and foster the professional growth of our newest Team members so they may mentor those who follow.
- We remember those nursing professionals who came before us and honor their legacy, determination, and sacrifice.
- We are fundamentally committed to provide exceptional care to past, present, and future generations who bravely defend and protect our Nation.
- The Army Nursing Team: Courage to Care, Courage to Connect, Courage to Change

[3] LTC Leigh McGraw

Health Care Ethics

Health care ethics (also known as *medical ethics*) is a system of moral principles that apply values and judgments to the practice of medicine. As a scholarly discipline, medical ethics encompasses its practical application in clinical settings as well as work on its history, philosophy, theology, and sociology.

History

Historically, Western medical ethics may be traced to guidelines on the duty of physicians in antiquity, such as the Hippocratic Oath, and early rabbinic and Christian teachings. In the medieval and early modern period, the field is indebted to Muslim medicine such as Ishaq bin Ali Rahawi (who wrote the Conduct of a Physician, the first book dedicated to medical ethics) and Muhammad ibn Zakariya ar-Razi (known as Rhazes in the West), Jewish thinkers such as Maimonides, Roman Catholic scholastic thinkers such as Thomas Aquinas, and the case-oriented analysis (casuistry) of Catholic moral theology. These intellectual traditions continue in Catholic, Islamic and Jewish medical ethics.

By the 18th and 19th centuries, medical ethics emerged as a more self-conscious discourse. For instance, authors such as Thomas Percival wrote about "medical jurisprudence" and reportedly coined the phrase "medical ethics." Percival's guidelines related to physician consultations have been criticized as being excessively protective of the home physician's reputation. Jeffrey Berlant is one such critic who considers Percival's codes of physician consultations as being an early example of the anti-competitive, "guild"-like nature of the physician community.[4, 5] In 1847, the American Medical Association adopted its first code of ethics, with this being based in large part upon Percival's work.[6] While the secularized field borrowed largely from Catholic medical ethics, in the 20th century a distinctively liberal Protestant approach was articulated by thinkers such as Joseph Fletcher. In the 1960s and 1970s, building upon liberal theory and procedural justice, much of the discourse of medical ethics went through a dramatic shift and largely reconfigured itself into bioethics.[7]

---

[4] Berlant, Jeffrey (1975). Profession and Monopoly: a study of medicine in the United States and Great Britain. University of California Press. ISBN 0520027345. http://www.pubmedcentral.nih.gov/articlerender.fcgi?artid=1081816.

[5] Percival, Thomas (1849). Medical ethics. John Henry Parker. pp. 49–57 esp section 8 pg.52. http://books.google.com/?id=yVUEAAAAQAAJ&printsec=frontcover&dq=medical+ethics.

[6] Lakhan SE, Hamlat E, McNamee T, Laird C (2009). "Time for a unified approach to medical ethics." Philosophy, Ethics, and Humanities in Medicine 4 (3): 13. doi:10.1186/1747-5341-4-13. PMC 2745426. PMID 19737406. http://www.pubmedcentral.nih.gov/articlerender.fcgi?tool=pmcentrez&artid=2745426.

[7] Walter, Klein eds. The Story of Bioethics: From seminal works to contemporary explorations.

Since the 1970s, the growing influence of ethics in contemporary medicine can be seen in the increasing use of Institutional Review Boards to evaluate experiments on human subjects, the establishment of hospital ethics committees, the expansion of the role of clinician ethicists, and the integration of ethics into many medical school curricula.[8]

Values in Medical Ethics

Six of the values that commonly apply to medical ethics discussions are:

1. **Autonomy** - the patient has the right to refuse or choose their treatment. (*Voluntas aegroti suprema lex.*)

2. **Beneficence** - a practitioner should act in the best interest of the patient. (*Salus aegroti suprema lex.*)

3. **Non-maleficence** - "first, do no harm" (*primum non nocere*).

4. **Justice** - concerns the distribution of scarce health resources, and the decision of who gets what treatment (*fairness and equality*).

5. **Dignity** - the patient (and the person treating the patient) have the right to dignity.

6. **Truthfulness and honesty** - the concept of informed consent has increased in importance since the historical events of the Doctors' Trial of the Nuremberg trials and Tuskegee Syphilis Study.

Values such as these do not give answers as to how to handle a particular situation, but provide a useful framework for understanding conflicts.

When moral values are in conflict, the result may be an ethical dilemma or crisis. Sometimes, no good solution to a dilemma in medical ethics exists, and occasionally, the values of the medical community (i.e., the hospital and its staff) conflict with the values of the individual patient, family, or larger non-medical community. Conflicts can also arise between health care providers, or among family members. Some argue for example, that the principles of autonomy and beneficence clash when patients refuse blood transfusions, considering them life-saving; and truth-telling was not emphasized to a large extent before the HIV era.

---

[8] Lakhan SE, Hamlat E, McNamee T, Laird C (2009). "Time for a unified approach to medical ethics." Philosophy, Ethics, and Humanities in Medicine 4 (3): 13. doi:10.1186/1747-5341-4-13. PMC 2745426. PMID 19737406. http://www.pubmedcentral.nih.gov/articlerender.fcgi?tool=pmcentrez&artid=2745426.

Army Medical Command

The U.S. Army Medical Command (MEDCOM) is a major command of the U.S. Army that provides command and control of the Army's fixed-facility medical, dental, and veterinary treatment facilities, providing preventive care, medical research and development and training institutions.

Structure and Subordinate Commands

MEDCOM is divided into Regional Medical Commands that oversee day-to-day operations in military treatment facilities, exercising command and control over the medical treatment facilities in their regions. There are currently five of these regional commands:

- Europe Regional Medical Command
- Southern Regional Medical Command
- Northern Regional Medical Command
- Pacific Regional Medical Command
- Western Regional Medical Command.

Additional subordinate commands of MEDCOM include:

- Army Medical Department Center & School (AMEDDC&S)
- U.S. Army Public Health Command (Provisional), (known as the U.S. Army Center for Health Promotion & Preventive Medicine prior to 1 October 2009 {USACHPPM or CHPPM})
- U.S. Army Medical Research and Materiel Command (USAMRMC)
- Warrior Transition Command (WTC)
- U.S. Army Dental Command (DENCOM)

Operations

In Garrison (Peacetime)

MEDCOM maintains day-to-day health care for soldiers, retired soldiers and the families of both. Despite the wide range of responsibilities involved in providing health care in traditional settings as well as on the battlefield, the Army Medical Department's quality of care compares very favorably with that of civilian health organizations, when measured by civilian standards. Many Army medical facilities report on their own quality-of-care standards on their individual Internet sites.

Deployments

When Army field hospitals deploy, most clinical professional and support personnel come from MEDCOM's fixed facilities. In addition to support of combat operations, deployments can be for humanitarian assistance, peacekeeping, and other stability and support operations. Under the Professional Officer Filler System (PROFIS), up to 26 percent of MEDCOM physicians and 43 percent of MEDCOM nurses are sent to field units during a full deployment. To replace PROFIS losses, Reserve units and Individual Mobilization Augmentees (non-unit reservists) are mobilized to work in medical treatment facilities. The department also provides trained medical specialists to the Army's combat medical units, which are assigned directly to combatant commanders.

Many Army Reserve and Army National Guard units deploy in support of the Army Medical Department. The Army depends heavily on its Reserve component for medical support—about 63 percent of the Army's medical forces are in the Reserve component.

Army Medical Department

The Army Medical Department of the U.S. Army (AMEDD) comprises the Army's six medical Special Branches (or "Corps") of officers and medical enlisted soldiers. It was established as the "Army Hospital" in July 1775 to coordinate the medical care required by the Continental Army during the Revolutionary War. The AMEDD is led by the Surgeon General of the U.S. Army, a lieutenant general.

The AMEDD is the U.S. Army's healthcare organization, not a U.S. Army command. The AMEDD is found in all three components of the Army: the Active Army, the U.S. Army Reserve, and the Army National Guard. Its headquarters are at Fort Sam Houston, San Antonio, Texas, which hosts the AMEDD Center and School. Equal numbers of AMEDD senior leaders can be found in Washington D.C., divided between the Pentagon and the Walter Reed Army Medical Center (WRAMC).

The Academy of Health Sciences, under the Army Medical Department Center & School, provides training to the officers and enlisted soldiers of the AMEDD. As a result of BRAC 2005, enlisted medical training was transferred to the new Medical Education and Training Campus, consolidating most military enlisted medical training at Fort Sam Houston.[9]

Medical Special Branches

- Medical Corps (MC)
- Nurse Corps (AN)
- Dental Corps (DC)
- Veterinary Corps (VC)
- Medical Service Corps (MS)
- Medical Specialist Corps (AMSC)

United States Army Training and Doctrine Command

Established 1 July 1973, the United States Army Training and Doctrine Command (TRADOC) is an army command of the United States Army headquartered at Fort Monroe, Virginia. It is charged with overseeing training of Army forces, the development of operational doctrine, and the development and procurement of new weapons systems. TRADOC operates 33 schools and centers at 16 Army installations. TRADOC schools conduct 2,734 courses (81 directly in support of mobilization) and 373 language courses. The 2,734 courses include 503,164 seats for 434,424 soldiers; 34,675 other-service personnel; 7,824 international soldiers; and 26,241 civilians.[10]

TRADOC MissionThe official mission statement for TRADOC states:

> TRADOC develops the Army's Soldiers and Civilian leaders and designs, develops and integrates capabilities, concepts and doctrine in order to build a campaign-capable, expeditionary Army in support of joint warfighting capability through Army Force Generation (ARFORGEN).[11]

---

[9] U.S. Army Medical Department AMEDD Center and School Portal available on the Internet at: http://www.cs.amedd.army.mil/. Additional information specific to the Fort Sam Houston consolidation is available n the Internet at: http://www.aetc.af.mil/shared/media/document/AFD-071026-035.pdf

[10] TRADOC fact sheet available at: http://www.tradoc.army.mil/about.htm

[11] TRADOC commander on ARFORGEN, and the US Army available at: http://www.tradoc.army.mil/about.htm

TRADOC is the official command component that is responsible for training and developing the United States Army.

TRADOC History

TRADOC was established as a major U.S. Army command on 1 July 1973. The new command, along with the U.S. Army Forces Command (FORSCOM), was created from the Continental Army Command (CONARC) located at Fort Monroe, VA. That action was the major innovation in the Army's post-Vietnam reorganization, in the face of realization that CONARC's obligations and span of control were too broad for efficient focus. The new organization functionally realigned the major Army commands in the continental United States. CONARC, and Headquarters, U.S. Army Combat Developments Command (CDC), situated at Fort Belvoir, VA, were discontinued, with TRADOC and FORSCOM at Fort Belvoir assuming the realigned missions. TRADOC assumed the combat developments mission from CDC, took over the individual training mission formerly the responsibility of CONARC, and assumed command from CONARC of the major Army installations in the United States housing Army training center and Army branch schools. FORSCOM assumed CONARC's operational responsibility for the command and readiness of all divisions and corps in the continental U.S. and for the installations where they were based.

Joined under TRADOC, the major Army missions of individual training and combat developments each had its own lineage. The individual training responsibility had belonged, during World War II, to Headquarters Army Ground Forces (AGF). In 1946 numbered Army areas were established in the U.S. under AGF command. At that time, the AGF moved from Washington, D.C. to Fort Monroe, VA. In March 1948, the AGR was replaced at Fort Monroe with the new Office, Chief of Army Field Forces (OCAFF). OCAFF, however, did not command the training establishment. That function was exercised by Headquarters, Department of the Army through the numbered Armies to the corps, division, and Army Training Centers. In February 1955, HQ Continental Army Command (CONARC) replaced OCAFF, assuming its missions as well as the training missions from DA. In January, HQ CONARC was redesignated U.S. Continental Army Command. Combat developments emerged as a formal Army mission in the early 1950s, and OCAFF assumed that role in 1952. In 1955, CONARC assumed the mission. In 1962, HQ U.S. Army Combat Development Command (CDC) was established to bring the combat developments function under one major Army command.[12]

[12] TRADOC history available at: http://www.tradoc.army.mil/about.htm

TRADOC Priorities

1. Leader Development
2. Initial Military Training
3. Concepts and Capabilities Integration
4. Human Capital Enterprise
5. Army Training and Learning Concept
6. Doctrine

This page intentionally left blank.

Pharmacology Math for the Practical Nurse

Subcourse MD0904

This page intentionally left blank.

U.S. ARMY MEDICAL DEPARTMENT CENTER AND SCHOOL
FORT SAM HOUSTON, TEXAS 78234-6100

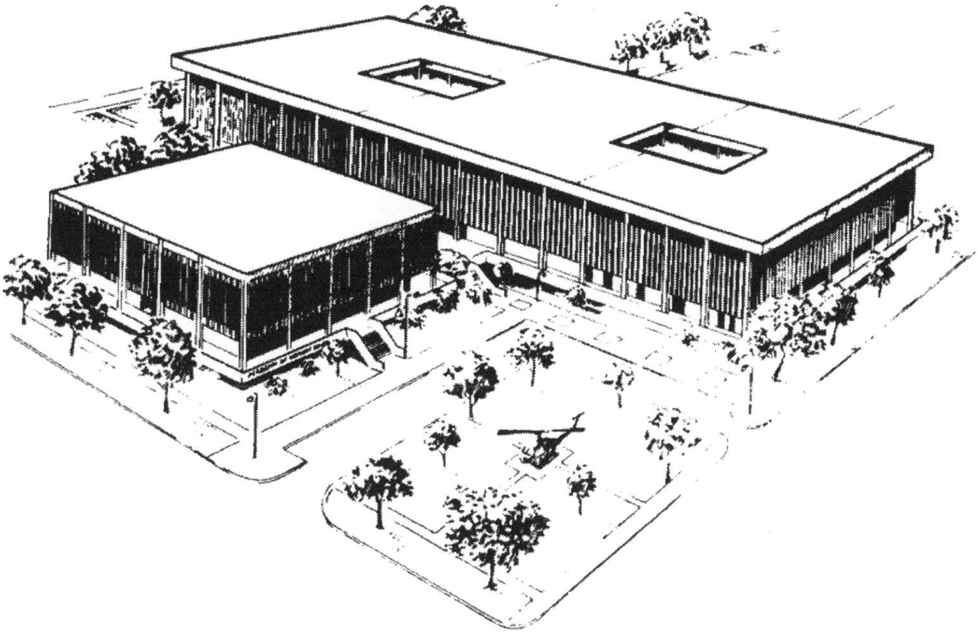

PHARMACOLOGY MATH FOR THE PRACTICAL NURSE

SUBCOURSE MD0904 EDITION 100

DEVELOPMENT

This subcourse is approved for resident and correspondence course instruction. It reflects the current thought of the Academy of Health Sciences and conforms to printed Department of the Army doctrine as closely as currently possible. Development and progress render such doctrine continuously subject to change.

ADMINISTRATION

For comments or questions regarding enrollment, student records, or shipments, contact the Nonresident Instruction Section at DSN 471-5877, commercial (210) 221-5877, toll-free 1-800-344-2380; fax: 210-221-4012 or DSN 471-4012, e-mail accp@amedd.army.mil, or write to:

COMMANDER
AMEDDC&S
ATTN MCCS HSN
2105 11TH STREET SUITE 4192
FORT SAM HOUSTON TX 78234-5064

Approved students whose enrollments remain in good standing may apply to the Nonresident Instruction Section for subsequent courses by telephone, letter, or e-mail.

Be sure your social security number is on all correspondence sent to the Academy of Health Sciences.

CLARIFICATION OF TRAINING LITERATURE TERMINOLOGY

When used in this publication, words such as "he," "him," "his," and "men" are intended to include both the masculine and feminine genders, unless specifically stated otherwise or when obvious in context.

TABLE OF CONTENTS

SUBCOURSE MD0904

Pharmacology Math for the Practical Nurse

INTRODUCTION

One of the 91WM6's most important responsibilities is the safe administration of medication. Used intelligently and accurately, drugs can surely save countless numbers of lives; used unwisely, they can have disastrous results. It is imperative that you have a thorough understanding of the basic concepts of math as well as the specific mathematical skills required for pharmaceutical calculations.

Subcourse Components:

This subcourse consists of two lessons and a pretest. The lessons and pretest are:

Lesson 1 Pretest.

Lesson 1, Basic Math.

Lesson 2, Pharmacology.

Credit Awarded:

To receive credit hours, you must be officially enrolled and complete an examination furnished by the Nonresident Instruction Section at Fort Sam Houston, Texas. Upon successful completion of the examination for this subcourse, you will be awarded 12 credit hours.

You can enroll by going to the web site http://atrrs.army.mil and enrolling under "Self Development" (School Code 555).

A listing of correspondence courses and subcourses available through the Nonresident Instruction Section is found in Chapter 4 of DA Pamphlet 350-59, Army Correspondence Course Program Catalog. The DA PAM is available at the following website: http://www.usapa.army.mil/pdffiles/p350-59.pdf.

PRETEST FOR LESSON 1

I. **COMMENTS**: This pretest is designed to help you identify the topics (if any) you need to review/study before going on to Lesson 2 of this subcourse.

You alone will know how you performed on the pretest. Your pretest results will not affect your score on the final examination for the subcourse.

Do your best. How well you perform on the pretest will determine how much of Lesson 1 you will need to study/review before you go on to Lesson 2.

II. **INSTRUCTIONS**: Please read and follow these instructions as closely as possible. The pay-off to you will be the wise use of your time.

STEP 1: Carefully read the instructions for the pretest.

STEP 2: Complete the 50-item pretest. Carefully read each item and write your answer in the space provided. Take as long as you need to complete the pretest.

STEP 3: Review your work. Be sure you wrote the correct answers.

STEP 4: Check your responses against the solutions following the pretest. Mark each of your responses as correct or incorrect.

STEP 5: Determine the number of items missed.

If you did not miss any items, you may skip Lesson 1 and proceed to Lesson 2.

If you missed only one or two items, read the paragraph(s) referenced to the right of the solution for each missed question to see why your answer was not correct. You may then proceed to Lesson 2.

If you missed more than two items, you should complete Lesson 1 before beginning Lesson 2.

NOTE: You may complete Lesson 1 even if you are not required to do so.

Continue with Exercises

PRETEST

NOTES

Throughout this subcourse, division may be indicated by " ÷ " or by " / " or by the phrase "divided by." For example "8 divided by 4" may be shown as " 8÷4" or "8/4."

"Divided into" may be represented by $\overline{)\quad}$. **NOTE**: 4 divided into 8 ($4\overline{)8}$) is the same as 8 divided by 4 (8 ÷ 4).

Fractions may be shown in linear (3/7) or vertical ($\frac{3}{7}$) form.

Mixed numbers (whole number plus a fraction) may be shown in linear or vertical form.

For example, 3 7/8 and $3\frac{7}{8}$. Both mean three and seven-eights.

1. $\begin{array}{r} 19 \\ +8 \\ \hline \end{array}$

2. $\begin{array}{r} 23 \\ 6 \\ +27 \\ \hline \end{array}$

3. $\begin{array}{r} 4391 \\ +3019 \\ \hline \end{array}$

4. $\begin{array}{r} 100 \\ -23 \\ \hline \end{array}$

5. $\begin{array}{r} 956 \\ -927 \\ \hline \end{array}$

6. $\begin{array}{r} 48 \\ \times 3 \\ \hline \end{array}$

7. $\begin{array}{r} 85 \\ \times 35 \\ \hline \end{array}$

8. 9873 ÷ 9 =

9. 175 ÷ 7 =

10. 2385 ÷ 25 =

11. Divide: $\frac{7}{8} \div \frac{1}{4} =$

12. Divide: $6 \div \frac{1}{3} =$

13. Multiply: $\frac{5}{6} \times \frac{2}{3} =$

14. Multiply: $8 \times \frac{2}{3} =$

15. Multiply: $2\frac{1}{2} \times 5\frac{1}{3} =$

16. Divide: $6\frac{1}{2} \div 1\frac{1}{3} =$

17. Change to a mixed number $\frac{6}{5}$ ____________

18. Change to a whole number $\frac{28}{7}$ ____________

19. Change to lowest terms $\frac{4}{8}$ ____________

20. Change to an improper fraction $2\frac{4}{5}$ ____________

21. Explain (put into words) 1.02 ______________________________

NOTE: In answering items 22 through 30, round off to the 2nd decimal point.

22. Solve: $2.5 \div 2 =$

23. Solve: $3.45 \div 10 =$

24. Solve: $15 \div 1.3 =$

25. Solve: $66 \div 2.5 =$

26. Solve: $5.75 \div 0.25 =$

27. Solve: $7.125 \times 1.3 =$

28. Solve: $6.01 \times 7 =$

29. Convert to decimals: $\frac{1}{6} =$

30. Convert to decimals: $\frac{3}{5} =$

31. Change 50% to a fraction. ____________

32. Change $3\frac{1}{2}$ % to a fraction. ____________

33. Change $\frac{1}{5}$ % to a fraction. ____________

34. Change $\frac{1}{8}$ to a percent. ____________

35. Change $\frac{1}{25}$ to a percent. ____________

36. Change 5% to a decimal. ____________

37. Change 2% to a decimal. ____________

38. Change $\frac{3}{4}$ % to a decimal. ____________

39. Change 0.1 to a percent. ____________

40. Change 0.05 to a percent. ____________

41. Write $\frac{1}{4}$ as a ratio. ____________

42. Write 1:3 as a percent. ____________ As a decimal. ____________

43. Write 1:150 as a percent. ____________ As a decimal. ____________

44. Change 10% to a ratio. ____________

45. Change 1% to a ratio. ____________

46. Change 80% to a ratio. ____________

47. Change 0.2 to a ratio. ____________

48. Change 0.025 to a ratio. ____________

49. Solve for x: 13:91 = x:14 ____________

50. Solve for z: $\frac{z}{21} = \frac{5}{12}$ ____________

Check Your Answers on Next Page

PRETEST ANSWERS

Following are the answers to the pretest you have just taken. Carefully check your pretest.

Basic Arithmetic

1. 27 (para 1-2)

2. 56 (para 1-2)

3. 7410 (para 1-2)

4. 77 (para 1-3)

5. 29 (para 1-3)

6. 144 (para 1-6)

7. 2975 (para 1-10)

8. 1097 (para 1-7)

9. 25 (para 1-7)

10. 95.4 or 95 2/5 (para 1-11)

Fractions

11. $3\frac{1}{2}$ (paras 1-26, 1-18)

12. 18 (paras 1-26, 1-18)

13. $\frac{5}{9}$ (paras 1-23, 1-18)

14. $5\frac{1}{3}$ (paras 1-24, 1-18)

15. $13\frac{1}{3}$ (paras 1-25, 1-21, 1-18)

16. $4\frac{7}{8}$ (paras 1-26, 1-21, 1-18)

17. $1\frac{1}{5}$ (para 1-18)

18. 4 (para 1-18)

19. $\frac{1}{2}$ (para 1-17)

20. $\frac{14}{5}$ (para 1-21)

Decimals

21. One and two hundredths (para 1-29)

22. 1.25 (para 1-31)

23. 0.345 = 0.35 (para 1-31)

24. 11.538 = 11.54 (para 1-31)

25. 26.4 (para 1-31)

26. 23 (para 1-31)

27. 9.2625 = 9.26 (para 1-34)

28. 42.07 (para 1-34)

29. 0.166 = 0.17 (para 1-36)

30. 0.6 (para 1-36)

Precentages

31. $\frac{50}{100} = \frac{1}{2}$ (para 1-40)

32. $\frac{7}{200}$ (para 1-40)

33. $\frac{1}{500}$ (para 1-40)

34. 12 $\frac{1}{2}$ percent or 12.5 percent (para 1-41)

35. 4 percent (para 1-41)

36. 0.05 (para 1-42)

37. 0.02 (para 1-42)

38. 0.0075 (para 1-42)

39. 10% (para 1-43)

40. 5% (para 1-43)

Ration and Proportion

41. 1:4 (para 1-46)

42. 33 $\frac{1}{3}$ percent ; 0.33 (para 1-47)

43. $\frac{2}{3}$% ; 0.0067 (para 1-47)

44. 1:10 (para 1-50)

45. 1:100 (para 1-50)

46. 4:5 (para 1-50)

47. 1:5 (para 1-51)

48. 1:40 (para 1-51)

49. x = 2 (para 1-55)

50. z = 8.75 (para 1-55)

End of Lesson 1 Pretest

LESSON ASSIGNMENT

LESSON 1 Basic Math.

TEXT ASSIGNMENT Paragraphs 1-1 through 1-57.

LESSON OBJECTIVES After completing this lesson, you should be able to:

1-1. Add, subtract, multiply, and divide whole numbers.

1-2. Reduce fractions to lowest terms.

1-3. Change improper fractions to mixed numbers or whole numbers and mixed numbers to improper fractions.

1-4. Add, subtract, multiply, and divide fractions and mixed numbers.

1-5. Add, subtract, divide, and multiply decimals.

1-6. Change decimals to fractions and fractions to decimals.

1-7. Solve problems using the ratio and proportion method.

SUGGESTION After completing the assignment, complete the exercises at the end of this lesson. These exercises will help you to achieve the lesson objectives.

LESSON 1

BASIC MATH

Section I. Basic Arithmetic

1-1. GENERAL

a. **Whole Numbers.** The number zero and the counting numbers (0, 1, 2, 3, 4, 5, 6, 7, 8, 9, 10, 11, 12, 13, 14, ...) are **whole numbers**. The first 10 whole numbers (0 through 9) are called **digits**.

b. **Powers of Ten.** Our number system is based upon the powers of ten. That is, the digit place to the immediate left of a given digit is worth ten times as much as the given digit place, and the digit place to the immediate right is worth one-tenth as much. For example, in the number 321, the one tells you how many ones (or units) are in the number, the two tells how many tens, and the three tells how many hundreds. See figure 1-1.

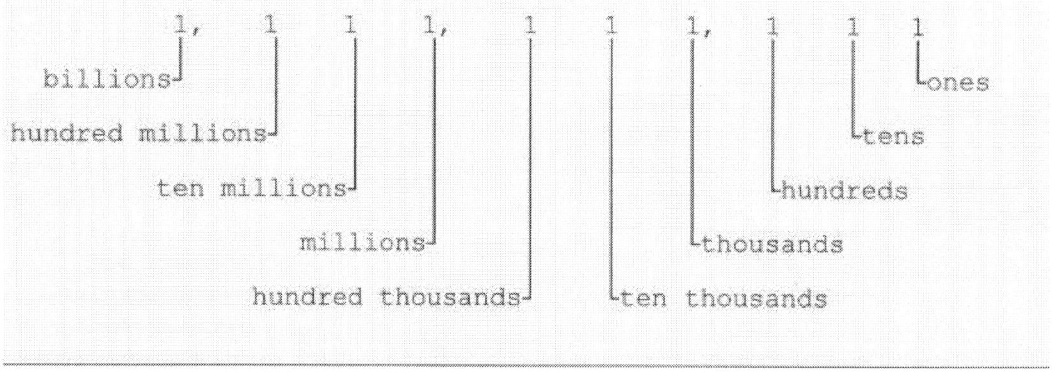

Figure 1-1. The number system.

1-2. SIMPLE ADDITION

a. The numbers to be added are the <u>addends</u>. The answer to an addition problem is the <u>sum</u>. When you are doing a problem in addition, work from right to left. Be sure to keep the columns of numbers in straight lines.

b. When you "carry" a number over to the next column to the left, you can jot it down at the top of the column.

EXAMPLE: Find the sum of 263, 19, and 1202.

```
   1           (the 1 is "carried")
  263  (addend)
   19  (addend)
+1202  (addend)
-----
 1484  (sum)
```

1-3. SIMPLE SUBTRACTION

a. The number "from which" another number is taken away is the "minuend." The number that is taken away is the "subtrahend." The answer is the "difference."

EXAMPLE: Subtract 4 from 17.

```
17 (minuend)
-4 (subtrahend)
13 (difference)
```

b. When you are doing a problem in subtraction, always remember to keep the columns of numbers in straight lines.

c. If the minuend in any column is smaller than the subtrahend, you can "borrow" from the next column to the left. This gives you ten more to work with in the right hand column but one less in the left hand column from which you have borrowed.

EXAMPLE: What is 35 minus 28?

```
 35
-28
```

To do the problem above, you have to change the 5 in the minuend to 15, and subtract 1 from 3 in the minuend.

```
 2 1 (10 is "borrowed")
 3 5
-2 8
   7
```

1-4. PRACTICE 1-1

DIRECTIONS: Complete the following problems. The answers are in paragraph 1-5 on the following page. If you miss two or more problems, review the section again before proceeding with the subcourse. Follow the same instructions for the other practice exercises in the lesson.

a. Find the sum of 29 and 13.

b. Add 8 and 49.

c. 109 + 309 =

d. Add 13, 318, and 5.

e. What is the sum of 1713 and 1694?

f. Subtract 19 from 73.

g. 83 - 47 =

h. Subtract 233 from 2011.

i. From 220, subtract 59.

j. What is 100 - 39?

1-5. ANSWERS TO PRACTICE 1-1

a.
$$\begin{array}{r} {\scriptstyle 1} \\ 29 \\ +13 \\ \hline 42 \end{array}$$

b.
$$\begin{array}{r} {}_{1}8 \\ +49 \\ \hline 57 \end{array}$$

c.
$$\begin{array}{r} {\scriptstyle 1} \\ 109 \\ +309 \\ \hline 418 \end{array}$$

d.
$$\begin{array}{r} {\scriptstyle 1} \\ 13 \\ 318 \\ +\ 5 \\ \hline 336 \end{array}$$

e.
$$\begin{array}{r} {\scriptstyle 1\,1} \\ 1713 \\ 1694 \\ \hline 3407 \end{array}$$

```
f.   6 1
      73
     -19
      54

g.   7 1
      83
     -47
      36

h.  1 9 10 1
     2 0 1 1
      - 2 3 3
     1 7 7 8

i.   1 11 1
      2 2 0
     -  5 9
      1 6 1

j.   0 9 1
      1 0 0
       - 3 9
         6 1
```

1-6. SIMPLE MULTIPLICATION

A number being multiplied is a "factor." The answer to a multiplication problem is a "product." When you multiply, a good habit is to keep the numbers in straight columns. This will help you in long multiplication problems.

EXAMPLE: Multiply 36 by 6.

```
 36 factor
x 6 factor
```

To work the problem above, follow these steps:

a. Multiply: 6 x 6 = 36. Write down the 6 and "carry" the 3.

```
 3
 36
x 6
  6
```

b. Multiply: 3 x 6 = 18. Add 3 (the number carried) to 18. 3+18 = 21.

$$\begin{array}{r} 36 \\ \underline{\times\ 6} \\ 216 \end{array}$$

1-7. SIMPLE DIVISION

a. The number "being divided" is the dividend. The number you are "dividing by" is the divisor. The answer is the quotient.

EXAMPLE:

$$\begin{array}{r} 2 \text{ (quotient)} \\ \text{(divisor) } 6\overline{)12} \text{ (dividend)} \end{array}$$

b. Anything left over is the remainder.

EXAMPLE:

$$\begin{array}{r} 2 \\ 6\overline{)13} \\ \underline{12} \\ 1 \text{ (remainder)} \end{array}$$

c. The remainder can always be written as a fraction. The remainder becomes the numerator and the divisor becomes the denominator. Thus, the remainder in the problem above is 1/6. The quotient is 2 1/6.

1-8. PRACTICE 1-2

a. What is 53 times 3?

b. Multiply 1139 x 2.

c. 209 x 6 =

d. What is the product of 27 and 8?

e. What is 120 x 7?

f. Divide 64 by 8.

g. What is the quotient when 315 is divided by 5?

h. $3\overline{)18}$

i. How many times does 8 go into 4248?

j. $4\overline{)139}$

1-9. ANSWERS TO PRACTICE 1-2

a.
$$\begin{array}{r} 53 \\ \underline{\times\ 3} \\ 159 \end{array}$$

b.
$$\begin{array}{r} {}^{1} \\ 1139 \\ \underline{\times\ 2} \\ 2278 \end{array}$$

c.
$$\begin{array}{r} {}^{5} \\ 209 \\ \underline{\times\ 6} \\ 1254 \end{array}$$

d.
$$\begin{array}{r} {}^{5} \\ 27 \\ \underline{\times\ 8} \\ 216 \end{array}$$

e.
$$\begin{array}{r} {}^{1} \\ 120 \\ \underline{\times\ 7} \\ 840 \end{array}$$

f.
$$\begin{array}{r} 8 \\ 8\overline{)64} \\ \underline{64} \\ 0 \end{array}$$

g.
$$\begin{array}{r} 63 \\ 5\overline{)315} \\ \underline{30} \\ 15 \\ \underline{15} \\ 0 \end{array}$$

h.

```
  6
3)18
  18
   0
```

i.

```
  531
8)4248
  40
   24
   24
    08
     8
     0
```

j.

```
  34 3/4
4)139
  12
   19
   16
    3
```

1-10. LONG MULTIPLICATION

a. The following procedure is used for multiplying factors with two or more digits.

EXAMPLE: Multiply 35 by 25.

```
  35 factors
x 25
 175 subproducts
 700
 875 product
```

STEPS followed in the problem above:

(1) Begin on the right and work left.

(2) First multiply 35 by 5. 5 x 5 is 25. Write down 5 in the unit column and carry the 2.

```
 2
 35
x25
  5
```

(3) 5 x 3 = 15. 15 + 2 = 17. Write down 17 to the left of the 5. The first subproduct is 175.

$$\begin{array}{r} 35 \\ \underline{\times 25} \\ 175 \end{array}$$

(4) Next, multiply 35 by 20. Place a zero in the ones (units) column and then multiply by 2. 2 x 5 = 10. Write down 0 and carry the 1.

$$\begin{array}{r} 35 \\ \underline{\times 25} \\ 175 \\ 00 \end{array}$$

(5) 2 x 3 is 6. 6 + 1 = 7. Write down 7 next to the 0. The second subproduct is 700.

$$\begin{array}{r} 35 \\ \underline{\times 25} \\ 175 \\ 700 \end{array}$$

(6) Add the two subproducts. 175 + 700 = 875. This is the product.

$$\begin{array}{r} 35 \\ \underline{\times 25} \\ 175 \\ \underline{700} \\ 875 \end{array}$$

b. When multiplying any factor by 10, 100, 1000 and so on, add to the factor the same number of zeros that are in the second factor.

EXAMPLE: Multiply 93 by 10. There is one zero in the 10.
Therefore, add one zero to 93.
93 x 10 = 930.

1-11. LONG DIVISION

There are several techniques for doing long division. You may be used to a different technique from the one shown below. If you prefer another way, use it.

EXAMPLE: Divide 875 by 25.

```
     35
25)875
   75
   125
   125
     0
```

STEPS followed in the problem above:

(1) Try to divide 25 into 87. About how many times will 25 go into 87? The answer is more than 3 but less than 4.

```
25)875
```

(2) Write down 3 in the space for the quotient, directly above the 7.

```
     3
25)875
```

(3) Now multiply 3 x 25 and write the answer under the 87. (3 x 25 = 75) Write 75 under the 87.

```
1    3
25)875
   75
```

(4) Subtract 75 from 87. The difference is 12. Write 12 directly under the 75.

```
     3
25)875
   75
   12
```

(5) Now "bring down" the 5 from the dividend. The 12 becomes 125.

```
     3
25)875
   75
   125
```

(6) Divide 125 by 25. The answer is 5. Write 5 in the space for the quotient, to the right of the 3.

```
   ___35
 25)875
    75
   125
```

(7) Multiply 5 x 25 and write the answer under the 125. (5 x 25 = 125)

```
 2 __35
 25)875
    75
   ____
    125
    125
```

(8) Subtract from 125. The difference is zero. Therefore, the quotient is exactly 35.

```
   ___35
 25)875
   75
   125
   125
     0
```

1-12. PRACTICE 1-3

a. Multiply 284 by 12. __________

b. What is the product of 310 and 219? __________

c. Multiply 112 by 82. __________

d. Multiply 527 by 277. __________

e. 331 x 105 = __________

f. Divide 612 by 12. __________

g. Divide 3928 by 491. __________

h. If 3000 is divided by 75, what is the quotient? __________

i. If 360 is divided by 25, what is the quotient? __________

j. Divide 1425 by 15. ____________

1-13. ANSWERS TO PRACTICE 1-3

a.
```
 1
   284
  x112
  ¹568
 ¹284
  3408
```

b.
```
   310
  x219
  2790
  310
 620
 67890
```

c.
```
   112
  x 82
   224
 ¹896
  9184
```

d.
```
    527
  x 277
   3689
   3689
  1054
 145979
```

e.
```
    331
  x 105
   1655
  3310
  34755
```

f.
```
      51
  12)612
     60
      12
      12
       0
```

g.
```
 7       8
  491)3928
      3928
         0
```

h.
```
       40
  75)3000
     300
      00
      00
       0
```

i.
```
      14.4 or       14     10 = 14 2
 ²25)360.0   ²25)360       25      5
     25          25
     110         110
     100         100
     100          10
     100
       0
```

j.
```
       95
  15)1425
     135
       75
       75
        0
```

Section II. FRACTIONS

1-14. DEFINITION

A fraction is less than a whole amount. A whole number may be divided into one or more equal parts. It is expressed by two numbers separated by a line.

EXAMPLES: $\frac{1}{2}$, $\frac{1}{3}$, $\frac{2}{3}$, $\frac{4}{5}$, $\frac{5}{6}$.

1-15. PARTS OF FRACTIONS

The parts of a fraction are the <u>numerator</u>, or upper number, and the <u>denominator</u>, or bottom number.

EXAMPLE: In the fraction $\frac{1}{3}$, the "1" is the numerator, and the "3" is the denominator.

1-16. KINDS OF FRACTIONS

a. A <u>proper fraction</u> has a numerator that is <u>smaller</u> than the denominator.

EXAMPLES: The fraction $\frac{1}{4}$ is a proper fraction because the numerator, "1" is smaller than the denominator. "4."

Other examples are: $\frac{1}{2}$, $\frac{3}{4}$, and $\frac{7}{8}$.

b. An improper fraction has a numerator that is <u>larger</u> than the denominator or <u>equal to</u> the denominator.

EXAMPLES: The fraction $\frac{4}{3}$ is an improper fraction because the numerator "4" is larger than the denominator "3."

Other examples are $\frac{9}{2}$, $\frac{5}{3}$, and $\frac{3}{3}$.

c. A <u>mixed number</u> is made up of a whole number and a fraction.

EXAMPLES: $2\frac{3}{4}$ is a mixed number because it has a whole number "2" and a fraction "3/4".

Other examples are: $3\frac{1}{4}$, $1\frac{1}{3}$, and 4 1/8.

1-17. CHANGING FRACTIONS TO LOWEST POSSIBLE TERMS

Some fractions can (and should) be changed (reduced) to their lowest terms. This is done by dividing the numerator and denominator by the same number. This should be the largest possible number that will go into the numerator and denominator. A fraction is said to be at its lowest terms when the numerator and denominator cannot be divided by the same number to arrive at a lower numerator and denominator.

EXAMPLE: Reduce the fraction $\frac{9}{12}$.

What number goes into 9 and 12 evenly?
The answer is 3.
Divide the numerator by 3. 9 divided by 3 = 3.

$$\frac{9}{12} = 3$$

Divide the denominator by 3. 12 divided by 3 = 4.

$$\frac{9}{12} = \frac{3}{4}$$

Therefore, $\frac{9}{12}$ can be reduced to $\frac{3}{4}$.

These two fractions are equal in value.

<u>Remember</u>, reducing does not change the value of a fraction.

1-18. CHANGING IMPROPER FRACTIONS TO MIXED NUMBERS OR WHOLE NUMBERS

Improper fractions are changed to mixed or whole numbers by dividing the numerator by the denominator.

EXAMPLES: $\frac{8}{4} = 8 \div 4 = 2$ (a whole number)

$\frac{6}{5} = 6 \div 5 = 1\frac{1}{5}$ (a mixed number)

1-19. PRACTICE 1-4

a. Identify the following as proper fractions, improper fractions, or mixed numbers:

(1) $7\frac{1}{5}$ ____________________

(2) $\frac{1}{3}$ ____________________

(3) $\frac{100}{150}$ ____________________

(4) $\frac{30}{10}$ ____________________

(5) $\frac{119}{200}$ ____________________

(6) $6\frac{1}{5}$ ____________________

b. Change these proper fractions to their lowest terms:

(1) $\frac{2}{8}$ =

(2) $\frac{25}{75}$ =

(3) $\frac{3}{9}$ =

(4) $\frac{8}{32}$ =

(5) $\frac{5}{15}$ =

(6) $\frac{6}{18}$ =

c. Change the following improper fractions to whole or mixed numbers:

(1) $\frac{4}{2}$ =

(2) $\frac{30}{5}$ =

(3) $\frac{14}{12}$ =

(4) $\frac{9}{7}$ =

(5) $\frac{15}{10}$ =

(6) $\frac{9}{6}$ =

1-20. ANSWERS TO PRACTICE 1-4

a. (1) Mixed

(2) Proper

(3) Proper

(4) Improper

(5) Proper

(6) Mixed

b. (1) $\frac{2}{8} = \frac{1}{4}$ $(2 \div 2 = 1)$ $(8 \div 2 = 4)$

(2) $\frac{25}{75} = \frac{1}{3}$ $(25 \div 25 = 1)$ $(75 \div 25 = 3)$

(3) $\frac{3}{9} = \frac{1}{3}$ $(3 \div 3 = 1)$ $(9 \div 3 = 3)$

(4) $\frac{8}{32} = \frac{1}{4}$ $(8 \div 8 = 1)$ $(32 \div 8 = 4)$

(5) $\frac{5}{15} = \frac{1}{3}$ $(5 \div 5 = 1)$ $(15 \div 5 = 3)$

(6) $\frac{6}{18} = \frac{1}{3}$ $(6 \div 6 = 1)$ $(18 \div 6 = 3)$

c. (1) $\frac{4}{2} = 2$ $(4 \div 2 = 2)$

(2) $\frac{30}{5} = 6$ $(30 \div 5 = 6)$

(3) $\frac{14}{12} = 1\frac{1}{6}$ $(14 \div 12 = 1\frac{1}{6})$

(4) $\frac{9}{7} = 1\frac{2}{7}$ $(9 \div 7 = 1\frac{2}{7})$

(5) $\frac{15}{10} = 1\frac{1}{2}$ $(15 \div 10 = 1\frac{1}{2})$

(6) $\frac{9}{6} = 1\frac{1}{2}$ $(9 \div 6 = 1\frac{1}{2})$

1-21. CHANGING MIXED NUMBERS TO IMPROPER FRACTIONS

Mixed numbers may be changed to improper fractions by:

a. Multiplying the whole number by the denominator of the fraction.

b. To this answer, adding the numerator of the fraction.

c. Placing this sum (or answer) over the denominator of the fraction.

EXAMPLE: Change $4\frac{2}{3}$ to an improper fraction.

STEPS: (1) 4 (whole number) x 3 (denominator) = 12

$$4\frac{2}{3} = \frac{12}{}$$

(2) 12 (answer from ABOVE) + 2 (numerator) = 14

$$4\frac{2}{3} = \frac{12}{} + 2 = \frac{14}{}$$

(3) 14 is placed over denominator = $\frac{14}{3}$

$$\text{Thus } 4\frac{2}{3} = \frac{12+2}{3} = \frac{14}{3}$$

1-22. ADDITION AND SUBTRACTION OF FRACTIONS

a. When you add and subtract fractions, the denominators of these fractions must be the same. To make the denominators of two fractions the same, you have to find the smallest denominator into which each of the original denominators will divide evenly. This is the lowest common denominator.

EXAMPLE: You are given the fractions $\frac{1}{2}$ and $\frac{1}{5}$ and are asked to find the lowest common denominator.

What is the smallest number into which 2 and 5 will divide evenly?

The answer is 10. 10 is the lowest common denominator.

You must now change your fractions to tenths.

$$\frac{1}{2} = \frac{1x5}{2x5} = \frac{5}{10} \qquad \frac{1}{5} = \frac{1x2}{5x2} = \frac{2}{10}$$

REMEMBER: The new fractions are the same in value as the old fractions.

b. To add fractions, find the lowest common denominator and change the fractions to fractions having the same denominator. Then add the numerators.

EXAMPLE: $\frac{1}{3} + \frac{3}{4} = ?$

Change fractions to the lowest common denominator.
Then add the numerators.

$$\frac{1}{3} = \frac{4}{12}$$

$$\frac{3}{4} = \frac{9}{12}$$

$$\frac{4}{12} + \frac{9}{12} = \frac{13}{12} \text{ or } 1\frac{1}{12}$$

c. To subtract fractions, again find the lowest common denominator and change the fractions to fractions having the same denominator. Then, subtract the second numerator from the first numerator.

EXAMPLE: $\frac{3}{4} - \frac{1}{3} = ?$

$$\frac{3}{4} = \frac{9}{12}$$

$$\frac{1}{3} = \frac{4}{12}$$

$$\frac{9}{12} - \frac{4}{12} = \frac{9-4}{12} = \frac{5}{12}$$

1-23. MULTIPLYING TWO FRACTIONS

Two fractions may be multiplied by:

a. Multiplying the numerators.

b. Multiplying the denominators.

c. Reducing the answer to lowest possible terms.

EXAMPLE: $\frac{3}{4} \times \frac{2}{5} = \frac{3 \times 2}{4 \times 5} = \frac{6}{20} = \frac{3}{10}$ (reduced to lowest possible terms).

1-24. MULTIPLYING WHOLE NUMBERS AND FRACTIONS

Whole numbers and fractions may be multiplied by:

a. Changing the whole number to an improper fraction.

b. Multiplying the two fractions.

c. Reducing the answer to a mixed number in its lowest possible terms.

EXAMPLE: $4 \times \frac{2}{3} = \frac{4}{1} \times \frac{2}{3} = \frac{8}{3} = 2\frac{2}{3}$

1-25. MULTIPLYING MIXED NUMBERS

Mixed numbers may be multiplied by:

a. Changing the mixed numbers to improper fractions.
b. Multiplying the two fractions.

c. Reducing the answer to a mixed number in its lowest possible terms.

EXAMPLE: $2\frac{1}{2} \times 4\frac{1}{3} = \frac{5}{2} \times \frac{13}{3} = 5 \times \frac{13}{2} \times 3 = \frac{65}{6} = 10\frac{5}{6}$

1-26. DIVIDING FRACTIONS

Fractions may be divided by:

a. Inverting the divisor (the number by which another number is divided). Inverting is done by reversing the upper number and the lower number of the fraction.

b. After inverting the divisor, multiplying.

c. Reducing the answer to lowest terms (and/or a mixed number).

EXAMPLES: $\frac{3}{4} \div \frac{2}{3} = \frac{3}{4} \times \frac{3}{2} = \frac{9}{8} = 1\frac{1}{8}$

$\frac{1}{3} \div \frac{1}{5} = \frac{1}{3} \times \frac{5}{1} = \frac{5}{3} = 1\frac{2}{3}$

$4\frac{1}{2} \div \frac{1}{3} = \frac{9}{2} \times \frac{3}{1} = \frac{27}{2} = 13\frac{1}{2}$

1-27. PRACTICE 1-5

NOTE: Remember to reduce answers to lowest terms when possible.

a. Change the following mixed numbers to improper fractions:

(1) $2\frac{3}{8}$ =

(2) $5\frac{1}{5}$ =

(3) $10\frac{2}{3}$ =

(4) $8\frac{1}{6}$ =

(5) $4\frac{1}{2}$ =

(6) 2 =

b. Multiply the following fractions:

(1) $\frac{5}{6} \times \frac{1}{.3}$ =

(2) $\frac{9}{10} \times \frac{3}{4}$ =

(3) $\frac{5}{8} \times \frac{1}{2}$ =

(4) $\frac{7}{8} \times \frac{2}{5}$ =

(5) $\frac{4}{5} \times \frac{3}{5} =$

(6) $\frac{1}{3} \times \frac{3}{8} =$

c. Multiply the following whole numbers and fractions:

(1) $7 \times \frac{1}{2} =$

(2) $10 \times \frac{1}{3} =$

(3) $11 \times \frac{1}{4} =$

(4) $9 \times \frac{2}{3} =$

(5) $15 \times \frac{2}{3} =$

(6) $6 \times \frac{1}{8} =$

d. Multiply the following mixed numbers:

(1) $3\frac{3}{5} \times 2\frac{1}{2} =$

(2) $9 \times 9\frac{1}{2} =$

(3) $3\frac{1}{8} \times 2\frac{1}{4} =$

(4) $2\frac{1}{4} \times 3\frac{1}{3} =$

(5) $5 \times 4\frac{1}{4} =$

(6) $8\frac{2}{3} \times 5\frac{1}{4} =$

e. Divide the following fractions and mixed numbers:

(1) $1\frac{1}{3} \div \frac{1}{2} =$

(2) $6 \div \frac{1}{3} =$

(3) $6\frac{1}{2} \div 2 =$

(4) $\frac{3}{4} \div \frac{1}{2} =$

(5) $7\frac{1}{2} \div 5\frac{1}{5} =$

(6) $8 \div \frac{1}{4} =$

1-28. ANSWERS TO PRACTICE 1-5

a. (1) $2\frac{3}{8} = \frac{19}{8}$ (2 x 8 = 16 + 3 = 19)

(2) $5\frac{1}{5} = \frac{26}{5}$ (5 x 5 = 25 + 1 = 26)

(3) $10\frac{2}{3} = \frac{32}{3}$ (10 x 3 = 30 + 2 = 32)

(4) $8\frac{1}{6} = \frac{49}{6}$ (8 x 6 = 48 + 1 = 49)

(5) $4\frac{1}{2} = \frac{9}{2}$ (4 x 2 = 8 + 1 = 9)

(6) $2 = \frac{2}{1}$

b. (1) $\frac{5}{6} \times \frac{1}{3} = \frac{5}{18}$ (5 x 1 = 5) (6 x 3 = 18)

(2) $\frac{9}{10} \times \frac{3}{4} = \frac{27}{40}$ (9 x 3 = 27) (10 x 4 = 40)

(3) $\frac{5}{8} \times \frac{1}{2} = \frac{5}{16}$ $\quad (5 \times 1 = 5)$ $(8 \times 2 = 16)$

(4) $\frac{7}{8} \times \frac{2}{5} = \frac{14}{40} = \frac{7}{20}$ $\quad (7 \times 2 = 14)$ $(8 \times 5 = 40)$ $\quad (14 \div 2 = 7)$ $(40 \div 2 = 20)$

(5) $\frac{4}{5} \times \frac{3}{5} = \frac{12}{25}$ $\quad (4 \times 3 = 12)$ $(5 \times 5 = 25)$

(6) $\frac{1}{3} \times \frac{3}{8} = \frac{3}{24} = \frac{1}{8}$ $\quad (1 \times 3 = 3)$ $(3 \times 8 = 24)$ $\quad (3 \div 3 = 1)$ $(24 \div 3 = 8)$

c. (1) $7 \times \frac{1}{2} = \frac{7}{2} = 3\frac{1}{2}$ $\quad (7 \times 1 = 7)$ $(1 \times 2 = 2)$ $\quad (7 \div 2 = 3\frac{1}{2})$

(2) $10 \times \frac{1}{3} = \frac{10}{3} = 3\frac{1}{3}$

(3) $11 \times \frac{1}{4} = \frac{11}{4} = 2\frac{3}{4}$

(4) $9 \times \frac{2}{3} = \frac{18}{3} = 6$ (or $\frac{\overset{3}{\cancel{9}}}{1} \times \frac{2}{\underset{1}{\cancel{3}}} = 6$)

(5) $15 \times \frac{2}{3} = \frac{30}{3} = 10$ (or $\frac{\overset{5}{\cancel{15}}}{1} \times \frac{2}{\underset{1}{\cancel{3}}} = 10$)

(6) $6 \times \frac{1}{8} = \frac{6}{8} = \frac{3}{4}$ (or $\frac{\overset{3}{\cancel{6}}}{1} \times \frac{1}{\underset{4}{\cancel{8}}} = \frac{3}{4}$)

d. (1) $3\frac{3}{5} \times 2\frac{1}{2} = \frac{18}{5} \times \frac{5}{2} = \frac{90}{10} = 9$ (or $\frac{\overset{9}{\cancel{18}}}{\underset{1}{\cancel{5}}} \times \frac{\overset{1}{\cancel{5}}}{\underset{1}{\cancel{2}}} = \frac{9}{1} = 9$)

(2) $9 \times 9\frac{1}{2} = \frac{9}{1} \times \frac{19}{2} = \frac{171}{2} = 85\frac{1}{2}$

(3) $3\frac{1}{8} \times 2\frac{1}{4} = \frac{25}{8} \times \frac{9}{4} = \frac{225}{32} = 7\frac{1}{32}$

(4) $2\frac{1}{4} \times 3\frac{1}{3} = \frac{9}{4} \times \frac{10}{3} = \frac{90}{12} = 7\frac{6}{12} = 7\frac{1}{2}$ (or $\frac{\overset{3}{\cancel{9}}}{\underset{2}{\cancel{4}}} \times \frac{\overset{5}{\cancel{10}}}{\underset{1}{\cancel{3}}} = \frac{15}{2}$)

(5) $5 \times 4\frac{1}{4} = \frac{5}{1} \times \frac{17}{4} = \frac{85}{4} = 21\frac{1}{4}$

(6) $8\frac{2}{3} \times 5\frac{1}{4} = \frac{26}{3} \times \frac{21}{4} = \frac{546}{12} = 45\frac{6}{12} = 45\frac{1}{2}$ or $\frac{\overset{13}{\cancel{26}}}{\underset{1}{\cancel{3}}} \times \frac{\overset{7}{\cancel{21}}}{\underset{2}{\cancel{4}}} = \frac{91}{2}$

e. (1) $1\frac{1}{3} \div \frac{1}{2} = \frac{4}{3} \times \frac{2}{1} = \frac{8}{3} = 2\frac{2}{3}$

(2) $6 \div \frac{1}{3} = \frac{6}{1} \times \frac{3}{1} = \frac{18}{1} = 18$

(3) $6\frac{1}{2} \div 2 = \frac{13}{2} \times \frac{1}{2} = \frac{13}{4} = 3\frac{1}{4}$

(4) $\frac{3}{4} \div \frac{1}{2} = \frac{3}{4} \times \frac{2}{1} = \frac{6}{4} = 1\frac{2}{4} = 1\frac{1}{2}$ (or $\frac{3}{\underset{2}{\cancel{4}}} \times \frac{\overset{1}{\cancel{2}}}{1} = \frac{3}{2} = 1\frac{1}{2}$)

(5) $7\frac{1}{2} \div 5\frac{1}{5} = \frac{15}{2} \times \frac{5}{26} = \frac{75}{52} = 1\frac{23}{52}$

(6) $8 \div \frac{1}{4} = \frac{8}{1} \times \frac{4}{1} = \frac{32}{1} = 32$

Section III. DECIMALS

1-29. DEFINITION

a. The word "decimal" means ten. A decimal is a fraction whose denominator is ten or a multiple of ten.

b. All the numbers written to the left of the "decimal point" (a dot) are whole numbers. The numbers written to the right of the decimal point are "decimals" (less than one).

c. The first place to the right of the decimal point is for tenths, the second place for hundredths, the third for thousandths, and so forth.

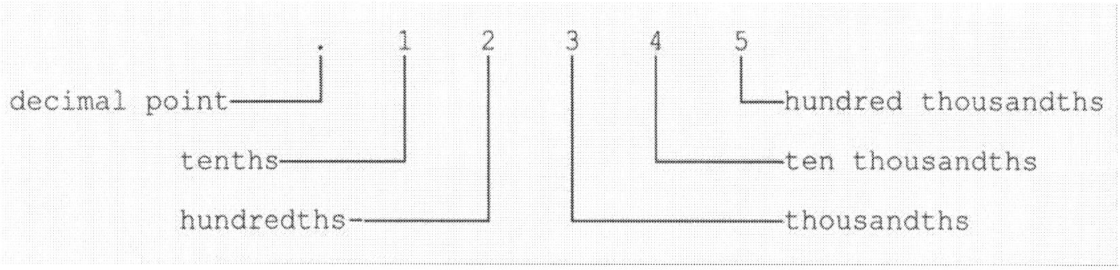

Figure 1-2. The decimal system.

EXAMPLES: 0.1 = one tenth

0.01 = one hundredth

0.001 = one thousandth

1.0 = one

10.0 = ten

100.0 = one hundred

1.1 = one and one tenth

10.01 = ten and one hundredth

1-30. ADDITION AND SUBTRACTION OF DECIMALS

When adding and subtracting decimals, remember to keep all the decimal points directly underneath each other.

EXAMPLE: Add 13.102, 1.73, and .47.

```
  13.102
   1.73
+   .47
  ------
  15.302
```

EXAMPLE: Subtract 4.56 from 8.2.

What you will need to do is change 8.2 to 8.20. (<u>Remember</u>, you can always add a zero to the <u>end</u> of a decimal without changing its value).

```
 8.20
-4.56
 ----
 3.64
```

1-31. DIVIDING DECIMALS

a. A decimal may be divided by a whole number by dividing in the usual manner and placing the decimal point in the answer directly above the decimal point in the number to be divided.

EXAMPLE: 5.5 ÷ 5 = 1.1

```
  1.1
5)5.5
  5
   5
   5
   0
```

b. A whole number may be divided by a decimal by:

(1) Making the divisor a whole number by moving the decimal point to the right as many places as necessary.

(2) Placing a decimal point after the whole number (dividend) and then moving the decimal point the same number of places to the right as the decimal point in the divisor was moved.

(3) Divide in the usual manner.

EXAMPLE: 55 ÷ 0.2

$0.2\overline{)55} = 0.2.\overline{)55.0.} = 02\overline{)550.}$

Thus, 55 ÷ 0.2 = 275

c. Now to divide a decimal by a decimal, all we do is:

(1) Make the divisor a whole number.

(2) Move the decimal point in the dividend the same number of places as the decimal in the divisor was moved.

(3) Place the decimal point in the quotient directly above the decimal point in the dividend.

(4) Divide in the usual manner.

EXAMPLE: 5.25 ÷ 2.5 =

$2.5.\overline{)5.2.5} = 25\overline{)52.5} = 2.1$

Thus 5.25 ÷ 2.5 = 2.1

d. If a decimal is to be divided by a multiple of ten (10, 100, 1000, etc.), move the decimal point as many places to the left as there are zeroes in the divisor.

EXAMPLE: When dividing .2 by 100, move the decimal point one place to the left for each of the zeros in the divisor (the number you are dividing into the other number). There are two zeros; therefore, you move the decimal two places to the left.

$.2 \div 100 = 0.00.2 = 0.002$

EXAMPLES:

(1)	$5 \div 10 = .5$	(4)	$1.8 \div 10 = .18$
(2)	$5 \div 100 = .05$	(5)	$1.8 \div 100 = .018$
(3)	$5 \div 1000 = .005$	(6)	$1.8 \div 1000 = .0018$

e. Did you remember how to round off numbers? Whenever instructed to round off to a specific decimal place, solve the problem to one more place and round off.

EXAMPLE: (round to 2d decimal place)

$52.5 - 5.2 = 10.096 = 10.10$

1-32. PRACTICE 1-6

Round the following numbers to two decimal places.

a. 10.333 =

b. 11.625 =

c. 12.611 =

d. 3.237 =

e. 2.621 =

f. 0.396 =

Divide the following decimals; round off to second decimal place.

g. $100.25 \div 50.5 =$

h. $40.5 \div 5.5 =$

i. 82.5 ÷ 0.02 =

j. 44 ÷ 2.2 =

k. 56 ÷ 4.3 =

l. 43.6 ÷ 5 =

m. 3.6 ÷ 3 =

Work the following problems:

n. 6.2. ÷ 1 00 =

o. 20 ÷ 10 =

p. 4.3 ÷ 1000 =

q. .08 ÷ 100 =

r. .7 ÷ 10 =

s. 12.324 ÷ 100 =

t. 65 ÷ 1000 =

u. .025 ÷ 10 =

v. 1.34 ÷ 1000 =

w. 65.0 ÷ 100 =

1-33. ANSWERS TO PRACTICE 1-6

a. 10.33

b. 11.63

c. 12.61

d. 3.24

e. 2.62

f. 0.40

g.

1.985
50.5.)100.2.500

50 5
49 7 5
45 4 5
4 3 00
4 0 40
2 600
2 525
75

h.

7.363 = 7.36
5.5.)40.5.000

38 5
2 0 0
1 6 5
3 50
3 30
200
165
35

i.

41 25.
0.02.)82.50.

8
02
2
0 5
4
10
10

j.

2 0.
2.2.)44.0.

44
0 0
0 0

k.

1 3.023 = 13.02
4.3.)56.0.000

43
13 0
12 9
1 0
0
1 00
86
140
129
11

l.

8.72
5)43.60
40
3 6
3 5
10
10
0

m.

1.2
3)3.6
3
0 6
6
0

n.	.062	o.	2
p.	.0043	q.	.0008
r.	.07	s.	.12324
t.	.065	u.	.0025
v.	.00134	w.	.65

1-34. MULTIPLYING DECIMALS

Decimals can be multiplied by whole numbers and decimals by:

a. Multiplying in the usual manner.

b. Pointing off the proper number of decimal places.

5.25 x 5 = 26.25

$$\begin{array}{r} 5.25 \\ \underline{\times\ \ 5} \\ 26.25 \end{array}$$

(Two decimal places pointed off for the two places in 5.25)

EXAMPLE: 5.25 x 5.5 = 28.875

$$\begin{array}{r} 5.25 \\ \underline{\times\ 5.5} \\ 2625 \\ \underline{2625\ } \\ 28.875 \end{array}$$

(Three decimal places pointed off for the three places in 5.25 and 5.5)

How many places would be pointed off in 3.24 x 3.56?

You are correct if you answered "four."

1-35. CHANGING DECIMALS TO FRACTIONS

Decimals can be changed to fractions by:

a. Removing the decimal point.

b. Placing the appropriate denominator under the number.

c. Reducing to lowest terms.

EXAMPLE: Change 0.05 to a fraction.

05 (decimal removed)

$\frac{05}{100}$ (note denominator) = $\frac{1}{20}$

1-36. CHANGING FRACTIONS TO DECIMALS

Fractions can be changed to decimals by dividing the numerator of the fraction by the denominator of the fraction.

EXAMPLE: Change $\frac{1}{2}$ to a decimal.

1 ÷ 2 (numerator ÷ denominator)

$$2\overline{)1.0}\ \ = .5$$

$\frac{1}{2}$ = 0.5

1-37. PRACTICE 1-7

Multiply the following:

a. 3.33 x 2.02 =

b. 40.1 x 4.01 =

c. 2.55 x 20.5 =

d. 5.25 x 3.5 =

e. 7.05 x 7.5 =

f. 85.05 x 3.05 =

Change the following to fractions:

g. 0.35 =

h. 0.3 =

i. 0.04 =

j. 0.005 =

k. 0.75 =

l. 0.55 =

Change the following to decimals:

m. $\frac{1}{4} =$

n. $\frac{1}{6} =$

o. $\frac{7}{8} =$

p. $\frac{5}{7} =$

q. $\frac{2}{5} =$

r. $\frac{1}{5} =$

1-38. ANSWERS TO PRACTICE 1-7

a.
```
   3.33
x  2.02
    666
  6660
 6.7266
```

b.
```
   40.1
 x 4.01
    401
160 40
160.801
```

c. 2.55
x 20.5
1 275
51 00
52.275

d. 5.25
x 3.5
2 625
15 75
18.375

e. 7.05
x 7.5
3 525
49 35
52.875

f. 85.05
x 3.05
4 2525
255 150
259.4025

g. $\frac{35}{100} = \frac{7}{20}$ $(35 \div 5 = 7)$ $(100 \div 5 = 20)$

h. $\frac{3}{10}$

i. $\frac{4}{100} = \frac{1}{25}$ $(4 \div 4 = 1)$ $(100 \div 4 = 25)$

j. $\frac{5}{1000} = \frac{1}{200}$ $(5 \div 5 = 1)$ $(1000 \div 5 = 200)$

k. $\frac{75}{100} = \frac{3}{4}$ $(75 \div 25 = 3)$ $(100 \div 25 = 4)$

l. $\frac{55}{100} = \frac{11}{20}$ $(55 \div 5 = 11)$ $(100 \div 5 = 20)$

m. .25
4)1.00
8
20
20

n.
```
   .166 = 0.17
6)1.000
  6
  40
  36
   40
   36
    4
```

o.
```
   .875 = 0.88
8)7.000
 6 4
  60
  56
   40
   40
```

p.
```
   .714 = 0.71
7)5.000
  4 9
    10
     7
     30
     28
      2
```

q.
```
   .4
5)2.0
  2 0
```

r.
```
    .2
5)1.0
  1 0
```

Section IV. PERCENTAGES

NOTE: The final exam will not include information from Section IV. This is for your information only.

1-39. DEFINITION

Percentage means parts in 100. The term "percent" is usually indicated by the symbol "%."

1-40. CHANGING PERCENTAGES TO FRACTIONS

When the percentage is a whole number, mixed number, or fraction, it can be changed to a fraction by:

a. Omitting the percent sign.

b. Writing the whole number, mixed number, or fraction as the numerator.

c. Writing 100 as the denominator.

d. Reducing the resulting fraction to lowest terms.

EXAMPLES: Change 5% to a fraction.

$$5\% = \frac{5}{100} = \frac{1}{20}$$

Change $\frac{1}{2}$% to a fraction.

$$\frac{1}{2}\% = \frac{\frac{1}{2}}{100} = \frac{1}{2} \div \frac{100}{1} = \frac{1}{2} \times \frac{1}{100} = \frac{1}{200}$$

Change 5 $\frac{1}{2}$% to a fraction.

$$5\frac{1}{2}\% = \frac{5\frac{1}{2}}{100} = \frac{11}{2} . \frac{100}{1} = \frac{11}{2} \times \frac{1}{100} = \frac{11}{200}$$

1-41. CHANGING FRACTIONS TO PERCENTAGES

Fractions can be changed to percentages by:

a. Multiplying by 100.

b. Adding the percent symbol.

EXAMPLE: Change $\frac{1}{2}$ to a percent.

$$\frac{1}{2} \times \frac{100}{1} = \frac{100}{2} \times 50\%$$

1-42. CHANGING PERCENTAGES TO DECIMALS

Percentages can also be changed to decimals by removing the percent sign; then:

a. If the percentage is a whole number, divide by 100 (this can be done quickly by moving the decimal point two places to the left).

EXAMPLE: Change 10% to a decimal.

$10\% \rightarrow 10. \rightarrow 0.1$

b. If the percentage is written as a fraction or mixed number, change to a decimal, and then move the decimal point two places to the left.

EXAMPLE: Change $\frac{1}{5}\%$ to a decimal.

$$\frac{1}{5}\% \rightarrow \frac{1}{5} \rightarrow 1 \div 5 = 0.2 \rightarrow 0.002$$

EXAMPLE: Change $3\frac{1}{2}\%$ to a decimal.

$$3\frac{1}{2}\% \rightarrow 3\frac{1}{2} = 7 \div 2 = 3.5 \rightarrow 0.035$$

1-43. CHANGING DECIMALS TO PERCENTAGES

A decimal can be changed to a percentage by:

a. Multiplying by 100 (this can be done by moving the decimal point two places to the right).

b. Adding a percent sign (%).

EXAMPLE: Change 0.5 to a percentage.

$0.5 \rightarrow 50. \rightarrow 50\%$

1-44. PRACTICE 1-8

a. Change the following percentages to fractions:

(1) 6 %

(2) $\frac{1}{8}\%$

(3) $3\frac{1}{2}\%$

(4) $\frac{4}{5}\%$

(5) $12\frac{1}{2}\%$

(6) 30%

b. Change the following fractions to percentages:

(1) $\frac{3}{5}$

(2) $\frac{1}{8}$

(3) $\frac{1}{4}$

(4) $\frac{1}{100}$

(5) $\frac{1}{50}$

(6) $\frac{1}{25}$

c. Change the following percentages to decimals:

(1) $\frac{3}{4}$ %

(2) 50 %

(3) 40 %

(4) $2\frac{1}{2}$ %

(5) 6 %

(6) $6\frac{1}{5}$ %

d. Change the following decimals to percentages:

(1) 0.25

(2) 0.125

(3) 3.5

(4) 7.5

(5) 0.75

(6) 0.4

1-45. ANSWERS TO PRACTICE 1-8

a. (1) $\frac{6}{100} = \frac{3}{50}$ (6 ÷ 2 = 3) (100 ÷ 2 = 50)

(2) $\frac{1/8}{100} = \frac{1}{8} \div \frac{100}{1} = \frac{1}{8} \times \frac{1}{100} = \frac{1}{800}$

(3) $\frac{3\frac{1}{2}}{100} = \frac{7}{2} \div \frac{100}{1} = \frac{7}{2} \times \frac{1}{100} = \frac{7}{200}$

(4) $\frac{\frac{4}{5}}{100} = \frac{4}{5} \div \frac{100}{1} = \frac{4}{5} \times \frac{1}{100} = \frac{4}{500} = \frac{1}{125}$ or $\frac{\overset{1}{\cancel{4}}}{5} \times \frac{1}{\underset{25}{\cancel{100}}} = \frac{1}{125}$

(5) $\frac{12\frac{1}{2}}{100} = \frac{25}{2} \div \frac{100}{1} = \frac{25}{2} \times \frac{1}{100} = \frac{25}{200} = \frac{1}{8}$ or $\frac{\overset{1}{\cancel{25}}}{2} \times \frac{1}{\underset{4}{\cancel{100}}} = \frac{1}{8}$

(6) $\frac{30}{100} = \frac{3}{10}$

b. (1) $\frac{3}{5} \times \frac{100}{1} = \underline{300}$ →60% (or $\frac{3}{\underset{1}{\cancel{5}}} \times \frac{\overset{20}{\cancel{100}}}{1} = 60$)

(2) $\frac{1}{8} \times \frac{100}{1} = \frac{100}{8}$ → 12 1/2% or 12.5%) (or $\times \frac{1}{\underset{2}{\cancel{8}}} \frac{\overset{25}{\cancel{100}}}{1} = \frac{25}{2} = 12.5$)

(3) $\frac{1}{4} \times \frac{100}{1} = \frac{100}{4} \rightarrow 25\%$ (or $\frac{1}{\cancel{4}_{1}} \times \frac{\cancel{100}^{25}}{1} = 25$)

(4) $\frac{1}{100} \times \frac{100}{1} = \frac{100}{100} \rightarrow 1\%$ (or $\frac{1}{\cancel{100}_{1}} \times \frac{\cancel{100}^{1}}{1} = 1$)

(5) $\frac{1}{50} \times \frac{100}{1} = \frac{100}{50} \rightarrow 2\%$ or ($\frac{1}{\cancel{50}_{1}} \times \frac{\cancel{100}^{2}}{1} = 2$)

(6) $\frac{1}{25} \times \frac{100}{1} = \frac{100}{25} \rightarrow 4\%$ (or $\frac{1}{\cancel{25}_{1}} \times \frac{\cancel{100}^{4}}{1} = 4$)

c. (1)

$$\begin{array}{r} .75 \\ 4\overline{)3.00} \\ \underline{2\,8} \\ 20 \\ \underline{20} \\ 0 \end{array} \rightarrow 0.0075$$

(2) 0.5

(3) 0.4

(4) $2\frac{1}{2}\% \rightarrow \frac{5}{2} = $

$$\begin{array}{r} 2.5 \\ 2\overline{)5.0} \\ \underline{4} \\ 1\,0 \\ \underline{1\,0} \\ 0 \end{array} \rightarrow 0.025$$

(5) 0.06

(6) $6\frac{1}{5}\% \rightarrow \frac{31}{5} = $

$$\begin{array}{r} 6.2 \\ 5\overline{)31.0} \\ \underline{30} \\ 1\,0 \\ \underline{1\,0} \\ 0 \end{array} \rightarrow 0.062$$

d. (1) 25%

(2) 12.5% or $12\frac{1}{2}\%$

(3) 350%

(4) 750%

(5) 75%

(6) 40%

Section V. RATIO AND PROPORTION

1-46. DEFINITION--RATIO

A ratio is a way of expressing a fractional part of a whole number. In a ratio, the numerator of the fraction is written in front of the denominator instead of over it.

EXAMPLE: In a ratio, the fraction $\frac{1}{2}$ would be written 1:2 or 1-2.

The symbol ":" or "-" is placed between the numbers of the ratio.

1-47. CHANGING A RATIO TO A PERCENTAGE OR DECIMAL

A ratio is changed to a percentage or decimal in the same way a fraction is changed to a percentage or decimal.

EXAMPLE: Change 1:50 to a percentage.

$$1:50 \rightarrow \frac{1}{50} \times \frac{100}{1} \rightarrow 2\%$$

EXAMPLE: Change 1:50 to a decimal.

$$1:50 = \frac{1}{50} = 1 \div 50 = 0.02$$

1-48. PRACTICE 1-9

a. Write the following as ratios:

(1) $\frac{1}{4}$ =

(2) $\frac{1}{100}$ =

(3) $\frac{1}{10}$ =

(4) $\frac{1}{1000}$ =

(5) $\frac{1}{50}$ =

(6) $\frac{1}{75}$ =

b. Change the following ratios to both decimals and percentages:

Ratio	Decimal	Percent
(1) 1:3	________	________
(2) 1:1000	________	________
(3) 1:150	________	________

1-49. ANSWERS TO PRACTICE 1-9

a. (1) 1:4

(2) 1:100

(3) 1:10

(4) 1:1000

(5) 1:50

(6) 1:75

b. (1) 0.33 $33\frac{1}{3}\%$

(2) 0.001 $\frac{1}{10}\%$

(3) 0.00666 or 0.0067 $\frac{2}{3}\%$

1-50. CHANGING PERCENTAGES TO RATIOS

Changing a percentage to a ratio is the same as changing a percentage to a fraction.

EXAMPLE: Change 50% to a ratio.

$$50\% = .50 = \frac{50}{100} = \frac{1}{2} = 1{:}2$$

1-51. CHANGING DECIMALS TO RATIOS

This is calculated in the same manner as changing a decimal to a fraction.

EXAMPLE: Change 0.5 to a ratio.

$$0.5 = \frac{5}{10} = \frac{1}{2} = 1{:}2$$

1-52. PRACTICE 1-10

a. Change the following percentages to ratios:

(1) 10% ________________

(2) $\frac{1}{2}\%$ ________________

(3) 80% ________________

(4) 40% ________________

(5) $\frac{1}{4}\%$ ________________

(6) 1% ________________

b. Change the following decimals to ratios:

(1) 0.2 ________________

(2) 0.025 ________________

(3) 0.05 ________________

(4) 0.001 ____________________

(5) 0.075 ____________________

(6) 0.1 ____________________

1-53. ANSWERS TO PRACTICE 1-10

a. (1) $.10 = \frac{10}{100} = \frac{1}{10} = 1{:}10$

(2) $\frac{\frac{1}{2}}{100} = \frac{1}{2} \div \frac{100}{1} = \frac{1}{2} \times \frac{1}{100} = \frac{1}{200} = 1{:}200$

(3) $.80 = \frac{80}{100} = \frac{8}{10} = \frac{4}{5} = 4{:}5$

(4) $.40 = \frac{40}{100} = \frac{4}{10} = \frac{2}{5} = 2{:}5$

(5) $\frac{1/4}{100} = \frac{1}{4} \div \frac{100}{1} = \frac{1}{4} \times \frac{1}{100} = \frac{1}{400} = 1{:}400$

(6) $.01 = \frac{1}{100} = 1{:}100$

b. (1) $\frac{2}{10} = \frac{1}{5} = 1{:}5$

(2) $\frac{25}{1000} = \frac{1}{40} = 1{:}40$

(3) $\frac{5}{100} = \frac{1}{20} = 1{:}20$

(4) $\frac{1}{1000} = 1{:}1000$

(5) $\frac{75}{1000} = \frac{3}{40} = 3{:}40$

(6) $\frac{1}{10} = 1{:}10$

1-54. DEFINITION--PROPORTION

An equation that tells us that one ratio is equal to another ratio is called a proportion.

EXAMPLE:

A baseball team wins 15 games out of 30 games played. If the team continues to win at the same rate, how many games will it win out of 40 games played?

a. Let N = number of games the team will win in 40 games played.

b. The ratio of games won to games already played is 15/30. Since the ratio of games won to games played is to remain the same, we may write this ratio as N/40. These ratios may also be written as 15:30 and N:40.

c. We may now write the equation 15/30 = N/40. This is our proportion.

1-55. PROPERTY OF PROPORTIONS

Proportions have a very useful property. Consider the proportion: $\frac{1}{3} = \frac{2}{6}$ or 1:3 =2:6.

a. The two inside terms (3 and 2) are called the "means" of the proportion, and the two outside terms (1 and 6) are called the "extremes" of the proportion.

b. Notice that if we multiply the two means, we obtain 3 x 2 = 6. Also, if we multiply the two extremes, we obtain 1 x 6 = 6. This illustrates the following property of proportions:

In a proportion, the product of the means is equal to the product of the extremes.

EXAMPLE: The ratio of alcohol to water in a certain type of antifreeze is 3:4. If a tank contains 24 quarts of alcohol, how many quarts of water must be added to make the antifreeze mixture?

Let X = the number of quarts needed.

$$\frac{\text{alcohol}}{\text{water}} \qquad \frac{3}{4} = \frac{24}{X}$$

Now, use the property of proportions to find "X."

$3:4 = 24:X$

$3X = 4 \times 24$

$3X = 96$

$\frac{1}{3}(3X) = \frac{1}{3}(96)$ or $\frac{3X}{3} = \frac{96}{3}$

$X = 32$ quarts of water

or

cross multiply

$\frac{3}{4} = \frac{24}{X}$

Multiply the numerator of the first ratio by the denominator of the second ratio. Then multiply the denominator of the first ratio by the numerator of the second ratio.

$3X = 4 \times 24$

$3X = 96$

$X = 32$ quarts of water

SECOND EXAMPLE:

If three ties cost $12.57, what is the cost of five ties at the same rate?

Let y = the cost of five ties.

$3:12.57 = 5:y$

$\frac{3}{12.57} = \frac{5}{y}$

$3y = 5 \times 12.57 = 62.85$

$\frac{1}{3}(3y) = \frac{1}{3}(62.85)$

y = $20.95

1-56. PRACTICE 1-11

a. $4:3 = 32:W$ W = __________

b. John earned $150 one week and spent $120. What is the ratio of the amount John saved to the amount John spent?

____

c. The ratio of a father's age to his son's age is 9:2. If the son's age is 12 years, what is the age of the father (in years)?

____

d. If three shirts cost $23, what is the cost of a dozen shirts at the same rate?

____

e. A gallon of paint covers 240 square feet of surface. If a living room contains 906 square feet of paintable surface and a kitchen contains 334 square feet of surface, what is the number of gallons of paint needed for the living room and kitchen?

____

1-57. ANSWERS TO PRACTICE 1-11

a. 4:3 = 32:W

4W = 3 x 32

4W = 96

W = 24

b. 30:120 = 1:4

c. 2:9 = 12:x

2X = 9 x 12

2X = 108

X = 54

d. 3:23 = 12:X

3X = 23 x 12

3X = 276

X = 92

e. 1:240 = X:1240 (1240 is the sum of 906 and 334)

$1 \times 1240 = 240X$

$1240 = 240X$

$X = 5\frac{1}{6}$

Continue with Exercises

EXERCISES, LESSON 1

INSTRUCTIONS: Answer the following items by writing the answer in the space provided.

After you have completed all of these items, turn to "Solutions to Exercises" at the end of the lesson and check your answers.

1. $\begin{array}{r} 2975 \\ \underline{\times\ 36} \end{array}$

2. $50\overline{)78340}$

3. $\begin{array}{r} 376 \\ \underline{-107} \end{array}$

4. $\begin{array}{r} 564 \\ \times\ \underline{231} \end{array}$

5. $\begin{array}{r} 4791 \\ \underline{+3208} \end{array}$

6. $\begin{array}{r} 4638 \\ \underline{-3135} \end{array}$

7. $6\overline{)726}$

8. $\begin{array}{r} 4372 \\ \underline{+6629} \end{array}$

9. $\begin{array}{r} 285 \\ \underline{-193} \end{array}$

10. $75\overline{)2625}$

11. Change to lowest terms: $\frac{16}{20}$

12. Change to mixed or whole number: $\frac{30}{5}$

13. Change to mixed or whole number: $\frac{16}{15}$

14. Change to improper fraction: $10\frac{1}{2}$

15. $8 \times \frac{2}{3} =$

16. $4 \times \frac{3}{8} =$

17. $\frac{3}{8} \times \frac{4}{5}$ =

18. $2 \times 1\frac{1}{2}$ =

19. $10\frac{1}{2} \times 3\frac{1}{4}$ =

20. $10 \div 1\frac{1}{2}$ =

21. $\frac{2}{3} \div \frac{3}{4}$ =

22. 100.25 ÷ 50.5 =

23. 30.3 ÷ 3.3 =

24. 65 ÷ 0.32 =

25. 5.63 ÷ 15 = ______________

26. 140 x 2.5 = ______________

27. 7.125 x 0.25 = ______________

28. Change 0.5 to a fraction ______________

29. Change 0.04 to a fraction ______________

30. Change $\frac{1}{3}$ to a decimal ______________

31. Change 0.5% to a decimal ______________

32. Change 0.8 to a percent ______________

33. Change 5.25 to a percent ______________

34. Change 75% to a fraction ______________

35. Change $7\frac{1}{2}$% to a decimal ______________

36. Change 15 $\frac{1}{2}$% to a fraction ______________

37. Change $\frac{4}{5}$ to a percent ______________

38. Change $\frac{3}{5}$% to a decimal ______________

39. Change 4.5 to a percent ______________

40. Change $\frac{1}{4}$% to a ratio ______________

41. Change 1:3 to a percent ______________

42. Change 1:2000 to a percent ______________

43. Change 1:2000 to a decimal ______________

44. Change 0.002 to a ratio ______________

45. Change 20% to a ratio ______________

46. Change 0.75 to a ratio ______________

47. Change 1:4 to a decimal ______________

48. Mr. Ash finds that he spends $47.50 for gas for each 1,000 miles that he drives his car. One month he drives his car 1,800 miles. The amount he spent on gas during that month is ______________.

49. On a map, the scale is 1" to 80 miles. The actual distance between two cities is 200 miles. The distance between the cities, on the map, is ______________.

50. A 25-acre field yields 375 bushels of wheat. How many acres should be planted to yield 525 bushels of wheat? ______________

Check Your Answers on Next Page

SOLUTIONS TO EXERCISES, LESSON 1

1.
$$\begin{array}{r} 2975 \\ \underline{\times\ 36} \\ 17850 \\ \underline{8925} \\ 107100 \end{array}$$

(para 1-10)

2.
$$\begin{array}{r} 1566.8 \\ 50\overline{)78340.0} \end{array}$$

$$\begin{array}{l} \underline{50} \\ 283 \\ \underline{250} \\ 334 \\ \underline{300} \\ 340 \\ \underline{300} \\ 400 \\ \underline{400} \end{array}$$

(para 1-11)

3.
$$\begin{array}{r} 376 \\ \underline{-107} \\ 269 \end{array}$$

(para 1-3)

4.
$$\begin{array}{r} 564 \\ \underline{\times\ 231} \\ 564 \\ 1692 \\ \underline{1128} \\ 130284 \end{array}$$

(para 1-10)

5.
$$\begin{array}{r} 4791 \\ \underline{+\ 3208} \\ 7999 \end{array}$$

(para 1-2)

6.
$$\begin{array}{r} 4638 \\ \underline{-3135} \\ 1503 \end{array}$$

(para 1-3)

7.
$$\begin{array}{r} 121 \\ 6\overline{)726} \end{array}$$

$$\begin{array}{l} \underline{6} \\ 12 \\ \underline{12} \\ 06 \\ \underline{6} \end{array}$$

(para 1-11)

8.
$$\begin{array}{r} 4372 \\ \underline{+6629} \\ 11001 \end{array}$$

(para 1-2)

9.
$$\begin{array}{r} 285 \\ \underline{-193} \\ 92 \end{array}$$

(para 1-3)

10.
$$\begin{array}{r} 35 \\ 75\overline{)2625} \end{array}$$

$$\begin{array}{l} \underline{225} \\ 375 \\ \underline{375} \end{array}$$

(para 1-11)

11. $\frac{16}{20} = \frac{4}{5}$

(para 1-17)

12. $\frac{30}{5} = 6$

(para 1-18)

13. $\frac{16}{15} = 1\frac{1}{15}$

(para 1-18)

14. $10\frac{1}{2} = \frac{21}{2}$

(para 1-21)

15. $\frac{8}{1} \times \frac{2}{3} = \frac{16}{3} = 5\frac{1}{3}$

(para 1-24)

16. $\frac{4}{1} \times \frac{3}{8} = \frac{12}{8} = 1\frac{1}{2}$

(para 1-24)

17. $\frac{3}{8} \times \frac{4}{5} = \frac{12}{40} = \frac{3}{10}$

(para 1-23)

18. $2 \times 1\frac{1}{2} = \frac{2}{1} \times \frac{3}{2} = \frac{6}{2} = 3$

(para 1-24)

19. $10\frac{1}{2} \times 3\frac{1}{4} = \frac{21}{2} \times \frac{13}{4} = \frac{273}{8} = 34\frac{1}{8}$

(para 1-25)

20. $10 \div 1\frac{1}{2} = \frac{10}{1} \times \frac{2}{3} = \frac{20}{3} = 6\frac{2}{3}$

(para 1-26)

21. $\frac{2}{3} \div \frac{3}{4} = \frac{2}{3} \times \frac{4}{3} = \frac{8}{9}$

(para 1-26)

22.
```
          1.985  = 1.99
 50.5.)100.2.500
   50 5
   49 7 5
   45 4 5
    4 3 00
    4 0 40
      2 600
      2 525
         75
```
(para 1-31)

23.
```
        9.181 = 9.18
 3.3.)30.3.000
   29 7
      6 0
      3 3
     2 70
     2 64
       60
       33
       27
```
(para 1-31)

24.
```
          2 03.125 = 203.13
 0.32.)65.00.000
       64
       1 0
         0
       1 00
         96
          40
          32
           80
           64
           160
           160
```
(para 1-31)

25.
$$\begin{array}{r} .375 \\ 15\overline{)5.630} \\ \underline{4\,5} \\ 1\,13 \\ \underline{1\,05} \\ 80 \\ \underline{75} \\ 5 \end{array} = 0.38$$

(para 1-31)

26.
$$\begin{array}{r} 140 \\ \underline{2.5} \\ 700 \\ \underline{280} \\ 350.0 \end{array}$$

(para 1-34)

27.
$$\begin{array}{r} 7.125 \\ \underline{0.25} \\ 35625 \\ \underline{14250} \\ 1.78125 \end{array} = 1.78$$

(para 1-34)

28. $0.5 = \frac{5}{10} = \frac{1}{2}$

(para 1-35)

29. $0.04 = \frac{4}{100} = \frac{1}{25}$

(para 1-35)

30. $\frac{1}{3} = 1 \div 3 = .33$

(para 1-36)

31. 0.5% = 0.005 (para 1-42)

32. 0.8 = 80% (para 1-43)

33. 5.25 = 525% (para 1-43)

34. $75\% = \frac{75}{100} = \frac{3}{4}$ (para 1-40)

35. $7\frac{1}{2}\% = \frac{15}{2} = 7.5 = .075$ (para 1-42)

36. $15\frac{1}{2}\% = \frac{15\frac{1}{2}}{100} = \frac{31}{2} \div \frac{100}{1} = \frac{31}{2} \times \frac{1}{100} = \frac{31}{200}$ (para 1-40)

37. $\frac{4}{5} = 4 \div 5 = .8 = 80\ \%$ (para 1-41)

38. $\frac{3}{5} = 3 \div 5 = .6 = 0.006$

(para 1-42)

39. 4.5 = 450% (para 1-41)

40. $\frac{1}{4}\% = \frac{\frac{1}{4}}{100} = \frac{1}{4} \div \frac{100}{1} = \frac{1}{4} \times \frac{1}{100} = \frac{1}{400} = 1{:}400$ (para 1-50)

41. $1{:}3 = \frac{1}{3} \times \frac{100}{1} = \frac{100}{3} = 33\frac{1}{3}\%$ (para 1-47)

42. $1{:}2000 = \frac{1}{2000} \times \frac{100}{1} = \frac{100}{2000} = \frac{1}{20}\%$ (para 1-47)

43. $1{:}2000 = \frac{1}{2000} = 1 \div 2000 = 0.0005$ (para 1-47)

44. $0.002 = \frac{2}{1000} = \frac{1}{500} = 1{:}500$ (para 1-51)

45. $20\% = .20 = \frac{20}{100} = \frac{1}{5} = 1{:}5$ (para 1-51)

46. $0.75 = \frac{75}{100} = \frac{3}{4} = 3{:}4$ (para 1-51)

47. $1{:}4 = \frac{1}{4} = 1 \div 4 = 0.25$ (para 1-47)

48. 47.50:1000 = X:1800

1000X = 85,500

X = $85.50 (para 1-55)

49. 1:80 = X:200

80X = 200

X = $2\frac{1}{2}$" or 2.5" (para 1-55)

50. 25:375 = X = 525

375X = 13,125

X = 35 (para 1-55)

End of Lesson 1

LESSON ASSIGNMENT

LESSON 2 Pharmacology

TEXT ASSIGNMENT Paragraphs 2-1 through 2-34.

LESSON OBJECTIVES After completing this lesson, you should be able to:

2-1. Compute medication dosages by the ratio and proportion method.

2-2. Convert from one unit to another, using the metric system, apothecary system, and houshold measurements.

2-3. Compute medication dosages for tablets, pills, and capsules.

2-4. Compute oral medication dosages for prepared strength liquids.

2-5. Compute dosages for parenteral medications.

2-6. Compute dosages for medications manufactured in standardized units.

2-7. Compute medication dosages based on body weight.

2-8. Compute continuous intravenous infusion rates.

2-9. Compute intravenous infusion rates for medication.

2-10. Given a medication label, identify the following information: generic name, trade name, strength of the medication, special storage considerations, and expiration date.

2-11. Given a physician's order for medication administration and the concentration of a drug solution, suspension, or dosage form, calculate the volume of the solution, suspension, tablet, or capsule to be given.

SUGGESTION After completing the assignment, complete the exercises at the end of this lesson.

LESSON 2

PHARMACOLOGY

Section I. RATIO AND PROPORTION OPERATIONS

2-1. DEFINITIONS

a. **Ratio**.

(1) The relationship of two quantities.

(2) May be expressed as a:

(a) Ratio 1:8, 1:200

(b) Fraction $\frac{1}{8}, \frac{1}{200}$

b. **Proportion**:

The equality of two ratios $\frac{1}{2} = \frac{3}{6}$

2-2. CROSS MULTIPLYING

A check as to the equality of two ratios can be made by cross multiplying.

a. Multiply the numerator of the first ratio times the denominator of the second ratio.

b. Then, multiply the denominator of the first ratio times the numerator of the second ratio.

c. If the ratios are the same or equal, the results of the cross multiplication will be the same.

<u>EXAMPLE</u>:

$$\frac{1}{2} = \frac{3}{6}$$

$$\frac{1}{2} \times \frac{3}{6}$$

(1) $1 \times 6 = 6$

(2) $2 \times 3 = 6$

(3) $6 = 6$ Therefore, the ratios are equal.

2-3. "X" AS THE UNKNOWN FACTOR

Because the products of the cross multiplications are always equal in a proportion, if one factor of either ratio is unknown, it may be solved by substituting "X" for the unknown factor in the proportion.

EXAMPLE:

$$\frac{1}{2} = \frac{X}{6}$$

$$\frac{1}{2} \times \frac{X}{6}$$

Cross multiply:

$$2\,(X) = 1\,(6)$$

$$2X = 6$$

$$\frac{2X}{2} = \frac{6}{2}$$

$$X = 3$$

2-4. RULES FOR RATIO AND PROPORTION OPERATIONS

a. The numerators must have the same units.

b. The denominators must have the same units.

c. Three of the four variables must be known.

2-5. SETTING UP THE PROPORTION

The expression of strength of a medication is usually the first ratio of the proportion, and this ratio is put in proportion to the amount of medication to be administered.

a. Example--If one aspirin tablet contains five grains of aspirin, then how many tablets will you give in order for the patient to receive 15 grains of aspirin?

NOTE: The EXPRESSION OF STRENGTH is "one tablet contains five grains of aspirin" and should be written as the first ratio of the proportion.

$$\underline{\text{IF}} \qquad \underline{\text{THEN}}$$

$$\frac{1 \text{ tablet}}{5 \text{ grains}} = \underline{\qquad\qquad}$$

b. Next, assign "X" its proper place in the second proportion. Because the question asks "How many tablets?" the "X" is placed opposite the tablets in the first ratio.

$$\underline{\text{IF}} \qquad \underline{\text{THEN}}$$

$$\frac{1 \text{ tablet}}{5 \text{ grains}} = \underline{X \text{ tablets}}$$

c. The question asks you to calculate the number of tablets required in order to give 15 grains of aspirin; therefore, the 15 grains will be placed opposite the grains in the first ratio.

$$\underline{\text{IF}} \qquad \underline{\text{THEN}}$$

$$\frac{1 \text{ tablet}}{5 \text{ grains}} = \frac{X \text{ tablets}}{15 \text{ grains}}$$

NOTE: Prior to cross-multiplying, be sure that corresponding units in each ratio are the same.

2-6. SOLVING for "X"

a. You have set up the proportion:

$$\underline{\text{IF}} \qquad \underline{\text{THEN}}$$

$$\frac{1 \text{ tablet}}{5 \text{ grains}} = \frac{X \text{ tablets}}{15 \text{ grains}}$$

b. Now, cross multiply:

$$5(X) = 1(15)$$

c. Solve for X:

$$\frac{5X}{5} = \frac{15}{5}$$

$$X = 3$$

d. Refer back to step a. to find the units of X. The units for X in this problem is tablets; therefore, the answer is 3 tablets.

NOTE: The most common mistake is the failure to label units. Labeling units will ensure that corresponding units of the proportion are the same.

2-7. ROUNDING OFF

a. When rounding answers to the nearest tenth, you must take your calculation out to the hundredth place and then round to the tenth place.

EXAMPLE: 3.91 = 3.9

b. When rounding answers to the hundredth place, you must take your calculation out to the thousandth place and then round to the hundredth place.

EXAMPLE: 3.846 = 3.85

c. *DO NOT ROUND UNTIL THE LAST STEP OF YOUR CALCULATION!!!!*

2-8. PRACTICE 2-1 (RATIO AND PROPORTION)

Round answers to the nearest tenth.

On Hand	Doctor's Order	Answer
a. Mellaril 100 mg/tab	50 mg.	__________
b. Gantrisin 0.5 Gm/cc	2 Gm	__________
c. Demerol 50 mg/cc	25 mg	__________
d. Dilantin 100 mg/cc	250 mg	__________
e. Valium 2.5 mg/tab	15 mg	__________
f. Ampicillin 0.5 Gm/tsp	1 Gm	__________
g. Lincocin 500 mg/0.5 cc	250 mg	__________

h.	Aldomet 0.1 Gm/cc	0.15 Gm	________
i.	Atropine gr 1/200/cc	gr 1/300	________
j.	Digoxin 0.125 mg/0.6 cc	0.25 mg	________
k.	Vistaril 100 mg/2 cc	75 mg	________
l.	Morphine 8 mg/cc	10 mg	________
m.	Polycillin 250 mg/ml	500 mg	________
n.	Digoxin 0.125 mg/tablet	0.250 mg	________
o.	Omnipen 125 mg/0.5 ml	350 mg	________
p.	Kantrex 1 gm/3 ml	0.5 gm	________
q.	Lanoxin Elixir 0.01 mg/ml	0.05 mg	________
r.	Lasix 20 mg/ml	70 mg	________
s.	Dilaudid 2 mg/tablet	3 mg	________
t.	Robitussin 10 mg/30 ml	30 mg	________
u.	Ativan 0.5 mg/tablet	2 mg	________
v.	Luminal 30 mg/tablet	90 mg	________
w.	Gantrisin 0.25 gm/tablet	1 gm	________
x.	Cedilanid 0.25 mg/2 cc	0.5 mg	________
y.	Scopolomine 0.6 mg/2 ml	0.3 mg	________
z.	Methicillin 500 mg/cc	750 mg	________

2-9. ANSWERS TO PRACTICE 2-1

a. $\frac{\text{1 tab}}{\text{100 mg}} = \frac{\text{X tabs}}{\text{50 mg}}$

$100 X = 50$

$= \frac{1}{2}$ tab

b. $\frac{1\ cc}{0.5\ Gm} = \frac{X\ cc}{2\ Gm}$

0.5 X = 2

X = 4 cc

c. $\frac{1\ cc}{50\ mg} = \frac{X\ cc}{25\ mg}$

50 X = 25

X = .5 cc

d. $\frac{1\ cc}{100\ mg} = \frac{X\ cc}{250\ mg}$

100 X = 250

X = 2.5 cc

e. $\frac{1\ tab}{2.5\ mg} = \frac{X\ tabs}{15\ mg}$

2.5 X = 15

X = 6 tabs

f. $\frac{1\ tsp}{0.5\ Gm} = \frac{X\ tsp}{1\ Gm}$

0.5X = 1

X = 2 tsp

g. $\frac{0.5\ cc}{500\ mg} = \frac{X\ cc}{250\ mg}$

500X = 125

X = 0.25 = 0.3 cc

h. $\frac{1 \text{ cc}}{0.1 \text{ Gm}} = \frac{X \text{ cc}}{0.15 \text{ Gm}}$

$0.1X = 0.15$

$X = 1.5$ cc

i. $\frac{1 \text{ cc}}{\text{gr } 1/200} = \frac{X \text{ cc}}{\text{gr } 1/300}$

$\frac{1}{200}X = \frac{1}{300}$

$X = \frac{1}{300} \div \frac{1}{200}$

$X = 0.66 = 0.7$ cc

j. $\frac{0.6 \text{ cc}}{0.125 \text{ mg}} = \frac{X \text{ cc}}{0.25 \text{ mg}}$

$0.125X = .150$

$X = 1.2$ cc

k. $\frac{2 \text{ cc}}{100 \text{ mg}} = \frac{X \text{ cc}}{75 \text{ mg}}$

$100X = 150$

$X = 1.5$ cc

l. $\frac{1 \text{ cc}}{8 \text{ mg}} = \frac{X \text{ cc}}{10 \text{ mg}}$

$8X = 10$

$X = 1.3$ cc

m. $\frac{1 \text{ ml}}{250 \text{ mg}} = \frac{X \text{ ml}}{500 \text{ mg}}$

$250X = 500$

$X = 2$ ml

n. $\frac{1 \text{ tablet}}{0.125 \text{ mg}} = \frac{X \text{ tablets}}{0.250 \text{ mg}}$

$0.125X = 0.250$

$X = 2$ tablets

o. $\frac{0.5 \text{ ml}}{125 \text{ mg}} = \frac{X \text{ ml}}{350 \text{ mg}}$

$125X = 175$

$X = 1.4$ ml

p. $\frac{3 \text{ ml}}{1 \text{ gm}} = \frac{X \text{ ml}}{0.5 \text{ gm}}$

$X = 1.5$ ml

q. $\frac{1 \text{ ml}}{0.01 \text{ mg}} = \frac{X \text{ ml}}{0.05 \text{ mg}}$

$0.01X = 0.05$

$X = 5$ ml

r. $\frac{1 \text{ ml}}{20 \text{ mg}} = \frac{X \text{ ml}}{70 \text{ mg}}$

$20X = 70$

$X = 3.5$ ml

s. $\frac{1 \text{ tablet}}{2 \text{ mg}} = \frac{X \text{ tablets}}{3 \text{ mg}}$

$2X = 3$

$X = 1\frac{1}{2}$ tablets

t. $\frac{30 \text{ ml}}{10 \text{ mg}} = \frac{X \text{ ml}}{30 \text{ mg}}$

$10X = 900$

$X = 90$ ml

u. $\frac{1 \text{ tablet}}{0.5 \text{ mg}} = \frac{X \text{ tablets}}{2 \text{ mg}}$

$0.5X = 2$

$X = 4$ tablets

v. $\frac{1 \text{ tablet}}{30 \text{ mg}} = \frac{X \text{ tablets}}{90 \text{ mg}}$

$30X = 90$

$X = 3$ tablets

w. $\frac{1 \text{ tablet}}{0.25 \text{ gm}} = \frac{X \text{ tablets}}{1 \text{ gm}}$

$0.25X = 1$

$X = 4$ tablets

x. $\frac{2 \text{ cc}}{0.25 \text{ mg}} = \frac{X \text{ cc}}{0.5 \text{ mg}}$

$0.25X = 1.0$

$X = 4$ cc

y. $\frac{2 \text{ ml}}{0.6 \text{ mg}} = \frac{X \text{ ml}}{0.3 \text{ mg}}$

$0.6X = 0.6$

$X = 1$ ml

z. $\frac{1 \text{ cc}}{500 \text{ mg}} = \frac{X \text{ cc}}{750 \text{ mg}}$

$500 X = 750$

$X = 1.5$ cc

Section II. SYSTEMS OF MEASUREMENT

2-10. NOTES

a. **The Metric System.**

(1) Units used in the metric system:

(a) Liter for volume (fluids).

(b) Gram for weight (solids).

(c) Meter for measure (length).

(2) Metric equivalents used in medicine:

(a) Volume--1000 milliliters (ml) = 1 liter (L).

(b) Weight:

1 1000 micrograms (mcg) = 1 milligram (mg).

2 1000 mg = 1 gram (gm).

3 1000 gm = 1 kilogram (kg).

(3) Procedure for conversion from one unit of the metric system to another:

(a) To change milligrams to grams (mg to gm), milliliters to liters (ml to L), or to change grams to kilograms, set up a ratio and proportion based on the equivalent.

EXAMPLE 1. Express 50 mg as grams.

50 mg = X gm

$$\frac{1000 \text{ mg}}{1 \text{ gm}} = \frac{50 \text{ mg}}{X \text{ gm}}$$

1000X = 50

X = .05 gm

EXAMPLE 2. Express 2200 ml as liters.

$$2200 \text{ ml} = X \text{ L}$$

$$\frac{1000 \text{ ml}}{1 \text{ L}} = \frac{2200 \text{ ml}}{X \text{ L}}$$

$$1000X = 2200$$

$$X = 2.2 \text{ L}$$

(b) To change liters to milliliters, kilograms to grams, grams to milligrams, set up a ratio and proportion based on the equivalent.

EXAMPLE 1. Express 3.5 liters as ml.

$$3.5 \text{ L} = X \text{ ml}$$

$$\frac{1 \text{ L}}{1000 \text{ ml}} = \frac{3.5 \text{ L}}{X \text{ ml}}$$

$$X = 3500 \text{ ml}$$

EXAMPLE 2. Express 0.5 gm as mg.

$$0.5 \text{ gm} = X \text{ mg}$$

$$\frac{1 \text{ gm}}{1000 \text{ mg}} = \frac{0.5 \text{ gm}}{X \text{ mg}}$$

$$X = 500 \text{ mg}$$

b. **The Apothecaries' System.**

(1) The apothecary system is the original system of medication measurement used by pharmacists and physicians. The system is still in use today to a limited extent. In general, drugs that continue to be ordered and dispensed in apothecary units are those that have been in use for many years. For most other drugs the metric system is the system of measurement commonly used.

(2) Apothecary equivalents to the metric system.

(a) Volume:

1 ounce (oz) = 30 ml
8 oz = 240 ml (approximate)
1 quart (qt) = 1000 ml (approximate) (4 cups)

(b) Weight:

1 grain (gr) = 60 mg
1 oz = 30 gm
2.2 lbs = 1 kg
1000 gm = 1 kg

(3) It is important to understand that the apothecary system is only approximately equivalent to the metric system and to the common household system.

(4) In the apothecary system, fractions and Roman numerals are commonly used to designate numbers. Morphine, for example, may be ordered as 1/4, 1/6, or 1/8 grain. In addition, atropine may be ordered as 1/150 grain or 1/200 grain.

(5) Roman numerals may or may not be capitalized and are often used in combination with "SS", which indicates 1/2. Therefore, the term ISS means 1 1/2, and iiss means 2 1/2.

c. **Household Measure.**

Approximate equivalents to household measure:

1 teaspoon (tsp) = 5 ml
1 tablespoon (tbsp) = 15 ml = 1/2 oz
3 teaspoons (tsp) = 1 tbsp
2 tablespoon (tbsp) = 30 ml = 1 oz

d. **Conversion Between Apothecaries' and Metric Systems.**

(1) Essential equivalents must be learned in order to convert between these two systems.

(2) Ratio and proportion is the easiest way to carry out these conversions.

(3) <u>EXAMPLES</u>:

(a) 45 mg = X gr

$$\frac{60\text{ mg}}{1\text{ gr}} = \frac{45\text{ mg}}{X\text{ gr}}$$

60X = 45

X = 3/4 gr

(b) gr V = X mg

$$\frac{1\ gr}{60\ mg} = \frac{5\ gr}{X\ mg}$$

X = 60(5)

X = 300 mg

(c) 5 tbsp = X ml

$$\frac{1\ tbsp}{15\ ml} = \frac{5\ tbsp}{X\ ml}$$

X = 75 ml

(d) 3 oz = X ml

$$\frac{1\ oz}{30\ ml} = \frac{3\ oz}{X\ ml}$$

X = 90 ml

(e) 7 lbs = X kg

$$\frac{2.2\ lbs}{1\ kg} = \frac{7\ lbs}{X\ kg}$$

2.2X = 7

X = 3.2 kg

(4) Rules for converting between systems.

(a) All units of measurement must be in the same system, that is, volume to volume, weight to weight.

(b) Label all units of measurement.

(c) BE SURE that the relationship between units is the same on both sides of the equation.

2-11. COMMON EQUIVALENTS

Metric	Apothecary	Household
1000 ml = 1 liter	equals approx. 1 quart = 4 cups	1 quart
500 ml	equals approx. 1 pint = 2 cups	1 pint
240 ml	equals approx. 8 ounces	1 cup
30 ml	equals approx. 1 ounce	

Approximate Common Equivalents

1 tbsp = 15 ml = 1/2 oz
1 tsp = 5 ml = 1/6 oz
3 tsp = 1 tbsp
2 tbsp = 6 tsp = 30 ml = 1 oz
8 oz = 240 ml = 1 cup

2.2 lbs = 1 kg

60 mg = 1 gr
1000 mcg = 1 mg
1000 mg = 1 gm
1000 gm = 1 kg

1 ml = 1 cc
1000 ml = 1 liter

1 unit whole blood = 500 ml
1 unit packed red blood cells = 250 ml

2-12. PRACTICE 2-2 (SYSTEMS OF MEASUREMENT)

a. Change the following measures to equivalents within the metric system:

(1) 1000 mg = ________ gm

(2) 500 mg = ________ gm

(3) 200 ml = ________ L

(4) 1500 mg = ________ gm

(5) 0.1 L = ________ ml

(6) 750 mg = ________ gm

(7) 1 kg = ________ gm

(8) 5 L = ________ ml

(9) 4 mg = ________ gm

(10) 100 gm = ________ kg

(11) 0.25 L = ________ ml

(12) 0.0006 gm = _______ mg

(13) 250 mg = ________ gm

(14) 2.5 L = _________ ml

(15) 0.05 gm = ________ mg

(16) 300 mcg = ________ mg

(17) 1 mg = _________ mcg

(18) 0.05 mg = ________ mcg

(19) 4700 ml = ________ L

(20) 0.75 gm = ________ mg

b. Change the following measures to approximate household measures:

(1) 10 ml = _______ tsp

(2) 120 ml = _______ tbsp

(3) 2 oz = ________ tsp

(4) 60 ml = _______ oz

(5) 20 tbsp = ______ oz

(6) 1/2 fl oz = _____ tbsp

(7) 60 ml = _______ tsp

(8) 6 tsp = _______ oz

(9) 1 oz = ________ tsp

(10) 16 tbsp = ______ oz

c. Change the following apothecary measures to the <u>metric</u> equivalent:

(1) gr XV = __________

(2) 6 fl oz = __________

(3) gr 1/6 = __________

(4) gr 1/8 = __________

(5) gr 1/4 = __________

(6) gr 1/10 = __________

(7) 11 lbs = __________

(8) 154 lbs = __________

(9) 8 fl oz = __________

(10) 1 pint = __________

(11) 1 oz = __________

(12) gr X = __________

d. Convert the following units of measure as indicated using the ratio and proportion method.

(1) 45 mg = X gr

(2) 10 ml = X tsp

(3) 5 tbsp = X ml

(4) 500 mcg = X mg

(5) 0.6 gm = X mg

(6) 30 ml = X tbsp

(7) 0.0004 mg = X mcg

(8) 400 mg = X gm

(9) 120 mg = X gr

(10) 400 mcg = X gm

(11) 80 mg = X gr

(12) 10 mg = X gr

(13) 1/4 gr = X mg

(14) 1/6 gr = X mg

2-13. ANSWERS TO PRACTICE 2-2 (SYSTEMS OF MEASUREMENT)

a. (1) 1000 mg = 1 gm

(2) 500 mg = .5 gm

(3) 200 ml = .2 L

(4) 1500 mg = 1.5 gm

(5) 0.1 L = 100 ml

(6) 750 mg = .75 gm

(7) 1 kg = 1000 gm

(8) 5 L = 5000 ml

(9) 4 mg = .004 gm

(10) 100 gm = .1 kg

(11) 0.25 L = 250 ml

(12) 0.0006 gm = .6 mg

(13) 250 mg = .25 gm

(14) 2.5 L = 2500 ml

(15) 0.05 gm = 50 mg

(16) 300 mcg = .3 mg

(17) 1 mg = 1000 mcg

(18) 0.05 mg = <u>50</u> mcg

(19) 4700 ml = <u>4.7</u> L

(20) 0.75 gm = <u>750</u> mg

b. (1) $\frac{1 \text{ tsp}}{5 \text{ ml}} = \frac{X \text{ tsp}}{10 \text{ ml}}$

$5X = 10$

$X = 2$ tsp

(2) $\frac{1 \text{ tbsp}}{15 \text{ ml}} = \frac{X \text{ tbsp}}{120 \text{ ml}}$

$15X = 120$

$X = 8$ tbsp

(3) $\frac{1 \text{ tsp}}{1/6 \text{ oz}} = \frac{X \text{ tsp}}{2 \text{ oz}}$

$1/6\ X = 2$

$X = 12$ tsp

(4) $\frac{1 \text{ oz}}{30 \text{ ml}} = \frac{X \text{ oz}}{60 \text{ ml}}$

$30X = 60$

$X = 2$ oz

(5) $\frac{1 \text{ oz}}{2 \text{ tbsp}} = \frac{X \text{ oz}}{20 \text{ tbsp}}$

$2X = 20$

$X = 10$ oz

(6) $\frac{1}{2}$ fl oz = 1 tbsp

(7) $\frac{1 \text{ tsp}}{5 \text{ ml}} = \frac{X \text{ tsp}}{60 \text{ ml}}$

$5X = 60$

$X = 12$ tsp

(8) $\frac{1/6 \text{ oz}}{1 \text{ tsp}} = \frac{X \text{ oz}}{6 \text{ tsp}}$

$\underline{X} = 1$ oz

(9) 1 oz = 6 tsp

(10) $\frac{1 \text{ oz}}{2 \text{ tbsp}} = \frac{X \text{ oz}}{16 \text{ tbsp}}$

$2X = 16$

$X = 8$ oz

c. (1) $\frac{60 \text{ mg}}{\text{gr } 1} = \frac{X \text{ mg}}{\text{gr } 15}$

$\underline{X} = 900$ mg

(2) $\frac{30 \text{ ml}}{1 \text{ fl oz}} = \frac{X \text{ ml}}{6 \text{ fl oz}}$

$X = 180$ ml

(3) $\frac{60 \text{ mg}}{\text{gr } 1} = \frac{X \text{ mg}}{\text{gr } \frac{1}{6}}$

$X = 10$ mg

(4) $\frac{60 \text{ mg}}{\text{gr } 1} = \frac{X \text{ mg}}{\text{gr } \frac{1}{8}}$

$X = 7.5$ mg

(5) $\frac{60 \text{ mg}}{\text{gr } 1} = \frac{X \text{ mg}}{\text{gr } \frac{1}{4}}$

$\underline{X} = 15$ mg

(6) $\frac{60 \text{ mg}}{\text{gr } 1} = \frac{X \text{ mg}}{\text{gr } \frac{1}{10}}$

$X = 6$ mg

(7) $\frac{1 \text{ kg}}{2.2 \text{ lbs}} = \frac{X \text{ kg}}{11 \text{ lbs}}$

$2.2X = 11$

$X = 5$ kg

(8) $\frac{1 \text{ kg}}{2.2 \text{ lbs}} = \frac{X \text{ kg}}{154 \text{ lbs}}$

$2.2X = 154$

$X = 70$ kg

(9) $\frac{30 \text{ ml}}{1 \text{ fl oz}} = \frac{X \text{ ml}}{8 \text{ fl oz}}$

$X = 240$ ml

(10) 1 pt = 500 ml

(11) 1 oz = 30 ml

(12) $\frac{60 \text{ mg}}{\text{gr } 1} = \frac{X \text{ mg}}{\text{gr } 10}$

$X = 600$ mg

d. (1) 45 mg = $\underline{X}$ gr

$\frac{60 \text{ mg}}{1 \text{ gr}} = \frac{45 \text{ mg}}{X \text{ gr}}$

$60X = 45$

$X = 3/4$ gr

(2) 10 ml = X tsp

$$\frac{5\text{ ml}}{1\text{ tsp}} = \frac{10\text{ ml}}{X\text{ tsp}}$$

5X = 10

X = 2 tsp

(3) 5 tbsp = X ml

$$\frac{1\text{ tbsp}}{15\text{ ml}} = \frac{5\text{ tbsp}}{X\text{ ml}}$$

X = 75 ml

(4) 500 mcg = X mg

$$\frac{1000\text{ mcg}}{1\text{ mg}} = \frac{500\text{ mcg}}{X\text{ mg}}$$

1000X = 500

X = .5 mg

(5) 0.6 gm = X mg

$$\frac{1\text{ gm}}{1000\text{ mg}} = \frac{0.6\text{ gm}}{X\text{ mg}}$$

X = 600 mg

(6) 30 ml = X tbsp

$$\frac{15\text{ ml}}{1\text{ tbsp}} = \frac{30\text{ ml}}{X\text{ tbsp}}$$

15X = 30

X = 2 tbsp

(7) 0.0004 mg = X mcg

$$\frac{1 \text{ mg}}{1000 \text{ mcg}} = \frac{0.0004 \text{ mg}}{X \text{ mcg}}$$

X = .4 mcg

(8) 400 mg = X gm

$$\frac{1000 \text{ mg}}{1 \text{ gm}} = \frac{400 \text{ mg}}{X \text{ gm}}$$

1000X = 400

X = .4 gm

(9) 120 mg = X gr

$$\frac{60 \text{ mg}}{1 \text{ gr}} = \frac{120 \text{ mg}}{X \text{ gr}}$$

60X = 120

X = 2 gr

(10) 400 mcg = X gm

$$\frac{1{,}000{,}000 \text{ mcg}}{1 \text{ gm}} = \frac{400 \text{ mcg}}{X \text{ gm}}$$

1,000,000X = 400

X = .0004 gm

(11) 80 mg = X gr

$$\frac{60 \text{ mg}}{1 \text{ gr}} = \frac{80 \text{ mg}}{X \text{ gr}}$$

60X = 80

X = 1 1/3 gr

(12) 10 mg = X gr

$$\frac{60 \text{ mg}}{1 \text{ gr}} = \frac{10 \text{ mg}}{X \text{ gr}}$$

60X = 10

$$X = \frac{1}{6} \text{ gr}$$

(13) 1/4 gr = X mg

$$\frac{1 \text{ gr}}{60 \text{ mg}} = \frac{1/4 \text{ gr}}{X \text{ mg}}$$

X = 15 mg

(14) 1/6 gr = X mg

$$\frac{1 \text{ gr}}{60 \text{ mg}} = \frac{1/6 \text{ gr}}{X \text{ mg}}$$

X = 10 mg

Section III. COMPUTING MEDICATION DOSAGES

2-14. INFORMATION REQUIRED IN EVERY PHYSICIAN'S MEDICATION ORDER

a. Date and time the order is written.

b. Name of the medication.

c. Dosage of the medication.

d. Directions for administration.

(1) Route:

(a) I.M.: intramuscular or intramuscularly.

(b) I.V.: intravenous or intravenously.

(c) P.O. or p.o.: by mouth.

(d) p.r.: per rectum or rectally.

(e) SC (or SQ): subcutaneous or subcutaneously.

(2) Time interval or frequency:

(a) q 4h: every 4 hours.

(b) b.i.d.: twice a day.

(c) p.r.n.: if needed, as needed.

(d) q.d.: every day, daily.

(e) q.i.d.: 4 times a day.

(f) q.o.d.: every other day.

(g) t.i.d.: 3 times a day.

2-15. FIVE "RIGHTS" OF MEDICATION ADMINISTRATION

a. The right patient.

b. The right drug.

c. The right dose.

d. The right route.

e. The right time.

2-16. COMPUTING DOSAGES FOR TABLETS, PILLS, AND CAPSULES

EXAMPLE: You are to give 0.5 gm of medication to a patient P.O. On hand are 250 mg capsules.

a. Set up the proportion. LABEL ALL UNITS.

$$\frac{1 \text{ capsule}}{250 \text{ mg}} = \frac{X \text{ capsules}}{0.5 \text{ gm}}$$

b. Convert the strength of the medication ordered and the strength of the medication stocked to the same unit of measurement.

$$0.5 \text{ gm} = X \text{ mg}$$

$$\frac{1 \text{ gm}}{1000 \text{ mg}} = \frac{0.5 \text{ gm}}{X \text{ mg}}$$

$$X = 500 \text{ mg}$$

c. Cross-multiply.

$$\frac{1 \text{ capsule}}{250 \text{ mg}} = \frac{X \text{ capsules}}{500 \text{ mg}}$$

250X = 500

d. Solve for "X." Label the answer.

X = 2 capsules

EXAMPLE: You are to give Ampicillin 375 mg P.O. Ampicillin is stocked in 250 mg scored tablets.

$$\frac{1 \text{ tablet}}{250 \text{ mg}} = \frac{X \text{ tablets}}{375 \text{ mg}}$$

250 X = 375

X = 1 1/2 tablets

PRACTICE: Try this one yourself. Then refer to the solution provided to check your work.

You are to administer phenobarbital gr 1/2 P.O. to a patient. On hand are 15 mg tablets.

SOLUTION:

$$\frac{1 \text{ tablet}}{15 \text{ mg}} = \frac{X \text{ tablets}}{\text{gr } 1/2}$$

$$\frac{\text{gr } 1}{60 \text{ mg}} = \frac{\text{gr } 1/2}{X \text{ mg}}$$

$$\frac{60 \text{ mg}}{\text{gr } 1} = \frac{X \text{ mg}}{\text{gr } 1/2}$$

X = 30 mg

$$\frac{1 \text{ tablet}}{15 \text{ mg}} = \frac{X \text{ tablets}}{30 \text{ mg}}$$

15 X = 30

X = 2 tablets

e. Round dosages for tablets, pills, and capsules to the whole or half.

2-17. COMPUTING DOSAGES FOR ORAL LIQUID MEDICATIONS (PREPARED-STRENGTH LIQUIDS)

NOTE: Remember that the size (total # of mls) of the bottle of medication has no influence on the Expression of Strength of the medication.

EXAMPLE #1: You are to give 125 mg of a liquid medication to a patient. The medication is stocked in a 100 ml bottle that contains 250 mg of the medication per 5 ml.

a. Set up the proportion. *LABEL ALL UNITS.*

$$\frac{250 \text{ mg}}{5 \text{ ml}} = \frac{125 \text{ mg}}{X \text{ ml}}$$

b. Convert the strength of the medication ordered and the strength of the medication stocked to the same unit of measurement.

(not applicable here)

c. Cross-multiply.

250X = 725

d. Solve for "X." Label the answer.

X = 2.5 ml

EXAMPLE #2: Administer ampicillin 125 mg P.O. to a pediatric patient. On hand is a 100 ml bottle of ampicillin suspension labeled 0.2 gm per 4 ml. How many ml will you give?

a. Set up the proportion. *LABEL ALL UNITS.*

$$\frac{0.2 \text{ gm}}{4 \text{ ml}} = \frac{125 \text{ mg}}{X \text{ ml}}$$

b. Convert the strength of the medication ordered and the medication stocked to the same unit of measurement.

$$\frac{1 \text{ gm}}{1000 \text{ mg}} = \frac{0.2 \text{ gm}}{X \text{ mg}}$$

X = 200 mg

$$\frac{200 \text{ mg}}{4 \text{ ml}} = \frac{125 \text{ mg}}{X \text{ ml}}$$

c. Cross-multiply.

200X = 500

d. Solve for "X." Label the answer.

X = 2.5 ml

NOTE: Round P.O. liquids to the nearest tenth place.

PRACTICE: The physician has ordered KCL 40 mEq P.O. for your patient. On hand is KCL 15 mEq per 5 ml. How many ml will you administer?

SOLUTION:

$$\frac{15 \text{ mEq}}{5 \text{ ml}} = \frac{40 \text{ mEq}}{X \text{ ml}}$$

15X = 200

X = 13.3 = 13.3 ml

PRACTICE: The physician's order reads: Tylenol elixir gr V P.O. q 4h p.r.n. for pain. The medication label reads: Tylenol elixir 60 mg per 0.5 ml. How many ml will you administer?

SOLUTION:

$$\frac{60\text{ mg}}{0.5\text{ ml}} = \frac{5\text{ gr}}{X\text{ ml}}$$

$$\frac{60\text{ mg}}{1\text{ gr}} = \frac{X\text{ mg}}{5\text{ gr}}$$

X = 300 mg

$$\frac{60\text{ mg}}{0.5\text{ ml}} = \frac{300\text{ mg}}{X\text{ ml}}$$

60X = 150

X = 2.5 ml

2-18. COMPUTING DOSAGE FOR PARENTERAL MEDICATIONS

a. **Parenteral Medication Calculations.** The procedure for computing parenteral medication dosages is the same as for oral liquid medications (prepared strength liquids).

EXAMPLE: The order is to give Demerol (meperidine) 35 mg I.M. q4h p.r.n. for pain. The medication is supplied in an ampule marked 50 mg per ml. How much of the medication should you give?

(1) Set up the proportion. Label all units.

$$\frac{50\text{ mg}}{1\text{ ml}} = \frac{35\text{ mg}}{X\text{ ml}}$$

(2) Convert the strength of the medication ordered and the strength of the medication stocked to the same unit of measurement.

(not applicable here)

(3) Cross-multiply.

50X = 35

(4) Solve for "X." Label answers.

X = .7 ml

NOTE: Round parenteral medications to the tenth, except for heparin and insulin, which are rounded to the hundredth.

PRACTICE: The order is to give morphine sulfate gr 1/8 I.M. q 4h p.r.n. for pain. On hand are ampules labeled 10 mg per ml. How much medication should you give?

SOLUTION:

$$\frac{10\text{ mg}}{1\text{ ml}} = \frac{\frac{1}{8}\text{ gr}}{X\text{ ml}}$$

$$\frac{60\text{ mg}}{1\text{ gr}} = \frac{X\text{ mg}}{\frac{1}{8}\text{ gr}}$$

$X = 7.5$ mg

$$\frac{10\text{ mg}}{1\text{ ml}} = \frac{7.5\text{ mg}}{X\text{ ml}}$$

$10X = 7.5$

$X = .75 = .8$ ml

PRACTICE: The order is to give 0.3 mg of atropine I.M. on call to surgery. The medication is stocked in a vial labeled gr 1/150 per ml. How much medication should you give?

SOLUTION:

$$\frac{\text{gr } 1/150}{1\text{ ml}} = \frac{0.3\text{ mg}}{X\text{ ml}}$$

$$\frac{60\text{ mg}}{\text{gr } 1} = \frac{X\text{ mg}}{\text{gr } 1/150}$$

$X = .4$ mg

$$\frac{.4\text{ mg}}{1\text{ ml}} = \frac{0.3\text{ mg}}{X\text{ ml}}$$

$.4\,X = 0.3$

$X = .75 = .8$ ml

PRACTICE: The physician orders Gentamicin 60 mg I.M. q 8h. The vial is labeled 80 mg per 2 ml. How much medication should you give?

SOLUTION:

$$\frac{80 \text{ mg}}{2 \text{ ml}} = \frac{60 \text{ mg}}{X \text{ ml}}$$

$80X = 120$

$X = 1.5$ ml

b. **Reconstitution of Medications for Injection.**

(1) Some medications will become unstable in solution over time. You may see these medications manufactured as dry powders.

(2) Prior to administration of these medications, an appropriate diluent (sterile water, normal saline, and so forth) must be added. The term used to describe the process of adding the diluent to the medication is reconstitution.

(3) Usually the volume of the diluent is expanded somewhat when added to the dry powder. For example, when 2 ml of diluent are added to a dry vial of 1 gram of Mefoxin, the resulting withdrawable volume is 2.5 ml.

(4) The directions for reconstitution of a medication may list a number of different amounts of diluent, each resulting in a different concentration. If that is the case, choose a concentration, which would provide an appropriate volume for the injection. When selecting a concentration, keep in mind that no more than 3-4 ml should be injected into one I.M. site. However, it may be necessary to divide the dose and inject it into two different sites.

EXAMPLE: The order is to give 300,000 units of Penicillin G Potassium I.M. A concentration of 200,000 units/ml should be used. The medication on hand is in a 1,000,000 unit vial. How many ml will you give? (Directions for reconstitution are listed below.)

1,000,000 unit vial:

Concentration	Diluent to be Added
100,000 units/ml	9.6 ml
200,000 units/ml	4.6 ml
250,000 units/ml	3.6 ml

NOTE: Figure 2-1 below illustrates the process of reconstitution of the medication in this example.

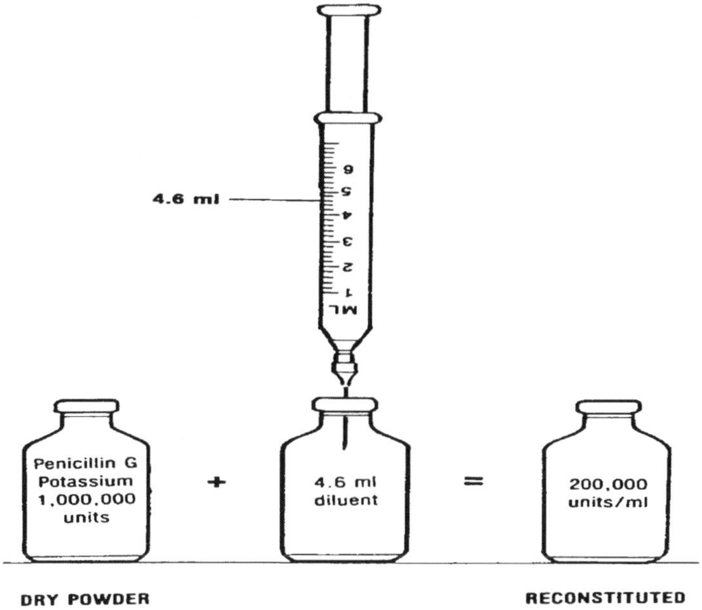

Figure 2-1. The process of reconstitution.

(a) Set up the proportion. Label all units.

$$\frac{200{,}000 \text{ units}}{1 \text{ ml}} = \frac{300{,}000 \text{ units}}{X \text{ ml}}$$

(b) Cross-multiply.

$200{,}000X = 300{,}000$

(c) Solve for X. Label answer.

$X = 1.5$ ml

PRACTICE: The physician has ordered 0.5 gm of Mefoxin I.M. b.i.d. You have a 1 gm vial available. Directions for reconstitution are:

Concentration	Amount of Diluent	Withdrawable Volume
400 mg/ml	2 ml for I.M. use	2.5 ml
95 mg/ml	10 ml for I.V. use	10.5 ml

1 Which concentration should be used?

2 How many ml should be administered?

a Set up the proportion. Label all units.

b. Convert the strength of the medication ordered and the strength of the medication stocked to the same unit of measurement.

c. Cross-multiply.

d. Solve for X. Round off to the nearest tenth. Label answer.

SOLUTION:

1. 400 mg/ml

2. a. $\frac{400\ mg}{1\ ml} = \frac{0.5\ gm}{X\ ml}$

b. $\frac{1\ gm}{1000\ mg} = \frac{0.5\ gm}{X\ mg}$

$X = 500\ mg$

$\frac{400\ mg}{1\ ml} = \frac{500\ mg}{X\ ml}$

c. $400X = 500$

d. $X = 1.25 = 1.3\ ml$

PRACTICE: The order is to give Cleocin Phosphate 300 mg I.V. Directions for reconstitution state: Add 50 ml of sterile water. Each ml will contain 12 mg of medication. How many ml will you give?

SOLUTION:

$\frac{1\ ml}{12\ mg} = \frac{X\ ml}{300\ mg}$

$12X = 300$

$X = 25\ ml$

c. **Heparin Calculations.**

(1) Heparin is supplied in various concentrations, labeled in units per ml.

(2) It is administered subcutaneously or intravenously.

(3) All heparin calculations should be carried out to the thousandth decimal place and rounded to the hundredth place.

(4) Subcutaneous injections of heparin should be administered using a tuberculin syringe.

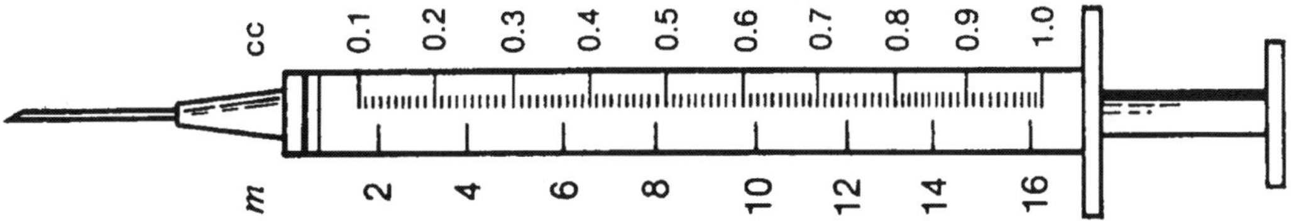

Figure 2-2. Tuberculin (T.B.) syringe.

EXAMPLE: The physician has ordered heparin 5,000 units SC q 8h. Using a vial labeled 40,000 units per ml, calculate the amount of heparin to give.

(a) Set up the proportion. Label all units.

$$\frac{40{,}000 \text{ units}}{1 \text{ ml}} = \frac{5{,}000 \text{ units}}{X \text{ ml}}$$

(b) Cross-multiply.

40,000X = 5,000

X = 0.125 ml

Give 0.13 ml

PRACTICE: The order is for 15,000 units of heparin SC q 12h. You have a vial labeled 20,000 units per ml. How much medication will you give?

SOLUTION:

$$\frac{20{,}000 \text{ units}}{1 \text{ ml}} = \frac{15{,}000 \text{ units}}{X \text{ ml}}$$

20,000X = 15,000

X = 0.75 ml

PRACTICE: The order is to give heparin 11,000 units SC q 8h. Available is a vial containing 20,000 units per ml. How much medication will you give?

SOLUTION:

$$\frac{20{,}000 \text{ units}}{1 \text{ ml}} = \frac{11{,}000 \text{ units}}{X \text{ ml}}$$

$$20{,}000X = 11{,}000$$

$$X = 0.55 \text{ ml}$$

d. **Insulin Calculations.**

(1) Insulin is supplied in 10 ml vials labeled in the number of units per ml. U-100 insulin is the most commonly used concentration.

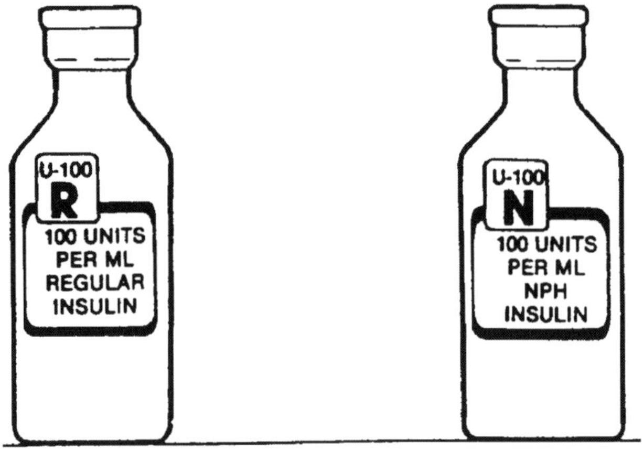

Figure 2-3. U-100 insulin.

(2) The simplest and most accurate way to measure insulin is with an insulin syringe. An insulin syringe is calibrated in units and the ordered dose is read directly on the syringe. Therefore, to measure 16 units of U-100 insulin, you would simply measure to the 16 unit mark on the U-100 insulin syringe.

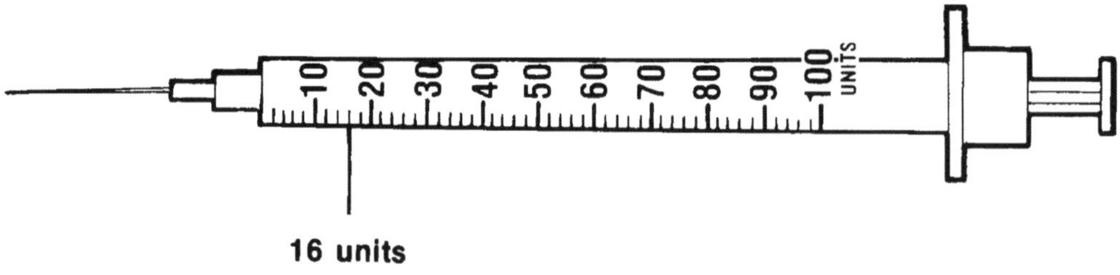

Figure 2-4. Measuring insulin in an insulin syringe.

(3) When measuring U-100 insulin (100 units per ml) in a 1 ml tuberculin syringe, the number of units ordered will always equal an equivalent number of hundredths of a milliliter. Therefore, to measure 16 units of U-100 insulin, measure to the 0.16 ml mark on the tuberculin syringe. Be sure to use the cc scale on the syringe.

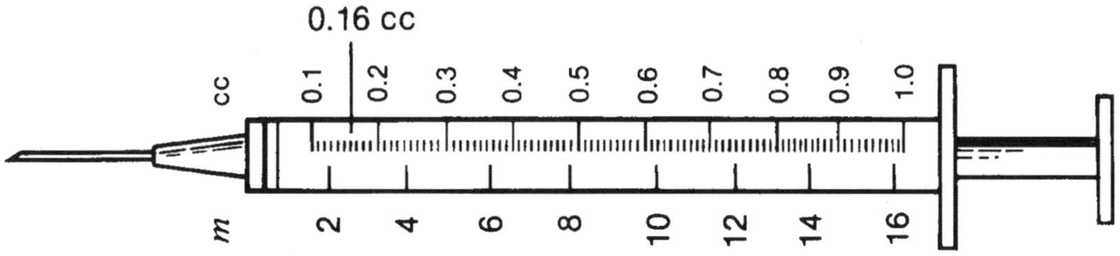

Figure 2-5. Measuring insulin in a tuberculin syringe.

(4) Calculations for insulin dosages are carried out in the same manner as for other parenteral medications. However, as with heparin, all insulin calculations should be rounded to the hundredth place.

EXAMPLE: The order is to give 20 units of Regular Insulin. You are using U-100 insulin and a tuberculin syringe. What is the required dose?

$$\frac{100 \text{ units}}{1 \text{ ml}} = \frac{20 \text{ units}}{X \text{ ml}}$$

$$100X = 20$$

$$X = 0.2 \text{ ml}$$

PRACTICE: The order is to give 30 units of NPH insulin SC. Available is a 10 ml vial labeled U-100 NPH insulin. Calculate the amount of insulin to give.

SOLUTION:

$$\frac{100 \text{ units}}{1 \text{ ml}} = \frac{30 \text{ units}}{X \text{ ml}}$$

$$100X = 30$$

$$X = 0.3 \text{ ml}$$

e. **Calculation of Medication Based on Body Weight.** Medication doses are often based on the patient's body weight, especially with infants and children. Although this is primarily a professional responsibility, you may use the manufacturer's recommendations to determine if a prescribed dose is a reasonable dose to administer.

EXAMPLE #1: The manufacturer's recommendation for pediatric Tylenol is 10 mg/kg/dose. How many mg are recommended for each dose for a 20 kg child?

Calculate the dosage (mg) of Tylenol the child is to receive, using the proportion method.

$$\frac{10 \text{ mg}}{1 \text{ kg}} = \frac{X \text{ mg}}{20 \text{ kg}}$$

1 X = 200 mg/dose for 20 kg child

EXAMPLE #2: The recommendation for Garamycin is 2 mg/kg/dose. The child weighs 15 kg. The Garamycin is supplied 10 mg/ml. How many mg are recommended for each dose for a 15 kg child? How many ml are required for a single dose?

a. Calculate the dosage (mg) of Garamycin to be given to the 15kg child for <u>one</u> <u>dose</u>.

$$\frac{2 \text{ mg}}{1 \text{ kg}} = \frac{X \text{ mg}}{15 \text{ kg}}$$

1 X = 30 mg for the 15 kg child.

b. Calculate the amount (ml) of Garamycin to be given for one dose.

$$\frac{10 \text{ mg}}{1 \text{ ml}} = \frac{30 \text{ mg}}{X \text{ ml}}$$

10 X = 30

X = 3 ml

Therefore, 3 ml will provide the recommended dose for a 15 kg child.

PRACTICE #1: A patient who weighs 154 pounds is to receive a medication that has a recommended one time dosage of 3 mg/kg. The medication is stocked in a vial labeled 50 mg/ml. Calculate the volume of the medication to be administered.

a. Convert the patient's body weight to kilograms.

$$\frac{1 \text{ kg}}{2.2 \text{ lbs}} = \frac{X \text{ kg}}{154 \text{ lbs}}$$

2.2 X = 154

X = 70 kg

b. Calculate the dosage of the medication based on the patient's body weight.

$$\frac{3 \text{ mg}}{1 \text{ kg}} = \frac{X \text{ mg}}{70 \text{ kg}}$$

1 X = 210 mg

c. Calculate the volume of the drug to be administered.

SOLUTION TO c.:

$$\frac{50 \text{ mg}}{1 \text{ ml}} = \frac{210 \text{ mg}}{X \text{ ml}}$$

50X = 210

X = 4.2 ml

PRACTICE #2: The order is for Depakene 15mg/kg/day for a patient who weighs 110 pounds. The medication is to be given in 3 divided doses. Depakene is stocked in 125 mg/capsules. Calculate the number of capsules to give per dose.

SOLUTION:

a. Convert the patient's body weight to kilograms.

$$\frac{1 \text{ kg}}{2.2 \text{ lbs}} = \frac{X \text{ kg}}{110 \text{ lbs}}$$

2.2 $\underline{X}$ = 110

$\underline{X}$ = 50 kg

b. Calculate the dosage (per day) of medication based on the patient's body weight.

$$\frac{15\text{ mg}}{1\text{ kg}} = \frac{X\text{ mg}}{50\text{ kg}}$$

X = 750 mg per day

c. Calculate the number of capsules to be administered per day.

$$\frac{125\text{ mg}}{1\text{ capsule}} = \frac{750\text{ mg}}{X\text{ capsules}}$$

125X = 750

X = 6 capsules per day

d. Calculate the number of capsules to be administered per dose.

6 ÷ 3 = 2 capsules per dose.

2-19. MODIFIED PROPORTION METHOD FOR COMPUTING DOSAGES

NOTE: The final examination at the end of the subcourse will not include information from paragraph 2-19. This alternative method of computing dosages is for your information only.

$$\frac{D}{H} \times Q \qquad \frac{\text{Desired Dose} \times \text{Quantity}}{\text{On Hand Dose}}$$

PRACTICE: You are to administer 300 mg of a medication to a patient. The medication is stocked in a vial labeled 250 mg per 2.5 ml. How many ml will you administer?

SOLUTION:

$$\frac{300\text{ mg}}{250\text{ mg}} \times 2.5\text{ ml} = \frac{750}{250} = 3\text{ ml}$$

2-20. PRACTICE 2-3 (COMPUTING MEDICATION DOSAGES)

1. You are to administer Dilantin 300 mg P.O. to a patient. Dilantin is stocked in 100 mg capsules. You will administer ____capsules.

2. Aspirin tablets are labeled 0.3 gm. How many tablets are needed for a dose of 600 mg?____________

3. The doctor has ordered Diabinese tablets 0.25 gm for your patient. You have available Diabinese 100 mg tablets. You will administer ______ tablets to your patient.

4. You are to administer Digoxin 0.375 mg P.O. to a patient. On hand are 0.25 mg tablets. You will administer _____ tablets.

5. You are to administer Phenobarbital gr 1/4 P.O. to a patient. On hand are 15 mg tablets. How many tablets will you give? _______

6. Your patient is to receive Digoxin 0.25 mg P.O. You have available a bottle labeled 0.05 mg per 1 ml. You will administer ___ ml to your patient.

7. The doctor has ordered Mellaril liquid 0.1 gm for your patient. You have available Mellaril liquid labeled 30 mg/ml. You will administer ____ ml to your patient.

8. The physician's order is KCL 40 mEq P.O. On hand is KCL 15 mEq per 5 ml. You will administer ______ml.

9. Administer Ampicillin 125 mg P.O. to a pediatric patient. On hand is a 100 ml bottle of Ampicillin suspension containing 200 mg per 4 ml. How many ml will you give? ____________

10. The order reads: Tylenol elixir gr X P.O., p.r.n. for pain. The medication label reads: Tylenol elixir 60 mg per 0.5 ml. You will administer _____ ml.

11. The physician has ordered Ritalin 30 mg P.O. t.i.d. On hand are 20 mg scored tablets. How many tablets will you give? _______

12. The order is for Mysoline 125 mg P.O. t.i.d. On hand are 250 mg tablets. How many tablets will you give per dose? ________ per day?________

13. You are to give the patient Ampicillin 250 mg P.O. q 6h. The suspension on hand contains 125 mg per 5 ml. How many ml will the patient receive per dose? _______

14. The order is to give Dilantin 100 mg P.O. t.i.d. The available suspension contains 30 mg per 5 ml. How many ml. will you give?______

15. The physician has ordered Tetracycline syrup 500 mg q 6h P.O. The available medication contains 125 mg per 5 ml. How many ml will you give? ______

16. The doctor has ordered 65 mg of Garamycin I.M. for your patient. You have available a multidose vial of Garamycin labeled 40 mg/ml. How much of the medication will the patient receive? ______

17. The doctor has ordered an injection of Atropine 0.3 mg I.M. for your patient. You have available a multi-dose vial labeled Atropine 1 mg/ml. You will administer ______ ml to your patient.

18. The doctor orders Morphine gr 1/4 I.M. for your patient. You have available Morphine 10 mg/ml. How much of the solution will you administer? ______

19. The doctor has ordered Digoxin 0.125 mg I.M. You have a vial of Digoxin labeled 0.5 mg/2 ml. How much of the medication should the patient receive? ______

20. You are to administer Atropine gr 1/200 I.M. to a patient. On hand is Atropine gr 1/150 per 0.8 ml. How many ml will you give?_______

21. The vial of powdered medication is labeled Staphcillin 1 gm. The directions say to add 1.5 ml of sterile saline. The solution will then equal 2 ml. How much of the solution should you give if the order is Staphcillin 500 mg I.M.?

____

22. The doctor has ordered Keflin 250 mg I.M. for a 5-year-old patient. You have available a vial of powdered drug labeled 1 gm Keflin. You read the manufacturer's directions and find you should add 4 ml of sterile water to dissolve the drug and produce a solution in which 2.2 ml equals 500 mg of Keflin. How many ml will you give?_______

23. The doctor has ordered Regular Insulin 46 units SC for your patient. Using Regular Insulin U-100, how many ml will you administer if the medication is drawn up in a tuberculin syringe? ______

24. You are to give 20 u of Regular Insulin. You have U-40 Regular Insulin available. How much will you give using a tuberculin syringe? ______

25. The physician has ordered Heparin 2000u SC for your patient. On hand is a 20 ml vial of Heparin labeled 10,000u per ml. You will give ________ ml.

26. The order is to give Prostaphlin 350 mg I.M. q 4h. Directions for reconstitution of the 1 gm vial state: Add 5.7 ml of sterile water. Each 1.5 ml will then contain 250 mg of medication. How many ml will you give? ___

27. The order is to give 0.25 gm Cefobid I.M. q 12h. Directions for reconstitution of the 1 gm vial state: Add 2.8 ml of sterile water to produce a concentration of 333 mg. per ml. How many ml will you give? ______

28. The order is to give Pipracil 750 mg I.M. q 8h. Directions for reconstitution of the 2 gm vial state: Add 4 ml of sodium chloride to produce a concentration of 1 gm per 2.5 ml. How many ml will you give?_______

29. The following refers to reconstitution of penicillin:

Diluent =	Concentration
3.2 ml =	1,000,000 units/ml
8.2 ml =	500,000 units/ml
18.2 ml =	250,000 units/ml

Using the 3.2 diluent, how much penicillin (ml) must be used to administer 1.5 million units? (1.5 million = 1,500,000)

30. The recommended dose of Penicillin G is 250,000 units/kg/day divided in 6 equal doses. The medication is available as 1,000,000 units per 10 ml. The child weighs 30 kg. Determine the number of ml to be administered per dose. ______.

31. The doctor has ordered 2000 units of Heparin SC. You have available a 5 ml vial labeled 10,000 units per ml. How many ml will you administer?

______

32. The order is to give Penicillin G 300,000 units I.M. for your patient. You have a vial that contains 200,000 units/ml. How much medication will you administer? ______

33. The order is to give Atropine gr 1/200 I.M. On hand is an ampule labeled gr 1/150 per 2 ml. How many ml will you give? _______

34. The order is to give Morphine 6 mg I.M. q 4h, p.r.n. The available vial is labeled 1/6 gr per ml. How many ml will you give?______

35. The order is to give Phenobarbital gr 1/4 I.M., q 4-6 h p.r.n. On hand is a tubex (prefilled syringe) labeled 30 mg/2 ml. How many ml will you give?

______

36. The order is to give Methicillin 0.6 gm I.M. q 6h. On hand is a vial labeled 150 mg per ml. How many ml should you give? ______

37. The order is to give Mylanta 45 ml P.O. q 2h. How many ounces will you administer? ______

38. The order is to give Erythromycin base 0.5 gm P.O. q 6h. On hand are 125 mg tablets. How many tablets will you give? ______

39. The physician has ordered Synthroid 25 mcg P.O. q AM. Available are 0.05 mg tablets. How many tablets will you give?_______

40. The order is for Slophyllin 60 mg P.O. q 8h. The medication is supplied in a syrup 80 mg/15 ml. How many ml will you give?_______

2-21. ANSWERS TO PRACTICE 2-3 (COMPUTING MEDICATION DOSAGES)

1. $$\frac{1 \text{ capsule}}{100 \text{ mg}} = \frac{X \text{ capsules}}{300 \text{ mg}}$$

   100 X = 300

   X = 3 capsules (paras 2-2, 2-3, 2-16)

2. (a) $$\frac{1 \text{ tablet}}{0.3 \text{ gm}} = \frac{X \text{ tablets}}{600 \text{ mg}}$$

   (b) 0.3 gm = X mg

   $$\frac{1 \text{ gm}}{1000 \text{ mg}} = \frac{0.3 \text{ gm}}{X \text{ mg}}$$

   X = 300 mg

   (c) $$\frac{1 \text{ tablet}}{300 \text{ mg}} = \frac{X \text{ tablets}}{600 \text{ mg}}$$

   300 X = 600

   X = 2 tablets (paras 2-2, 2-3, 2-7, 2-16)

3. (a) $$\frac{1 \text{ tablet}}{100 \text{ mg}} = \frac{X \text{ tablets}}{0.25 \text{ gm}}$$

   (b) 0.25 gm = X mg

   $$\frac{1 \text{ gm}}{1000 \text{ mg}} = \frac{0.25 \text{ gm}}{X \text{ mg}}$$

   X = 250 mg

   (c) $$\frac{1 \text{ tablet}}{100 \text{ mg}} = \frac{X \text{ tablets}}{250 \text{ mg}}$$

   100 X = 250

   X = 2.5 or 2 1/2 tablets (paras 2-2, 2-3, 2-7, 2-16)

4. $\frac{\text{1 tablet}}{\text{0.25 mg}} = \frac{\text{X tablets}}{\text{0.375 mg}}$

0.25 X = 0.375

X = 1.5 or 1 1/2 tablets (paras 2-2, 2-3, 2-16)

5. (a) $\frac{\text{1 tablet}}{\text{15 mg}} = \frac{\text{X tablets}}{\text{gr 1/4}}$

(b) $\frac{\text{gr 1}}{\text{60 mg}} = \frac{\text{gr 1/4}}{\text{X mg}}$

X = 15 mg

(c) $\frac{\text{1 tablet}}{\text{15 mg}} = \frac{\text{X tablets}}{\text{15 mg}}$

15 X = 15

X = 1 tablet (paras 2-2, 2-3, 2-7, 2-16)

6. $\frac{\text{0.05 mg}}{\text{1 ml}} = \frac{\text{0.25 mg}}{\text{X ml}}$

0.05 X = 0.25

X = 5 ml (para 2-14)

7. (a) $\frac{\text{30 mg}}{\text{1 ml}} = \frac{\text{0.1 gm}}{\text{X ml}}$

(b) 0.1 gm = X mg

$\frac{\text{1 gm}}{\text{1000 mg}} = \frac{\text{0.1 gm}}{\text{X mg}}$

X = 100 mg

(c) $\frac{\text{30 mg}}{\text{1 ml}} = \frac{\text{100 mg}}{\text{X ml}}$

30 X = 100

X = 3.3 ml (paras 2-2, 2-3, 2-7, 2-17)

8. $\frac{15 \text{ mEq}}{5 \text{ ml}} = \frac{40 \text{ mEq}}{X \text{ ml}}$

15 X = 200

X = 13.3 ml (paras 2-2, 2-3, 2-17)

9. $\frac{200 \text{ mg}}{4 \text{ ml}} = \frac{125 \text{ mg}}{X \text{ ml}}$

200 X = 500

X = 2.5 ml (paras 2-2, 2-3, 2-17)

10. (a) $\frac{60 \text{ mg}}{0.5 \text{ ml}} = \frac{\text{gr } 10}{X \text{ ml}}$

(b) gr 10 = X mg

$\frac{\text{gr } 1}{60 \text{ mg}} = \frac{\text{gr } 10}{X \text{ mg}}$

X = 600 mg

(c) $\frac{60 \text{ mg}}{0.5 \text{ ml}} = \frac{600 \text{ mg}}{X \text{ ml}}$

60 X = 300

X = 5 ml (paras 2-2, 2-3, 2-7, 2-17)

11. $\frac{1 \text{ tablet}}{20 \text{ mg}} = \frac{X \text{ tablets}}{30 \text{ mg}}$

20 X = 30

X = 1.5 or 1 1/2 tablets (paras 2-2, 2-3, 2-14, 2-16)

12. $\frac{1 \text{ tablet}}{250 \text{ mg}} = \frac{X \text{ tablets}}{125 \text{ mg}}$

250 X = 125

X = 1/2 tablet per dose

1/2 X 3 = 1 1/2 tablets per day (paras 2-2, 2-3, 2-14, 2-16)

13. $\frac{125 \text{ mg}}{5 \text{ ml}} = \frac{250 \text{ mg}}{X \text{ ml}}$

$125 X = 1250$

$X = 10$ ml (paras 2-2, 2-3, 2-17)

14. $\frac{30 \text{ mg}}{5 \text{ ml}} = \frac{100 \text{ mg}}{X \text{ ml}}$

$30 X = 500$

$X = 16.7$ ml (paras 2-2, 2-3, 2-10, 2-14, 2-17)

15. $\frac{125 \text{ mg}}{5 \text{ ml}} = \frac{500 \text{ mg}}{X \text{ ml}}$

$125 X = 2500$

$X = 20$ ml per day (paras 2-2, 2-3, 2-17)

16. $\frac{40 \text{ mg}}{1 \text{ ml}} = \frac{65 \text{ mg}}{X \text{ ml}}$

$40 X = 65$

$X = 1.6$ ml (paras 2-2, 2-3, 2-18a)

17. $\frac{1 \text{ mg}}{1 \text{ ml}} = \frac{0.3 \text{ mg}}{X \text{ ml}}$

$X = 0.3$ ml (paras 2-2, 2-3, 2-18a)

18. (a) $\frac{10 \text{ mg}}{1 \text{ ml}} = \frac{\text{gr } 1/4}{X \text{ ml}}$

(b) $\frac{60 \text{ mg}}{\text{gr } 1} = \frac{X \text{ mg}}{\text{gr } 1/4}$

$X = 15$ mg

(c) $\frac{10 \text{ mg}}{1 \text{ ml}} = \frac{15 \text{ mg}}{X \text{ ml}}$

$10 X = 15$

$X = 1.5$ ml (paras 2-2, 2-3, 2-10, 2-18a)

19. $\frac{0.5 \text{ mg}}{2 \text{ ml}} = \frac{0.125 \text{ mg}}{X \text{ ml}}$

$0.5 X = 0.250$

$X = 0.5$ ml (paras 2-2, 2-3, 2-18a)

20. $\frac{\text{gr } 1/150}{0.8 \text{ ml}} = \frac{\text{gr } 1/200}{X \text{ ml}}$

$\frac{1}{150} X = .004$ ml

$X = 0.6$ ml (paras 2-2, 2-3, 2-15a)

21. (a) $\frac{1 \text{ gm}}{2 \text{ ml}} = \frac{500 \text{ mg}}{X \text{ ml}}$

(b) 1 gm = 1000 mg

(c) $\frac{1000 \text{ mg}}{2 \text{ ml}} = \frac{500 \text{ mg}}{X \text{ ml}}$

$1000 X = 1000$

$X = 1$ ml (paras 2-2, 2-3, 2-10, 2-18a)

22. $\frac{2.2 \text{ ml}}{500 \text{ mg}} = \frac{X \text{ ml}}{250 \text{ mg}}$

$500 X = 550$

$X = 1.1$ ml (paras 2-2, 2-3, 2-18b)

23. $\frac{100 \text{ units}}{1 \text{ ml}} = \frac{46 \text{ units}}{X \text{ ml}}$

$100 X = 46$

$X = 0.46$ ml (paras 2-2, 2-3, 2-18d)

24. $\frac{40 \text{ units}}{1 \text{ ml}} = \frac{20 \text{ units}}{X \text{ ml}}$

$40X = 20$

$X = 0.5$ ml (paras 2-2, 2-3, 2-18d)

25. $\frac{10{,}000 \text{ units}}{1 \text{ ml}} = \frac{2000 \text{ units}}{X \text{ ml}}$

$10{,}000X = 2000$

$X = 0.2$ ml (paras 2-2, 2-3, 2-18c)

26. $\frac{250 \text{ mg}}{1.5 \text{ ml}} = \frac{350 \text{ mg}}{X \text{ ml}}$

$250X = 525$

$X = 2.1$ ml (paras 2-2, 2-3, 2-18b)

27. (a) $\frac{333 \text{ mg}}{1 \text{ ml}} = \frac{0.25 \text{ gm}}{X \text{ ml}}$

(b) $\frac{1 \text{ gm}}{1000 \text{ mg}} = \frac{0.25 \text{ gm}}{X \text{ mg}}$

$X = 250$ mg

(c) $\frac{333 \text{ mg}}{1 \text{ ml}} = \frac{250 \text{ mg}}{X \text{ ml}}$

$333X = 250$

$X = 0.8$ ml (paras 2-2, 2-3, 2-10, 2-18b)

28. (a) $\frac{1 \text{ gm}}{2.5 \text{ ml}} = \frac{750 \text{ mg}}{X \text{ ml}}$

(b) $\frac{1 \text{ gm}}{1000 \text{ mg}} = \frac{X \text{ gm}}{750 \text{ mg}}$

$1000X = 750$

$X = .75$ gm

(c) $\frac{1 \text{ gm}}{2.5 \text{ ml}} = \frac{.75 \text{ gm}}{X \text{ ml}}$

X = 1.875 = 1.9 ml (paras 2-2, 2-3, 2-10, 2-18b)

29. $\frac{1{,}000{,}000 \text{ units}}{1 \text{ ml}} = \frac{1{,}500{,}000 \text{ units}}{X \text{ ml}}$

1,000,000 X = 1,500,000

X = 1.5 ml (paras 2-2, 2-3, 2-18b)

30. (a) $\frac{250{,}000 \text{ units}}{1 \text{ kg}} = \frac{X \text{ units}}{30 \text{ kg}}$

X = 7,500,000 units per day

(b) $\frac{1{,}000{,}000 \text{ units}}{10 \text{ ml}} = \frac{7{,}500{,}000 \text{ units}}{X \text{ ml}}$

1,000,000 X = 75,000,000

X = 75 ml per day

75. 6 = 12.5 ml per dose (paras 2-2, 2-3, 2-18e)

31. $\frac{10{,}000 \text{ units}}{1 \text{ ml}} = \frac{2000 \text{ units}}{X \text{ ml}}$

10,000 X = 2,000

X = 0.2 ml (paras 2-2, 2-3, 2-18c)

32. $\frac{200{,}000 \text{ units}}{1 \text{ ml}} = \frac{300{,}000 \text{ units}}{X \text{ ml}}$

200,000 X = 300,000

X = 1.5 ml (paras 2-2, 2-3, 2-18a)

33. $\dfrac{\text{gr } \frac{1}{150}}{2 \text{ ml}} = \dfrac{\text{gr } \frac{1}{200}}{X \text{ ml}}$

$\dfrac{1X}{150} = \dfrac{1}{100}$

X = 1.5 ml (paras 2-2, 2-3, 2-18a)

34. (a) $\dfrac{\frac{1}{6} \text{ gr}}{1 \text{ ml}} = \dfrac{6 \text{ mg}}{X \text{ ml}}$

(b) $\dfrac{\frac{1}{1} \text{ gr}}{60 \text{ mg}} = \dfrac{6 \text{ gr}}{X \text{ mg}}$

X = 10 mg

(c) $\dfrac{10 \text{ mg}}{1 \text{ ml}} = \dfrac{6 \text{ mg}}{X \text{ ml}}$

10 X = 6

X = 0.6 ml (paras 2-2, 2-3, 2-10, 2-18a)

35. (a) $\dfrac{30 \text{ mg}}{2 \text{ ml}} = \dfrac{\text{gr } 1/4}{X \text{ ml}}$

(b) $\dfrac{\text{gr } 1}{60 \text{ mg}} = \dfrac{\text{gr } 1/4}{X \text{ ml}}$

X = 15 mg

(c) $\dfrac{30 \text{ mg}}{2 \text{ ml}} = \dfrac{15 \text{ mg}}{X \text{ ml}}$

30 X = 30

X = 1 ml (paras 2-2, 2-3, 2-10, 2-18a)

36. (a) $\frac{150 \text{ mg}}{1 \text{ ml}} = \frac{0.6 \text{ gm}}{X \text{ ml}}$

(b) $\frac{1 \text{ gm}}{1000 \text{ mg}} = \frac{0.6 \text{ gm}}{X \text{ mg}}$

X = 600 mg

(c) $\frac{150 \text{ mg}}{1 \text{ ml}} = \frac{600 \text{ mg}}{X \text{ ml}}$

150 X = 600

X = 4 ml (paras 2-2, 2-3, 2-10, 2-18a)

37. $\frac{1 \text{ oz}}{30 \text{ ml}} = \frac{X \text{ oz}}{45 \text{ ml}}$

30 X = 45

X = 1.5 oz (paras 2-2, 2-3, 2-11, 2-17)

38. (a) $\frac{1 \text{ tablet}}{125 \text{ mg}} = \frac{X \text{ tablets}}{0.5 \text{ gm}}$

(b) $\frac{1 \text{ gm}}{1000 \text{ mg}} = \frac{0.5 \text{ gm}}{X \text{ mg}}$

X = 500 mg

(c) $\frac{1 \text{ tablet}}{125 \text{ mg}} = \frac{X \text{ tablets}}{500 \text{ mg}}$

125 X = 500

X = 4 tablets (paras 2-2, 2-3, 2-10, 2-16)

39. (a) $\frac{1 \text{ tablet}}{0.05 \text{ mg}} = \frac{X \text{ tablets}}{25 \text{ mcg}}$

(b) $\frac{1 \text{ mg}}{1000 \text{ mcg}} = \frac{X \text{ mg}}{25 \text{ mcg}}$

1000 X = 25

X = 0.025 mg

(c) $\frac{1 \text{ tablet}}{0.05 \text{ mg}} = \frac{X \text{ tablets}}{0.025 \text{ mg}}$

$0.05 X = 0.025$

$X = 0.5$ or 1/2 tablet (paras 2-2, 2-3, 2-10, 2-16)

40. $\frac{80 \text{ mg}}{15 \text{ ml}} = \frac{60 \text{ mg}}{X \text{ ml}}$

$80 X = 900$

$X = 11.3$ ml (paras 2-2, 2-3, 2-17)

Section IV. COMPUTING INTRAVENOUS INFUSION RATES

2-22. INFORMATION REQUIRED ON AN ORDER FOR I.V. FLUIDS

a. Type of fluid to be infused.

b. Volume of the fluid to be infused.

c. Time period over which the fluid is to be infused.

2-23. I.V. ADMINISTRATION SET CALIBRATIONS

a. I.V. flow rates are regulated in drops per minute (gtts/min).

b. The size of the drop (drop factor) varies from large to small, and depending on the manufacturer and type of set used, it will require 10, 15, or 20 gtts to equal 1 ml in standard macrodrip sets, and 60 gtts to equal 1 ml in micro- or minidrip sets. (See examples in figure 2-6.)

2-24. OBJECTIVES OF I.V. THERAPY

a. To supply fluids when patients are unable to take adequate fluids by mouth.

b. To provide salts needed to maintain electrolyte balance: KCL, calcium, magnesium.

c. To provide glucose for metabolism.

(1) D_5W = 5% Dextrose.

(2) $D_{10}W$ = 10% Dextrose.

(3) D_5 $_{1/2}$NS = 5% Dextrose, .45% Normal Saline.

(4) D_5NS = 5% Dextrose, .9% Normal Saline.

(5) D_5 $_{1/4}$NS = 5% dextrose, .23% Normal Saline.

d. To provide water-soluble vitamins.

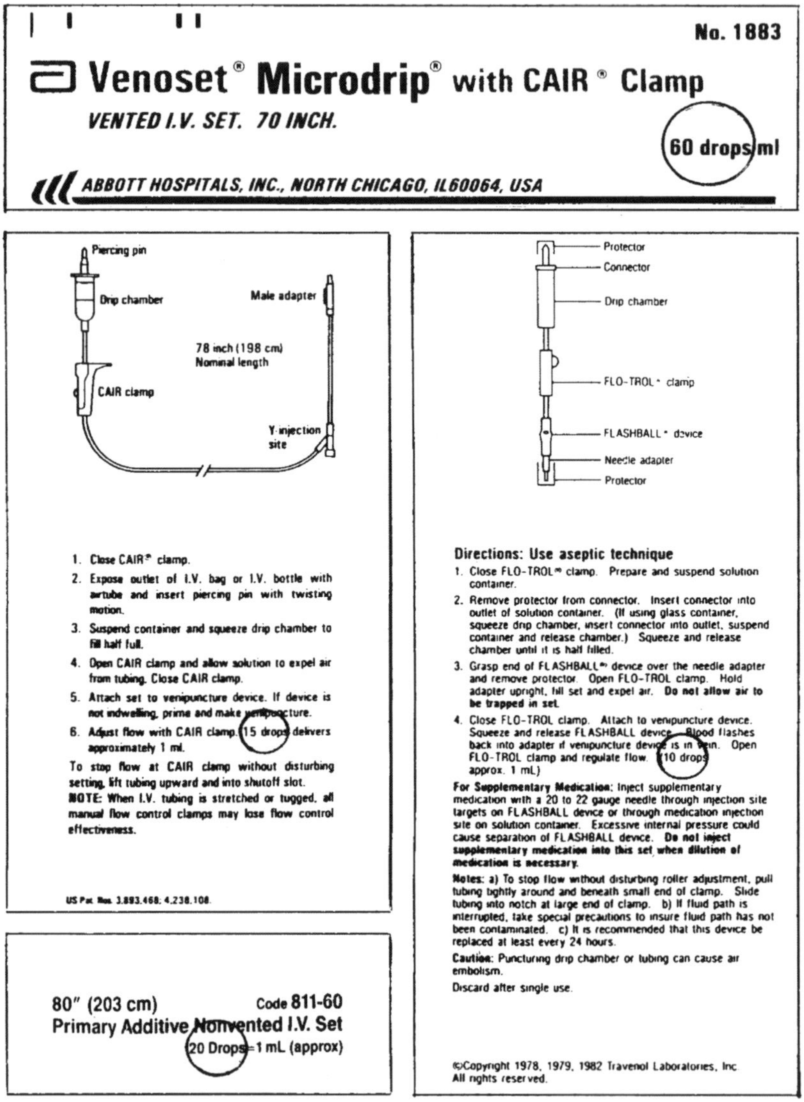

Figure 2-6. I.V. set calibrations.

2-25. FACTORS THAT INFLUENCE VOLUME DETERMINATION

a. Patient's daily maintenance requirements.

b. Volume losses prior to therapy.

c. Concurrent losses; gastric suction, vomiting, or diarrhea.

d. Patient's metabolic requirements.

2-26. COMPUTING CONTINUOUS I.V. INFUSION RATES

a. **I.V. Formula.**

EXAMPLE #1: The order is for D_5 $_{1/2}$NS 1000 ml to be infused over eight hours. Calculate the infusion rate using an I.V. set calibrated to deliver 20 gtts/ml.

$$\frac{\text{Volume (ml) x drop factor (gtts/ml)}}{\text{Time (minutes)}}$$

$$\frac{\text{1000 ml x 20 gtts/ml}}{480}$$

$$\frac{20{,}000}{480} = 41.67 = 42 \text{ gtts/min.}$$

NOTE: For I.V.'s, round off to the nearest whole number.

EXAMPLE #2: The patient is to receive 1000 ml of 0.45% sodium chloride over the next 10 hours. The drop factor of the tubing is 15 gtts/ml. Determine the rate in gtts/min.

$$\frac{\text{1000 ml x 15 gtts/ml}}{\text{600 minutes}}$$

$$\frac{15{,}000}{600} = 25 \text{ gtts/min.}$$

EXAMPLE #3: The order is to infuse D_5 $_{1/2}$NS at <u>125 ml/hr</u> for the next 24 hours. The I.V. administration set is calibrated 20 gtts/ml. Calculate the infusion rate.

$$\frac{\text{Volume x drop factor}}{\text{Time (min.)}}$$

$$\frac{\text{125 ml/hr x 20 gtts/ml}}{\text{60 min.}}$$

$$\frac{2500}{60} = \text{42 gtts/min.}$$

PRACTICE 1: The order is to infuse 1500 ml of Ringer's lactate over the next 24 hours. The drop factor of the tubing is 60 gtts/ml. Determine the rate in gtts/min.

SOLUTION:

$$\frac{\text{1500 ml x 60 gtts/ml}}{1440}$$

$$\frac{90{,}000}{1440} = \text{63 gtts/min}$$

PRACTICE 2: The order is to give 250 ml of Rheomacrodex (dextran 40) over 45 minutes. The drop factor of the tubing is 10 gtts/ml. Determine the rate in gtts/min.

SOLUTION:

$$\frac{\text{250 ml x 10 gtts/ml}}{45}$$

$$\frac{2500}{45} = \text{56 gtts/min}$$

b. **Practice Problems.**

(1) The patient is to receive 2000 ml of D_5NS over 12 hours. The drop factor of the tubing is 15 gtts/ml. Determine the infusion rate.

SOLUTION:

$$\frac{2000 \text{ ml} \times 15 \text{ gtts/ml}}{720}$$

$$\frac{30{,}000}{720} = 42 \text{ gtts/ml}$$

(2) The physician has ordered 2000 ml of NS at a rate of 125 ml/hr for the next 16 hours. The drop factor of the tubing is 20 gtts/ml. Determine the rate in gtts/min.

SOLUTION:

$$\frac{125 \text{ ml} \times 20 \text{ gtts/ml}}{60}$$

$$\frac{2500}{60} = 42 \text{ gtts/min}$$

(3) The order is to infuse 1500 ml of Ringer's lactate over the next 24 hours. The drop factor of the tubing is 20 gtts/ml. Determine the rate in gtts/min.

SOLUTION:

$$\frac{1500 \text{ ml} \times 20 \text{ gtts/ml}}{1440}$$

$$\frac{30{,}000}{1440} = 21 \text{ gtts/min.}$$

(4) The patient is to receive Intralipid 10% at a rate of 500 ml over 4 hours. The drop factor of the tubing is 10 gtts/ml. Determine the infusion rate.

SOLUTION:

$$\frac{500 \text{ ml} \times 10 \text{ gtts/ml}}{240}$$

$$\frac{5000}{240} = 21 \text{ gtts/min.}$$

(5) The order is to infuse 1000 ml of D_5W over 24 hours to keep the vein open. Using I.V. with a drop factor of 60 gtts/ml, determine the infusion rate.

SOLUTION:

$$\frac{1000 \text{ ml} \times 60 \text{ gtts/ml}}{1440}$$

$$\frac{60{,}000}{1440} = 42 \text{ gtts/min.}$$

2-27. ADMINISTRATION OF MEDICATIONS BY IVPB (INTERMITTENT INFUSION)

NOTE: Intermittent infusion of medications requires giving a drug through an in-progress I.V. or through a special I.V. catheter called a heparin lock.

a. The terms piggyback and I.V. piggyback (IVPB) are commonly used when referring to any intermittent infusion that requires more than 5 minutes to complete.

b. The medication is usually diluted in 50 to 100 ml of I.V. fluid and infused over about 30 minutes.

EXAMPLE: The order is to give Cimetidine 300 mg IVPB q 6h. It is recommended that this medication be dissolved in 100 ml of I.V. solution (D_5W) and infused over 30 minutes. Using a drop factor of 20 gtts/ml, determine the infusion rate.

$$\frac{100 \text{ ml} \times 20 \text{ gtts/ml}}{30}$$

$$\frac{2000}{30} = 67 \text{ gtts/min.}$$

PRACTICE #1: The order is to give 6,000,000 units of Penicillin G IVPB q 4h. The medication is to be dissolved in 150 ml of I.V. fluid, and the recommended infusion time is 1 1/2 hours. Using a drop factor of 20 gtts/ml, determine the infusion rate.

SOLUTION:

$$\frac{150 \text{ ml} \times 20 \text{ gtts/ml}}{90}$$

$$\frac{3000}{90} = 33 \text{ gtts/min.}$$

PRACTICE #2: The order is to give Solu-Medrol 125 mg IVPB q.4h. The medication is to be dissolved in 50 ml of I.V. fluid and the recommended administration time is 15 minutes. Using a drop factor of 20 gtts/ml, determine the infusion rate.

SOLUTION:

$$\frac{50 \text{ ml} \times 20 \text{ gtts/ml}}{15}$$

$$\frac{1000}{15} = 67 \text{ gtts/min.}$$

2-28. ADMINISTRATION OF MEDICATIONS BY CONTINUOUS INFUSION

NOTE: With continuous I.V. infusions of medications, the physician will order a medication dosage and not fluid volume. For example, the order may specify mg/hr or units/hr.

EXAMPLE: The order is to administer a continuous I.V. Heparin drip at a rate of 1200 units per hour. The pharmacy sends up a 250 ml bag of Normal Saline with 25,000 units of Heparin added. Using a drop factor of 60 gtts/ml, determine the infusion rate to deliver the ordered amount of medication.

a. Determine the amount of drug in the solution.

$$\frac{25{,}000 \text{ units}}{250 \text{ ml}}$$

b. Determine the number of ml/hr to be administered to give the ordered dosage.

$$\frac{25{,}000 \text{ units}}{250 \text{ ml}} = \frac{1200 \text{ units}}{X \text{ ml}}$$

$$25{,}000 X = 300{,}000$$

$$X = 12 \text{ ml/hr}$$

c. Determine the infusion rate in gtts/min.

$$\frac{12 \text{ ml} \times 60 \text{ gtts/ml}}{60}$$

$$\frac{720}{60} = 12 \text{ gtts/min}$$

PRACTICE #1: The physician has ordered a continuous infusion of Aminophylline at a rate of 25 mg/hr. The pharmacy sends up a 500 ml bag of D_5W with 500 mg of Aminophylline added. Using a drop factor of 60 gtts/ml, determine the infusion rate.

SOLUTION:

a. $\frac{500 \text{ mg}}{500 \text{ ml}}$

b. $\frac{500 \text{ mg}}{500 \text{ ml}} = \frac{25 \text{ mg}}{X \text{ ml}}$

$500X = 12{,}500$

$X = 25 \text{ ml/hr}$

c. $\frac{25 \text{ ml} \times 60 \text{ gtts/ml}}{60}$

$\frac{1500}{60} = 25 \text{ gtts/min}$

PRACTICE #2: The patient is to receive a regular insulin drip of 10 units/hr. The pharmacy sends up a 250 ml bag of normal saline with 100 units of regular insulin added. The I.V. administration set delivers 60 gtts/ml. How many gtts/min will you administer?

SOLUTION:

a. $\frac{100 \text{ units}}{250 \text{ ml}}$

b. $\frac{100 \text{ units}}{250 \text{ ml}} = \frac{10 \text{ units}}{X \text{ ml}}$

$100X = 2500$

$X = 25 \text{ ml/hr}$

c. $\frac{25 \text{ ml} \times 60 \text{ gtts/ml}}{60}$

$\frac{1500}{60} = 25 \text{ gtts/min}$

2-29. PRACTICE 2-4 (COMPUTING INTRAVENOUS INFUSION RATES)

a. The order is to infuse an I.V. of D_5W 1000 ml over 12 hours. Calculate the infusion rate using an I.V. set that delivers 20 gtts/ml.

b. The order is to infuse a 0.9% normal saline 250 ml over 45 minutes. Calculate the infusion rate using an I.V. set that delivers 10 gtts/ml.

c. The order is to infuse D_5RL 1000 ml q 8h for 24 hours. Calculate the infusion rate using a drop factor of 15 gtts/ml.

d. The order is for 2000 ml of hyperalimentation to infuse over 24 hours. The I.V. set delivers 60 gtts/ml. The solution should be administered at a rate of _______ gtts/min.

e. The patient is to receive 1200 ml of D_5RL over 10 hours. The I.V. set delivers 20 gtts/ml. The infusion rate will be ______ gtts/min.

f. Administer 150 ml of Normal Saline over 30 minutes using an I.V. set that delivers 10 gtts/ml. The infusion rate will be ______.

g. The order is for Amikacin Sulfate 100 mg to be dissolved in 150 ml of D_5W to run over 1 hour. Using an I.V. set that delivers 20 gtts/ml, determine the infusion rate.

h. The order is for Gentamycin 180 mg IVPB q 8h. The medication is dissolved in 100 ml of D_5W and should infuse over 45 minutes. Using a drop factor of 20 gtts/ml, determine the infusion rate.

i. The order is to infuse 500 ml of 0.9% NS over 2 hours. The I.V. administration set delivers 15 gtts/ml. How many gtts/min will you administer?

j. You are to infuse D_5W at 15 ml/hr to a pediatric patient. The I.V. administration set delivers 60 gtts/ml. Determine the infusion rate.

k. The order is to give two units of whole blood (1 unit is 500 ml). The blood is to infuse over the next 4 hours and the drop factor of the tubing is 10 gtts/ml. Determine the infusion rate in gtts/min.

l. The patient is to receive 3 units of packed red blood cells (1 unit equals 250 ml) to be infused over the next 4 hours. The drop factor is 10 gtts/ml. Determine the infusion rate in gtts/min.

m. The order is to infuse 1000 ml D_5NS with 40 mEq KCl* over the next 8 hours. Using I.V. tubing with a drop factor of 20 gtts/ml, determine the infusion rate.

* KCl (potassium chloride) is always measured in milliequivalents (mEq).

n. The physician orders an I.V. of 1000 ml of D_5 $_{1/4}NS$ to have 20 mEq of KCl added. The KCl is available in multiple dose vials with 2 mEq per ml. How many ml of KCl should be added to the I.V. solution?

o. An I.V. of D_5W with 20 mEq KCl is ordered to run at 20 ml/hr using a microdrop set calibrated at 60 gtts/ml. Determine the infusion rate.

p. The order is to infuse Intralipids 500 ml over 6 hours using a drop factor of 10 gtts/ml. Determine the infusion rate.

q. The order is for 0.45% NaC1 500 ml to infuse in 4 hours. The I.V. set drop factor is 20 gtts/min. Determine the infusion rate.

r. The order is to give Geopen 2 gm IVPB q 6h. The recommended dilution is 2 gm in 50 ml of I.V. solution to be administered over 15 minutes. Using a drop factor of 20 gtts/ml, determine the infusion rate.

s. The patient is to receive Aldomet 500 mg IVPB q 6h. The medication is dissolved in 100 ml of I.V. fluid. Each 500 mg is to be run in over 1 hour. Using a drop factor of 15 gtts/ml, determine the infusion rate.

t. The order is to give 100 mg of Aminophyllin in a total of 35 ml of fluid over the next 45 minutes. Using a drop factor of 60 gtts/ml, determine the rate in gtts/min.

u. The patient is to receive Heparin at a rate of 1500 units per hour. The I.V. has 30,000 units per 500 ml of D_5W. Using a drop factor of 60 gtts/ml, determine the infusion rate in gtts/min and ml/hr.

v. The patient is to receive Heparin 1400 units per hour. The pharmacy sends up a 250 ml bag of 0.9 normal saline with 25,000 units of heparin added. The I.V. set delivers 60 gtts/ml. Determine the infusion rate in gtts/min and ml/hr.

w. The order is for a continuous Regular Insulin drip of 15 units/hr. The pharmacy sends up a 250 ml bag of normal saline with 150 units of regular insulin. The I.V. administration set delivers 60 gtts/ml. Determine the infusion rate in gtts/min and ml/hr.

x. The order is for Aminophylline at 20 mg/hr. The pharmacy sends up a 500 ml bag of D_5W with 500 mg of Aminophylline added. Using a drop factor of 60 gtts/ml, determine the infusion rate in gtts/min and ml/hr.

2-30. ANSWERS TO PRACTICE 2-4 (COMPUTING INTRAVENOUS INFUSION RATES)

a. $\frac{1000 \text{ ml} \times 20 \text{ gtts/ml}}{720}$

$\frac{20,000}{720} = 28 \text{ gtts/min}$

b. $\frac{250 \text{ ml} \times 10 \text{ gtts/ml}}{45}$

$\frac{2500}{45} = 56 \text{ gtts/min}$

c. $\frac{1000 \text{ ml} \times 15 \text{ gtts/ml}}{480}$

$\frac{15,000}{480} = 31 \text{ gtts/min}$

d. $\frac{2000 \text{ ml} \times 60 \text{ gtts/ml}}{1440}$

$\frac{120,000}{1440} = 83 \text{ gtts/min}$

e. $\frac{1200 \text{ ml} \times 20 \text{ gtts/ml}}{600}$

$\frac{24,000}{600} = 40 \text{ gtts/min}$

f. $\frac{150 \text{ ml} \times 10 \text{ gtts/ml}}{30}$

$\frac{1500}{30} = 50 \text{ gtts/min}$

g. $\frac{150 \text{ ml} \times 20 \text{ gtts/ml}}{60}$

$\frac{3000}{60} = 50$ gtts/min

h. $\frac{100 \text{ ml} \times 20 \text{ gtts/ml}}{45}$

$\frac{2000}{45} = 44$ gtts/min

i. $\frac{500 \text{ ml} \times 15 \text{ gtts/ml}}{120}$

$\frac{7500}{120} = 63$ gtts/min

j. $\frac{15 \text{ ml} \times 60 \text{ gtts/ml}}{60}$

$\frac{900}{60} = 15$ gtts/min

k. $\frac{1000 \text{ ml} \times 10 \text{ gtts/ml}}{240}$

$\frac{10,000}{240} = 42$ gtts/min

l. $\frac{750 \text{ ml} \times 10 \text{ gtts/ml}}{240}$

$\frac{7500}{240} = 31$ gtts/min

m. $\frac{1000 \text{ ml} \times 20 \text{ gtts/ml}}{480}$

$\frac{20,000}{480} = 42$ gtts/min

n. $\frac{2 \text{ mEq}}{1 \text{ ml}} = \frac{20 \text{ mEq}}{X \text{ ml}}$

$2X = 20$

$X = 10$ ml

o. $\frac{20 \text{ ml} \times 60 \text{ gtts/ml}}{60}$

$\frac{1200}{60} = 20$ gtts/min

p. $\frac{500 \text{ ml} \times 10 \text{ gtts/ml}}{360}$

$\frac{5000}{360} = 14$ gtts/min

q. $\frac{500 \text{ ml} \times 20 \text{ gtts/min}}{240}$

$\frac{10{,}000}{240} = 42$ gtts/min

r. $\frac{50 \text{ ml} \times 20 \text{ gtts/ml}}{15}$

$\frac{1000}{15} = 67$ gtts/min

s. $\frac{100 \text{ ml} \times 15 \text{ gtts/ml}}{60}$

$\frac{1500}{60} = 25$ gtts/min

t. $\frac{35 \text{ ml} \times 60 \text{ gtts/ml}}{45}$

$\frac{2100}{45} = 47$ gtts/min

u. (1) $\frac{30{,}000 \text{ units}}{500 \text{ ml}} = \frac{1500 \text{ units}}{X \text{ ml}}$

$30{,}000 X = 750{,}000$

$X = 25$ ml/hr

(2) $\frac{25 \text{ ml} \times 60 \text{ gtts/ml}}{60}$

$\frac{1500}{60} = 25$ gtts/min

v. (1) $\frac{25{,}000 \text{ units}}{250 \text{ ml}} = \frac{1400 \text{ units}}{X \text{ ml}}$

25,000 X = 350,000

X = 14 ml/hr

(2) $\frac{14 \text{ ml} \times 60 \text{ gtts/ml}}{60}$

$\frac{840}{60} = 14$ gtts/min

w. (1) $\frac{150 \text{ units}}{250 \text{ ml}} = \frac{15 \text{ units}}{X \text{ ml}}$

150 X = 3750

X = 25 ml/hr

(2) $\frac{25 \text{ ml} \times 60 \text{ gtts/ml}}{60}$

$\frac{1500}{60} = 25$ gtts/ml

x. (1) $\frac{500 \text{ mg}}{500 \text{ ml}} = \frac{20 \text{ mg}}{X \text{ ml}}$

500 X = 10,000

X = 20 ml/hr

(2) $\frac{20 \text{ ml} \times 60 \text{ gtts/ml}}{60}$

$\frac{1200}{60} = 20$ gtts/min

2-31. INTERPRETING INFORMATION FROM A MEDICATION LABEL

a. Generic name--the chemical name for a drug.

b. Trade name--a drug company's name for a particular drug.

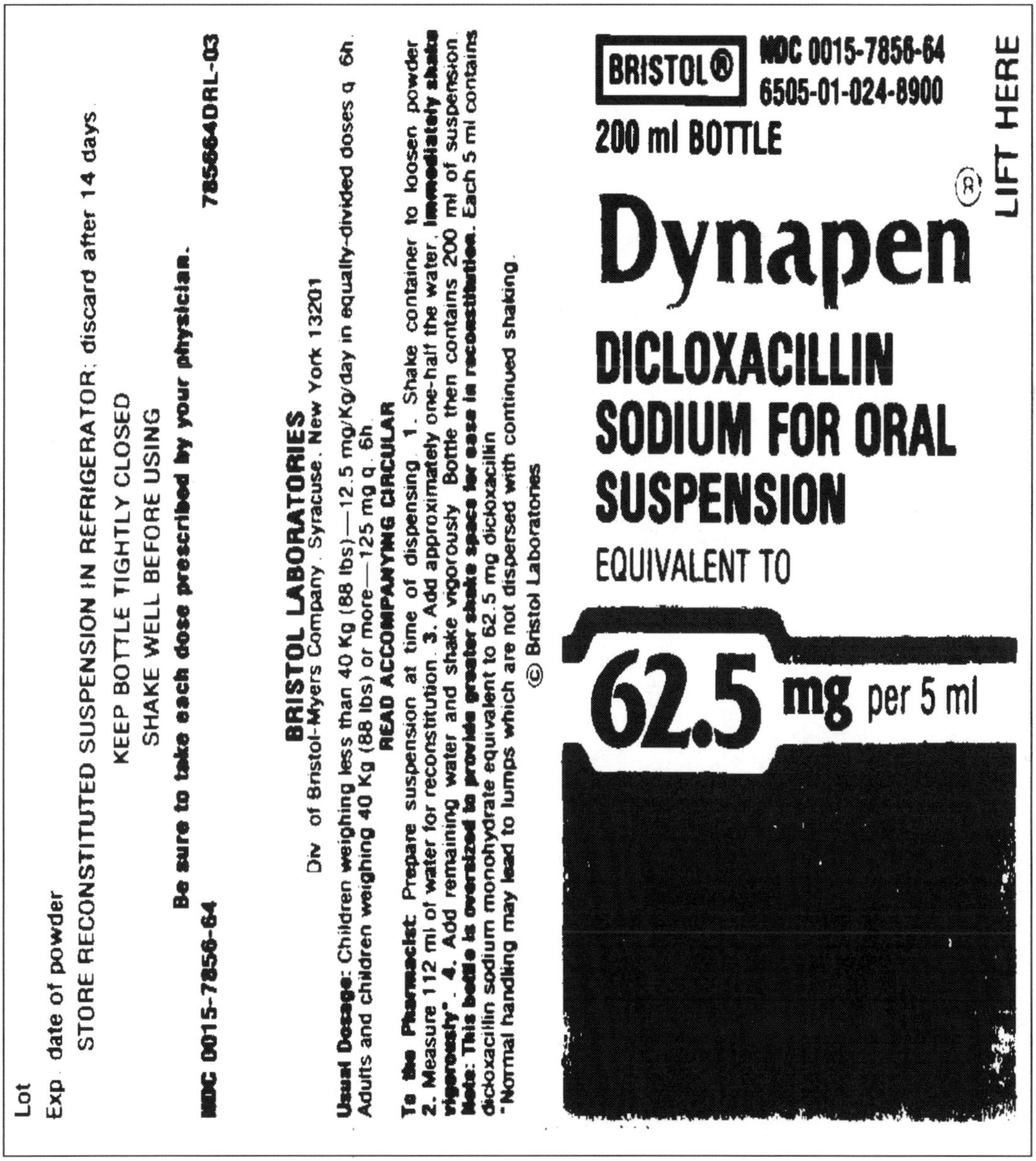

c. Strength of the medication.

(1) Instructions for reconstitution.

(2) Concentration of the drug in a given volume of solution.

d. Special storage considerations--temperature.

e. Expiration date interpretation.

2-32. PRACTICE EXERCISE--LABEL INTERPRETATION (PART 1)

Directions: Read the labels provided to calculate the indicated doses (next page). All medications are in oral form, either tablet, pill, suspension, or capsules. Fill in the blanks; then check the solutions provided in paragraph 2-33.

a. Prepare a 20 mg dosage of Inderal _____ tab(s)

b. The order is for Ampicillin susp. 375 mg _____ ml

c. The order is for Benadryl 100 mg _____ cap(s)

d. Prepare 500 mg of penicillin V potassium _____ tab(s)

e. Prepare 500 mg of Amoxicillin susp _____ ml

f. Isosorbide dinitrate 40 mg _____ cap(s)

g. Prepare 150,000 u. of nystatin oral suspension . _____ ml

h. Acetaminophen 325 mg is ordered _____ tab(s)

i. The order is for allopurinol 300 mg _____ tab(s)

j. Prepare sulfasalazine 1000 mg _____ tab(s)

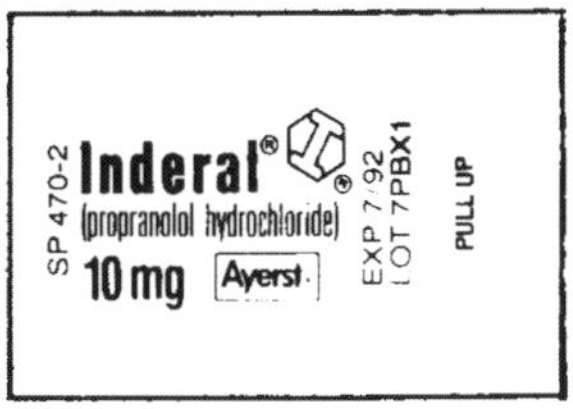
SP 470-2
Inderal®
(propranolol hydrochloride)
10 mg
Ayerst
EXP 7/92
LOT 7PBX1
PULL UP

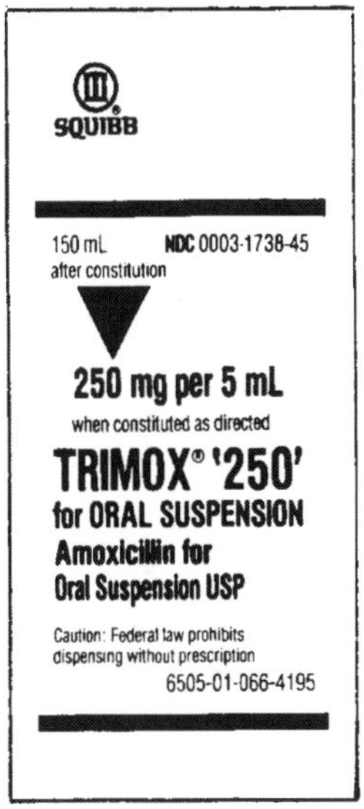
SQUIBB
150 mL
NDC 0003-1738-45
after constitution
250 mg per 5 mL
when constituted as directed
TRIMOX® '250'
for ORAL SUSPENSION
Amoxicillin for
Oral Suspension USP
Caution: Federal law prohibits
dispensing without prescription
6505-01-066-4195

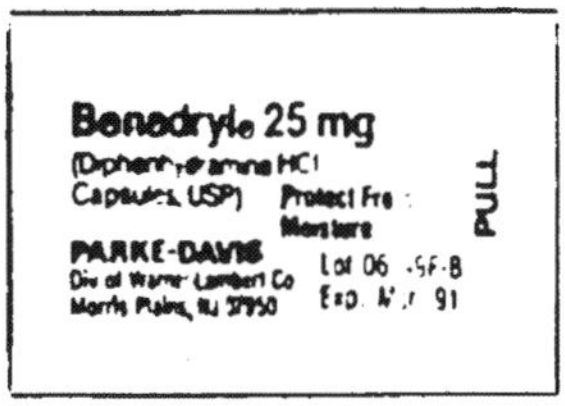
Benadryl® 25 mg
PARKE-DAVIS
PULL

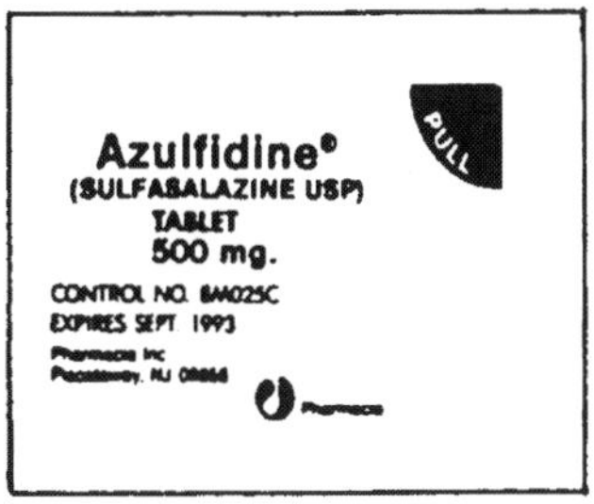
Azulfidine®
(SULFASALAZINE USP)
TABLET
500 mg.
EXPIRES SEPT 1993
PULL

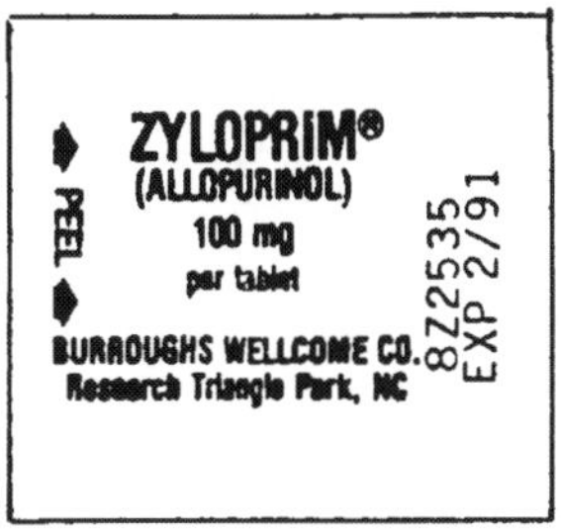
PEEL
ZYLOPRIM®
(ALLOPURINOL)
100 mg
per tablet
BURROUGHS WELLCOME CO.
Research Triangle Park, NC
8Z2535
EXP 2/91

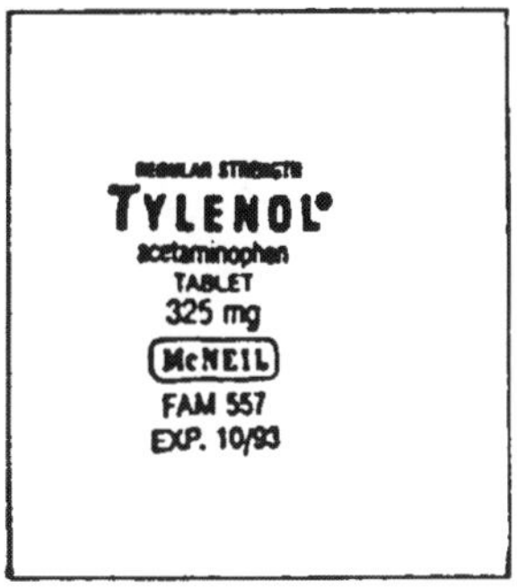
TYLENOL®
acetaminophen
TABLET
325 mg
McNEIL
FAM 557
EXP. 10/93

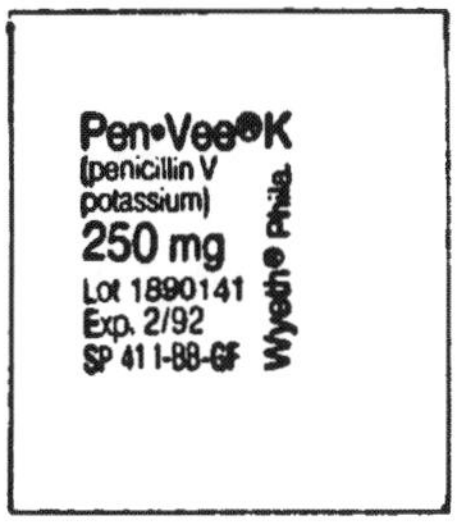
Pen•Vee®K
(penicillin V
potassium)
250 mg
Lot 1890141
Exp. 2/92
SP 411-88-GF
Wyeth® Phila.

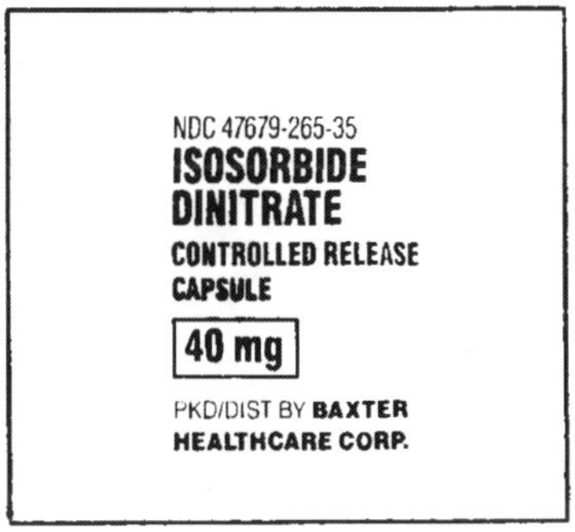
NDC 47679-265-35
ISOSORBIDE
DINITRATE
CONTROLLED RELEASE
CAPSULE
40 mg
PKD/DIST BY BAXTER
HEALTHCARE CORP.

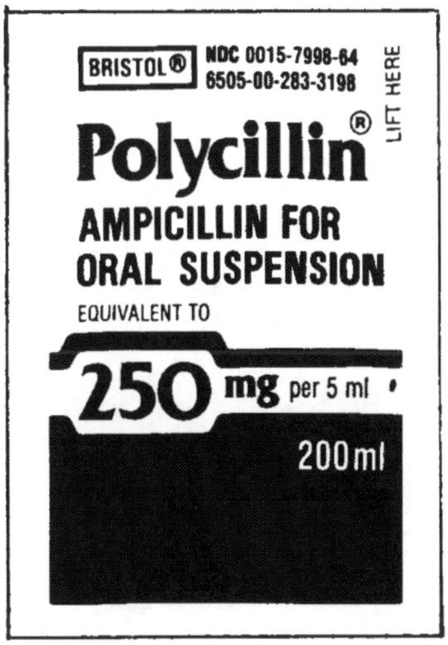
BRISTOL®
NDC 0015-7998-64
6505-00-283-3198
LIFT HERE
Polycillin®
AMPICILLIN FOR
ORAL SUSPENSION
EQUIVALENT TO
250 mg per 5 ml
200 ml

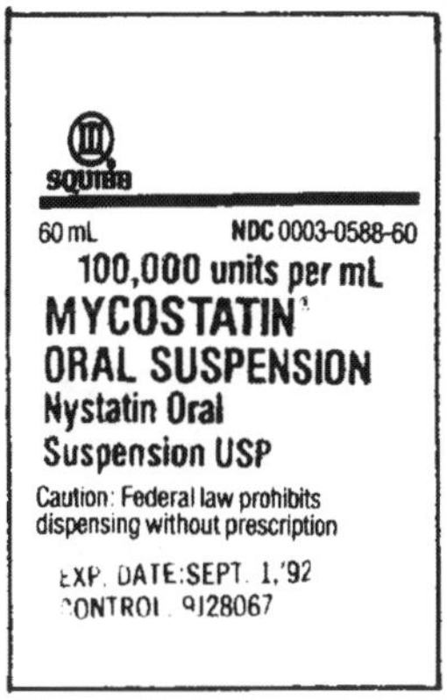
SQUIBB
60 mL
NDC 0003-0588-60
100,000 units per mL
MYCOSTATIN®
ORAL SUSPENSION
Nystatin Oral
Suspension USP
Caution: Federal law prohibits
dispensing without prescription
EXP. DATE:SEPT. 1,'92

2-33. ANSWERS TO PRACTICAL EXERCISE--LABEL INTERPRETATION (PART I)

a. $\frac{1 \text{ tab}}{10 \text{ mg}} = \frac{X \text{ tabs}}{20 \text{ mg}}$

10 X = 20

X = 2 tabs

b. $\frac{250 \text{ mg}}{5 \text{ ml}} = \frac{375 \text{ mg}}{X \text{ ml}}$

250 X = 1875

X = 7.5 ml

c. $\frac{1 \text{ cap}}{25 \text{ mg}} = \frac{X \text{ caps}}{100 \text{ mg}}$

25 X = 100

X = 4 caps

d. $\frac{1 \text{ tab}}{250 \text{ mg}} = \frac{X \text{ tabs}}{500 \text{ mg}}$

250 X = 500

X = 2 tabs

e. $\frac{250 \text{ mg}}{5 \text{ ml}} = \frac{500 \text{ mg}}{X \text{ ml}}$

250 X = 2500

X = 10 ml

f. 40 mg = 1 cap

g. $\frac{100{,}000 \text{ units}}{1 \text{ ml}} = \frac{150{,}000 \text{ units}}{X \text{ ml}}$

100,000 X = 150,000

X = 1.5 ml

h. 325 mg = 1 tab

i. $\frac{1 \text{ tab}}{100 \text{ mg}} = \frac{X \text{ tabs}}{300 \text{ mg}}$

100 X = 300

X = 3 tabs

j. $\frac{1 \text{ tab}}{500 \text{ mg}} = \frac{X \text{ tabs}}{1000 \text{ mg}}$

500 X = 1000

X = 2 tabs

2-34. PRACTICAL EXERCISE--LABEL INTERPRETATION (PART II)

DIRECTIONS. Read the labels provided to prepare the indicated dosages. Round oral dosages to the nearest tenth, and parenteral dosages to the nearest hundredth. Fill in the blanks on items a through j; then check the solutions provided.

a. Aminophylline 200 mg P.O. q 6h ______ ml

b. Ampicillin 400 mg P.O. q 6h ______ ml

c. Sulfamethoxazole 350 mg (trimethoprim 70 mg) P.O. ______ ml

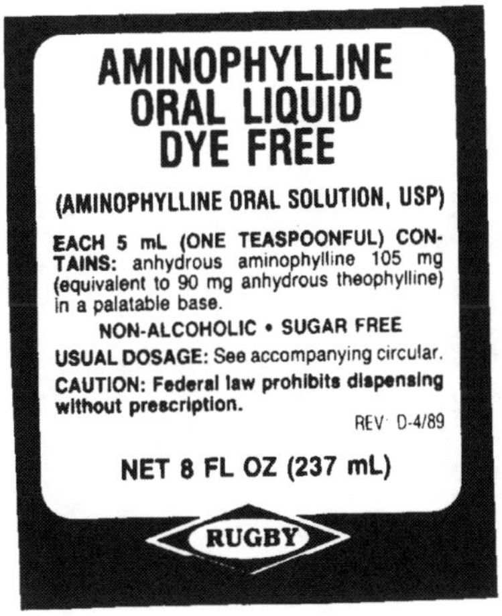

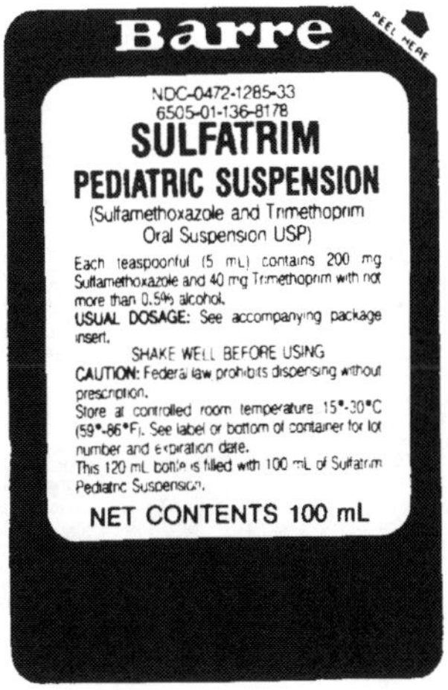

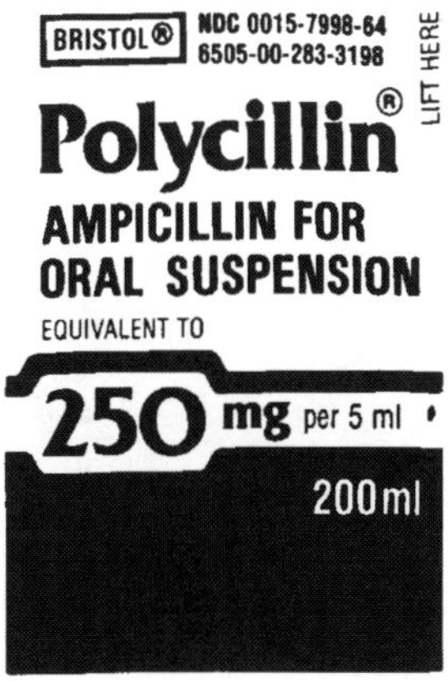

d. Digoxin elixir 0.08 mg P.O. ______ ml

e. Ceftriaxone 250 mg I.M. q 12h ______ ml

f. Dicloxicillin 150 mg P.O. q 8h ______ ml

g. Acetaminophen elixir 240 mg P.O. q 4h ______ ml

	Vial Strength	Concentration (units/ml)	Amount of Diluent
h.	Penicillin G Potassium 20,000,000 units	500,000	______ ml

* Refer to the Penicillin G Potassium vial label and package insert to answer question h.

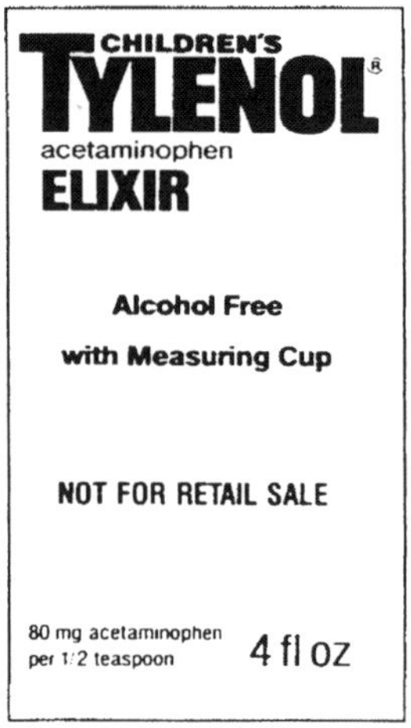

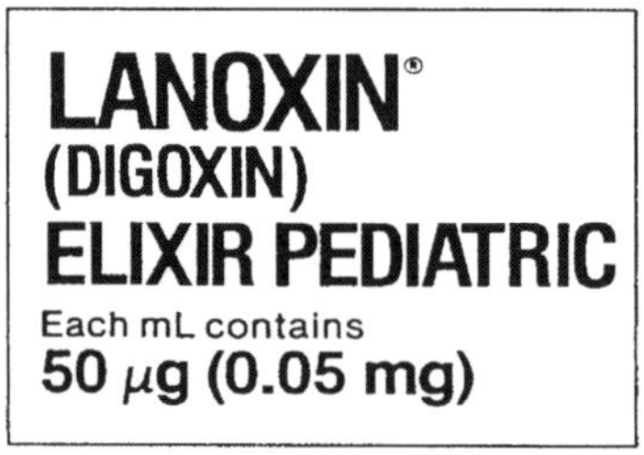

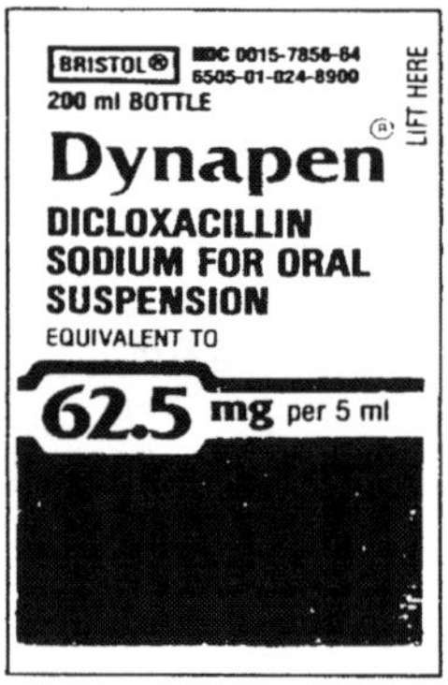

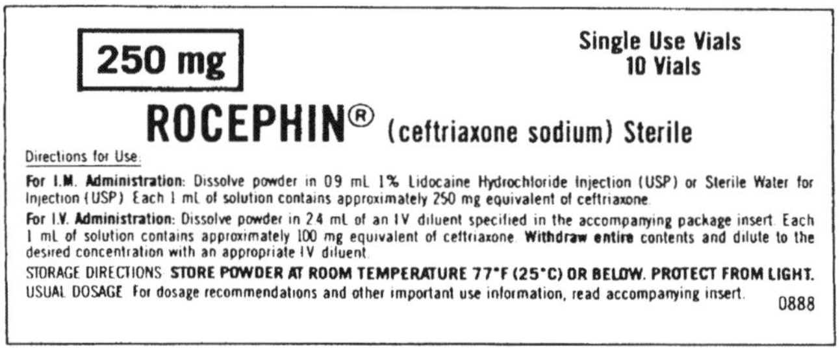

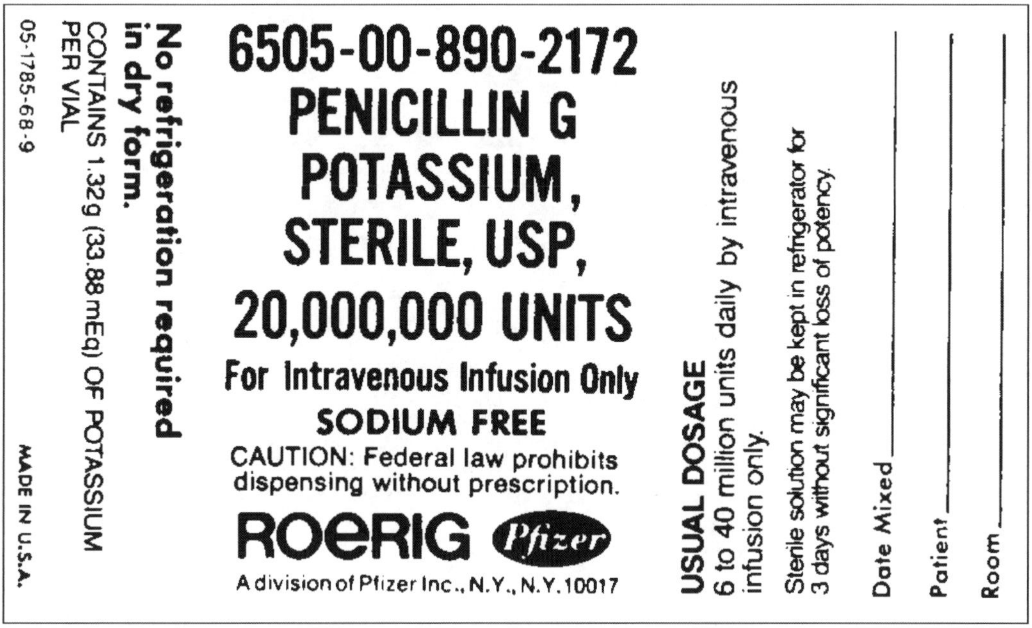

The following table shows the amount of solvent required for solution of various concentrations of 20,000,000 units:

Desired Concentration (units/ml)	For Intravenous Infusion Only 20,000,000 units Approximate Volume (ml) of Solvent
250,000	72.0
500,000	32.0
1,000,000	12.0

	Vial Strength	Amount of Diluent	Dosage Strength of Prepared Solution
i.	cefotaxime 2 g (prepare for I.M. injection)	(1) ______ ml	(2) ______ mg/ml

* Refer to the cefotaxime vial label and package insert to answer question i.

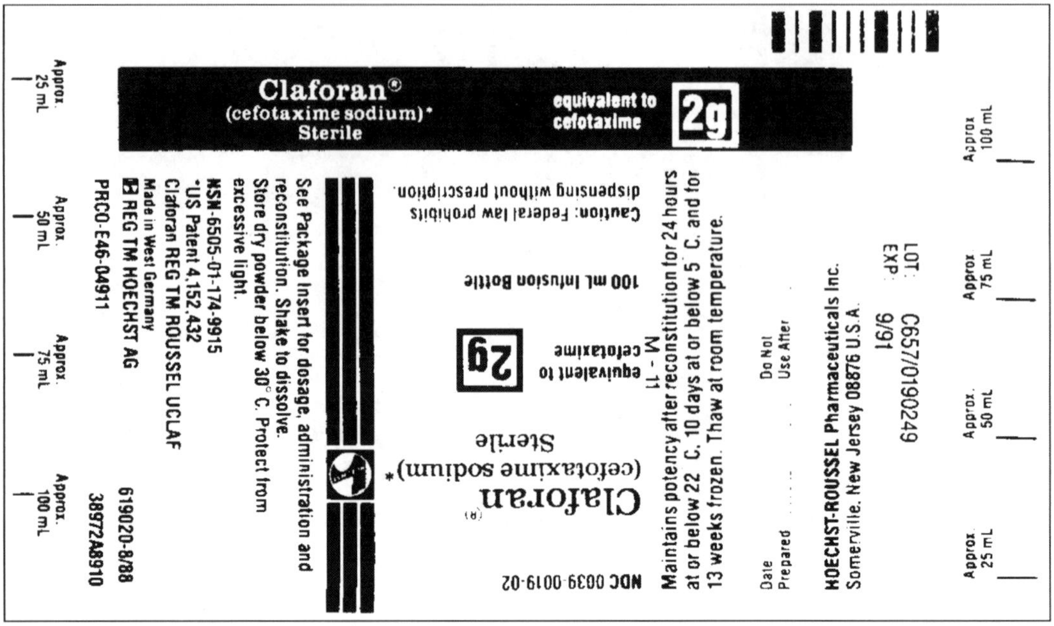

Preparation of Solution: Claforan for IM or IV administration should be reconstituted as follows:

Strength	Amount of Diluent To Be Added (ml)	Approximate Withdrawable Volume (ml)	Approximate Average Concentration (mg/ml)
Intramuscular			
1 g vial	3	3.4	300
2 g vial	5	6.0	330
Intravenous			
1 g vial	10	10.4	95
2 g vial	10	11.0	180

Shake to dissolve; inspect for particulate matter and discoloration prior to use. Solutions of Claforan range from very pale yellow to light amber, depending on concentration, diluent used, and length and condition of storage. For intramuscular use: Reconstitute VIALS with Sterile Water for Injection or Bacteriostatic Water for Injection as described above.

2-35. ANSWERS TO PRACTICAL EXERCISE--LABEL INTERPRETATION (PART II)

a. $\frac{105 \text{ mg}}{5 \text{ ml}} = \frac{200 \text{ mg}}{X \text{ ml}}$

105 X = 1000

X = 9.5 ml

b. $\frac{250 \text{ mg}}{5 \text{ ml}} = \frac{400 \text{ mg}}{X \text{ ml}}$

250 X = 2000

X = 8 ml

c. $\frac{200 \text{ mg}}{5 \text{ ml}} = \frac{350 \text{ mg}}{X \text{ ml}}$ or $\frac{40 \text{ mg}}{5 \text{ ml}} = \frac{70 \text{ mg}}{X \text{ ml}}$

200 X = 1750 or 40 X = 350

X = 8.8 ml X = 8.8 ml

d. $\frac{0.05 \text{ mg}}{1 \text{ ml}} = \frac{0.08 \text{ mg}}{X \text{ ml}}$

0.05 X = 0.08

X = 1.6 ml

e. 250 mg/1 ml

f. $\frac{62.5 \text{ mg}}{5 \text{ ml}} = \frac{150 \text{ mg}}{X \text{ ml}}$

62.5 X = 750

X = 12 ml

g. $\frac{80 \text{ mg}}{1/2 \text{ tsp}} = \frac{240 \text{ mg}}{X \text{ ml}}$

$\frac{1 \text{ tsp}}{5 \text{ ml}} = \frac{1/2 \text{ tsp}}{X \text{ ml}}$

X = 2.5 ml

$\frac{80 \text{ mg}}{2.5 \text{ ml}} = \frac{240 \text{ mg}}{X \text{ ml}}$

80 X = 600

X = 7.5 ml

h. 32.0 ml

i. (1) 5 ml (2) 330 mg/ml

2-36. SUMMARY OF ROUNDING RULES FOR MEDICATION CALCULATIONS

a. Express IV DRIP RATES in <u>WHOLE NUMBERS</u>.

b. Express TABLETS in <u>WHOLE OR HALVES</u>.

c. INJECTABLES should be rounded to <u>TENTHS</u>, except for HEPARIN AND INSULIN, which are rounded to <u>HUNDREDTHS</u>.

d. P.O. LIQUIDS should be rounded to <u>TENTHS</u>.

e. Round KILOGRAMS to <u>TENTHS</u>.

Continue with Exercises

EXERCISES, LESSON 2

INSTRUCTIONS: Answer the following items by writing the answer in the space provided.

After you have completed all of these items, turn to "Solutions to Exercises" at the end of the lesson and check your answers with the solutions.

1. You wish to administer a dose of 15 mg of a particular drug to a patient. The drug is supplied in a multidose vial labeled 5 mg/ml. Calculate the volume (ml) of the drug to be administered.

2. A patient has been given five capsules. Each capsule contained 250 mg of a particular drug. Calculate the total number of mg of drug the patient received.

3. The mother of a pediatric patient tells you that she has given her child a total of 7 tsp of cough syrup over the past 24 hours. The amount of 7 tsp equals ____ ml.

4. The physician has ordered Chlorpromazine 20 mg I.M. for your patient. Chlorpromazine is labeled 25 mg/ml. Determine how many mls you will give.

5. The order is for Morphine gr 1/6 I.M. On hand is a Morphine tubex labeled 15 mg/ml. You will give ___ ml.

6. Convert the following weights to their equivalents:

   a. 1650 gm = ____ kg

   b. 19 lbs = _____ kg

   c. 14.5 lbs = ____ kg

   d. 70 lbs = _____ kg

   e. 200 mg = ____ gm

   f. 5 mg = ____ gr

   g. 10 mg = _____ gr

   h. 2 gm = _____ mg

   i. 40 gm = _____ mg

   j. 2.2 lbs = ____ kg

7. Your patient is to receive Lasix 40 mg P.O. q AM. Lasix is stocked in 20 mg tablets. How many tablets will you administer?

8. Your patient is to receive Digoxin 0.25 mg P.O. q AM. Digoxin is stocked in 0.125 mg tablets. How many tablets will you administer?

9. The physician has ordered Heparin 10,000 units SQ for your patient. Heparin is stocked in a multidose vial labeled 20,000 units/ml. How many ml's will you give?

10. The order is to give Atropine 0.6 mg. I.M. on call to surgery. On hand is a vial labeled Atropine 0.4 mg/ml. How many ml's will you give?

11. The order is to give Morphine 4 mg I.M. stat. Available is a vial labeled morphine 10 mg/ml. How many ml's will you give?

12. The order is to give Demerol 35 mg I.M. q 4h p.r.n. pain. The medication is supplied in a tubex labeled 50 mg/ml. How many ml's will you give?

13. The order is to give Valium 8 mg I.M. on call to surgery. The Valium stocked is labeled 10 mg/2 ml. How many ml's will you give?

14. The order is to give Prostaphlin 350 mg I.M. q 4h. Directions for reconstitution of the 1 gm vial state: Add 5.7 ml of sterile water. Each 1.5 ml will then contain 250 mg of medication. How many ml's will you give?

15. The order is to give Polycillin-N 700 mg I.M. q 4h. The directions for reconstitution of each 1-gm vial of Polycillin state: Add 3.4 ml of sodium chloride to produce a concentration of 250 mg/ml. How many ml's will you give?

16. The patient is to receive Vistaril 75 mg I.M. q 4h p.r.n. nausea. On hand is a vial containing 100 mg/2 ml. How many ml's will you give?

17. The order is to give Omnipen 350 mg I.M. q 6h. The directions on the vial state: Add 1.9 ml to produce a concentration of 125 mg/0.5 ml. How many ml will you give?

18. The patient is to receive 3 units of whole blood over the next 6 hours. Each unit contains 500 ml. Using a drop factor of 10 gtts/ml, determine the infusion rate.

19. The order is for 1000 ml D_5W with 20 mEq KCl to alternate with 1000 ml $D_{51/2}NS$ with 20 mEq KCl over the next 24 hours at a rate of 150 ml/hr. Using a drop factor of 15 gtts/ml, determine the infusion rate.

20. The order is to give Cimetidine 300 mg IVPB q 6h. The medication is dissolved in 100 ml of D_5W and is to infuse in 30 minutes. Using a drop factor of 20 gtts/ml, determine the infusion rate.

21. The order is to give Tobramycin 80 mg IVPB q 12h. The medication is added to 100 ml of D_5W and is to infuse in 60 minutes. Using a drop factor of 15 gtts/ml, determine the infusion rate.

22. The order is to infuse 1500 ml of Ringer's lactate over the next 24 hours. The drop factor of the tubing is 60 gtts/ml. Determine the rate in gtts/min.

23. The patient is to receive 1000 ml of $D_{51/4}NS$ at 125 ml/hr. Using a drop factor of 20 gtts/ml, determine the infusion rate.

24. Your patient is to receive heparin 1500 units/hr by a continuous I.V. infusion. The pharmacy sends up a 500 ml bag of 0.9% sodium chloride with 25,000 units of heparin added. The I.V. set delivers 60 gtts/ml. The solution should be administered at a rate of ___gtts/min and ____ml/hr.

25. Case Study.

Mr. K. was admitted with shortness of breath; rule out left lower lobe pneumonia. His current diagnosis is chronic obstructive pulmonary disease (COPD). Among his medical orders are the following: oxygen at 2 liters/min via nasal prongs; pulmonary toilet q 2h, out of bed as tolerated; Brethine 5 mg P.O. t.i.d.; Erythromycin 400 mg q 6h P.O.; Potassium Chloride solution 30 mEq P.O. b.i.d., dilute each tablespoon in 4 oz water or fruit juice.

Refer to the labels of the ordered medications to answer the questions that follow.

a. How many mg's does each Brethine tablet contain?

b. How many Brethine tablets will you administer per dose? ____ per day?

c. How many mg are in 1 ml of Erythromycin?

d. How many ml's of Erythromycin will you administer per dose?
____ per day ?

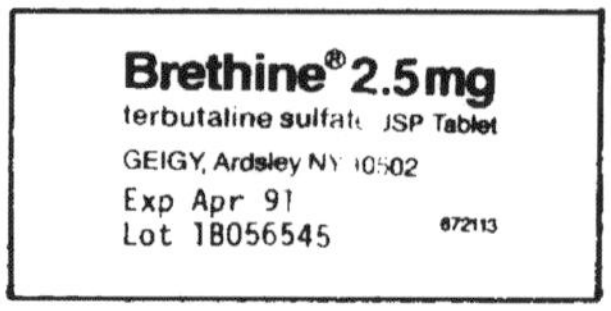

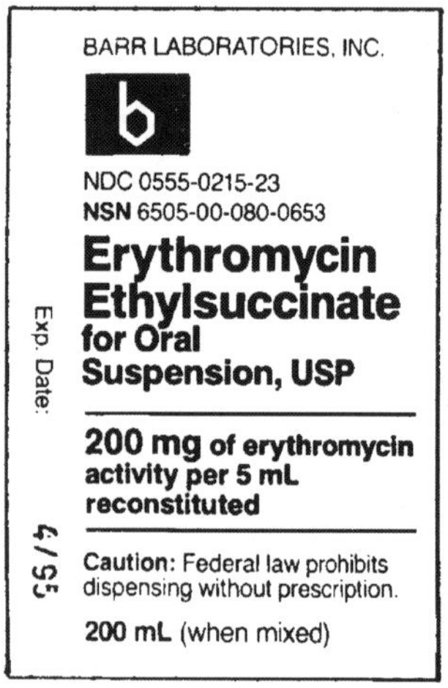

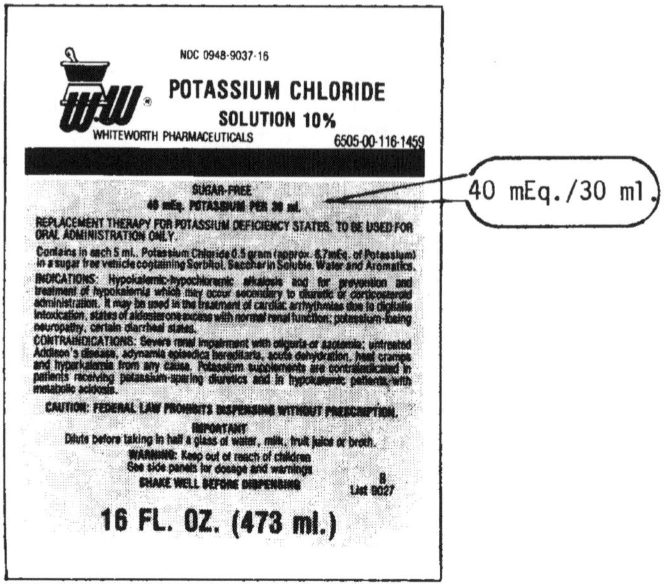

e. How many days will one bottle of Erythromycin last?

f. How many ml's of Potassium Chloride should you give?

g. How many ounces of fruit juice should be used to dilute one dose of Potassium Chloride?

26. Case Study

G.W. is a 9-month-old child admitted with a chronic urinary tract infection. G.W. weighs 22 lbs. Currently, G.W. has a temperature of 104□R. Among her medical orders are foley catheterization to straight drainage; force fluids; urine for culture and sensitivity; Tylenol elixir q.i.d. p.r.n. for temp 101□ or greater; vital signs q 4h; I.V. of D_5RL at 30°ml/hr; Sulfatrim suspension 10 mg q 6h; intake and output (weigh all diapers).

Refer to the dosage guidelines and medication labels to answer the questions which follow.

Dosage guidelines for Children's Tylenol Elixir:

4-11 months	one-half teaspoon
12-23 months	three-quarters teaspoon
2-3 years	one teaspoon
4-5 years	one and one-half teaspoons
6-8 years	two teaspoons
9-10 years	two and one-half teaspoons
11-12 years	three teaspoons

Dosage guidelines for Sulfatrim

The recommended dosage of Sulfatrim for children with urinary tract infections is 8 mg/kg trimethoprim and 40 mg/kg sulfamethoxazole per 24 hours, given in two divided doses every 12 hours for 10 days. Use the following table as a guide for children two months of age or older.

Weight		Dose--every 12 hours
lb	kg	Teaspoonfuls
22	10	1 (5 ml)
44	20	2 (10 ml)
66	30	3 (15 ml)
88	40	4 (20 ml)

a. Does the baby need a dose of Tylenol now? If so, how many cc's should you give?

b. How many mg of acetaminophen are in each dose of Tylenol?

c. Should you administer another dose of Tylenol later in the day?

d. It is 1400 hours and you have just checked vital signs. What time should you check again?

e. How many ml's of Sulfatrim should you administer?

f. How many mg of each of the two active ingredients are contained in each dose of Sulfatrim?

27. How many tablets of Tylenol would you administer if the physician ordered 600 mg for pain? On hand are 10 gr tablets.

28. The order is to give 1 oz of Maalox. How many tbsp's would you give?

29. The order is for 2.0 gm of Neomycin. On hand are 500 mg tablets. How many tablets will you give?

30. How many ounces of Maalox will you give if the order is for 45 ml?

31. The physician orders gr 1/32 of Dilaudid P.O. q 3-4h p.r.n. for pain. On hand are tablets gr 1/64 each. How many tablets will you give?

32. The order is for Erythromycin base 0.5 gm q 6h. On hand are 125 mg tablets. How many tablets will you give?

33. The order is to give 250 mcg of Lanoxin P.O. q AM using 0.125 mg tablets. How many tablets will you give?

34. The physician orders Fiorinal 30 mg P.O. On hand are gr 1/8 capsules. How many capsules will you give?

35. The order is to give Achromycin (tetracycline) syrup 0.25 gm P.O. q.i.d. The medication is available in syrup form, 125 mg per 5 ml. How many tsp's will you give?

36. The physician ordered Synthroid 25 mcg q AM. Available are 0.05 mg tablets. How many tablets will you give?

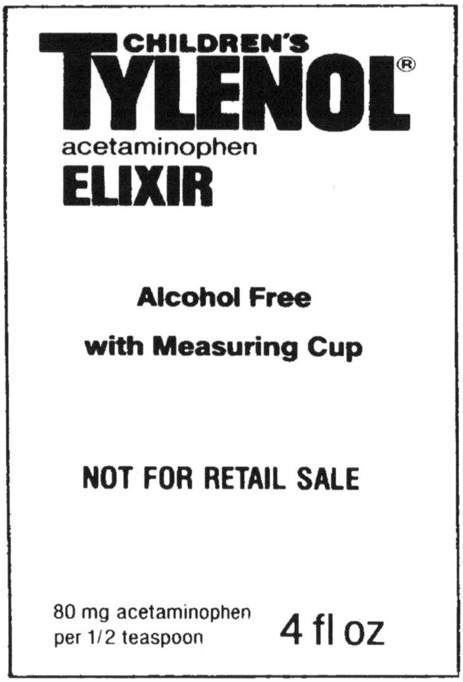

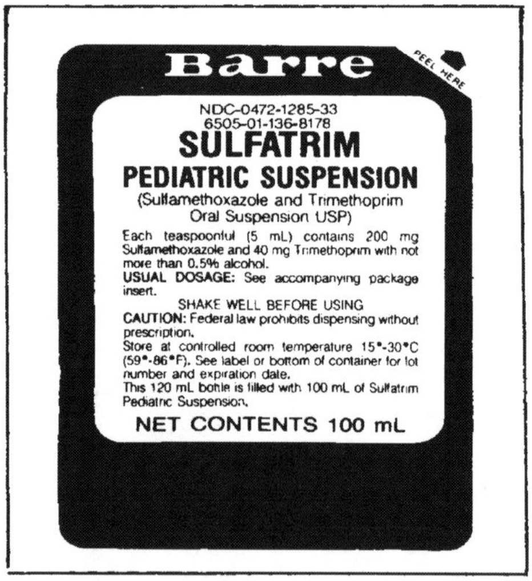

37. Case Study

H.B., a 64-year-old male, was re-admitted with a post-operative wound infection. He was discharged three days earlier after having his appendix removed. He is seven days post-op. He has consistently had a temperature of 103°; wound is red with foul-smelling purilent drainage. Among his current medical orders are: Wet to dry dressing changes q 4h; vitals q 4h; antibiotic Prostaphlin IVPB 250 mg to be given q 6h; Tylenol 2 tabs q 4h prn for temp greater than 101°; up ad lib.

Refer to the reconstitution guidelines and label to answer the questions that follow.

Reconstitution guidelines for Prostaphlin IV

Vial Size	Diluent	Resulting Concentration
250 mg	1.4 cc	250 mg/1.5 cc
500 mg	2.7 cc	250 mg/1.5 cc
1 gm	5.7 cc	250 mg/1.5 cc

Reconstitute with sterile water or sodium chloride injection.

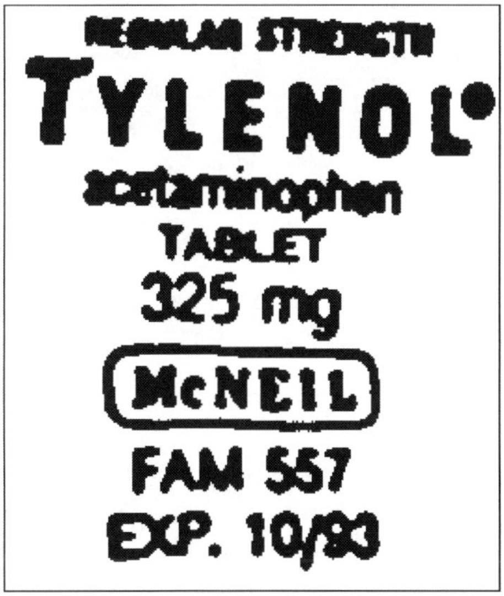

a. What diluent(s) can be used to reconstitute the Prostaphlin?

b. How many ml of diluent should be added to the vial of Prostaphlin for reconstitution?

c. After reconstituting the vial of Prostaphlin, the 250 mg is further diluted in 100 ml of D_5W. Using minidrop (60 gtts/ml) tubing, how many gtts/min are needed to administer the Prostaphlin if the IV is to run for 1 1/2 hours?

d. How many mg of acetaminophen will each dose of Tylenol contain?

e. What is the maximum number of mg of Tylenol you can administer per day?

38. The physician ordered Cleocin 120 mg IVPB q 8h. The antibiotic is supplied in vials with 300 mg/2 ml. The guidelines for administration of Cleocin are to dilute the medication in 50 ml of D_5W and infuse over 30 minutes.

    a. How many ml's of Cleocin will you add to 50 ml of D_5W for the ordered dose?

    b. Using a drop factor of 60 gtts/ml, determine the infusion rate.

39. The order is to give 0.3 mg of Atropine I.M. on call to surgery. The medication is provided in a vial labeled gr 1/150 per ml. How many ml's should you give?

40. The order is to administer Regular Insulin at a rate of 7 u/hr via a continuous I.V. infusion. The pharmacy sends a 500-ml bag of 0.9% sodium chloride with 250 units of Regular insulin added. Using a drop factor of 60 gtts/ml, calculate the infusion rate in gtts/min and ml/hr.

41. The order is to give Mandol (Cefamandole) 1 gm q 6h IVPB. Recommended dilution is 100 ml of D_5W or NS. Recommended rate of infusion is over 30 minutes. Using a drop factor of 20 gtts/ml, determine the infusion rate in gtts/min.

42. The order is to give Keflin 480 mg IVPB q 6h to a 19 kg child. The medication is supplied in a 500 mg vial. Reconstitution directions are: Add 5 ml of diluent to give a concentration of 500 mg/2.7 ml. You are to administer the Keflin in 25 ml of I.V. fluid over 30 minutes.

    a. How many ml of medication will you add to the I.V. fluid?

    b. Using a drop factor of 60 gtts/ml, determine the infusion rate.

43. The order is to administer 47 units of NPH insulin SQ q AM. You have a 10°ml vial of U100 NPH insulin. Using a tuberculin syringe, determine how many ml's to give.

44. The physician has ordered 700 units per hour of Heparin. The pharmacy sends 500 ml of D_5NS with 20,000 u of Heparin. Using a drop rate factor of 60 gtts/ml, determine the infusion rate.

45. The physician has ordered 11,000 units of Heparin SQ q 12h. On hand is a vial labeled 40,000 units/ml. How many ml's will you give?

46. The order is for Decadron 5 mg I.M. Decadron is stocked in multiple dose vials labeled 4 mg/ml. How many ml's will you give?

47. The order is to give Atarax 30 mg I.M. Atarax is stocked in vials labeled 50 mg/ml. How much will you give?

48. The order is for Elixophyllin 100 mg P.O. q 6h. Elixophyllin is stocked 80 mg/15 ml. How many ml's will you administer?

49. The order is for Amoxicillin 375 mg P.O. q 8h. Amoxicillin is stocked as an oral suspension with 250 mg per 5 ml. How many ml's will you give?

50. The order is to infuse 1000 ml of $D_5$1/2NS at 125 ml/hr for the next 24 hours. Using a drop factor of 15 gtts/ml, determine the infusion rate.

Check Your Answers on Next Page

SOLUTIONS TO EXERCISES, LESSON 2

1. $\frac{5 \text{ mg}}{1 \text{ ml}} = \frac{15 \text{ mg}}{X \text{ ml}}$

   5 X = 15

   X = 3 ml (paras 2-5, 2-6, 2-17)

2. $\frac{1 \text{ cap}}{250 \text{ mg}} = \frac{5 \text{ caps}}{X \text{ mg}}$

   X = 1250 mg (para s 2-5, 2-6, 2-16)

3. $\frac{1 \text{ tsp}}{5 \text{ ml}} = \frac{7 \text{ tsp}}{X \text{ ml}}$

   X = 35 ml (para 2-5,2-6, 2-10)

4. $\frac{25 \text{ mg}}{1 \text{ ml}} = \frac{20 \text{ mg}}{X \text{ ml}}$

   25 X = 20

   X = 0.8 ml (para 2-5, 2-6, 2-18)

5. $\frac{15 \text{ mg}}{1 \text{ ml}} = \frac{\text{gr } 1/6}{X \text{ ml}}$

   $\frac{\text{gr } 1}{60 \text{ mg}} = \frac{\text{gr } 1/6}{X \text{ mg}}$

   X = 10 mg

   $\frac{15 \text{ mg}}{1 \text{ ml}} = \frac{10 \text{ mg}}{X \text{ ml}}$

   15 X = 10

   X = 0.7 ml (paras 2-5, 2-6, 2-7, 2-10, 2-18)

6. a. $\frac{1000 \text{ gm}}{1 \text{ kg}} = \frac{1650 \text{ gm}}{X \text{ kg}}$

$1000 X = 1650$

$X = 1.65$ kg or 1.7 kg

b. $\frac{2.2 \text{ lbs}}{1 \text{ kg}} = \frac{19 \text{ lbs}}{X \text{ kg}}$

$2.2 X = 19$

$X = 8.6$ kg

c. $\frac{2.2 \text{ lbs}}{1 \text{ kg}} = \frac{14.5 \text{ lbs}}{X \text{ kg}}$

$2.2 X = 14.5$

$X = 6.6$ kg

d. $\frac{2.2 \text{ lbs}}{1 \text{ kg}} = \frac{70 \text{ lbs}}{X \text{ kg}}$

$2.2 X = 70$

$X = 31.8$ kg

e. $\frac{1000 \text{ mg}}{1 \text{ gm}} = \frac{200 \text{ mg}}{X \text{ gm}}$

$1000 X = 200$

$X = 0.2$ gm

f. $\frac{1 \text{ gr}}{60 \text{ mg}} = \frac{X \text{ gr}}{5 \text{ mg}}$

$60 X = 5$

$X = 1/12$ gr

g. $\frac{1 \text{ gr}}{60 \text{ mg}} = \frac{X \text{ gr}}{10 \text{ mg}}$

60 X = 10

X = 1/6 gr

h. $\frac{1 \text{ gm}}{1000 \text{ mg}} = \frac{2 \text{ gm}}{X \text{ mg}}$

X = 2000 mg

i. $\frac{1 \text{ gm}}{1000 \text{ mg}} = \frac{40 \text{ gm}}{X \text{ mg}}$

X = 40,000 mg

j. 2.2 lbs = 1 kg (para 2-10)

7. $\frac{1 \text{ tablet}}{20 \text{ mg}} = \frac{X \text{ tablets}}{40 \text{ mg}}$

20 X = 40

X = 2 tablets (paras 2-5, 2-6, 2-16)

8. $\frac{1 \text{ tablet}}{0.125 \text{ mg}} = \frac{X \text{ tablets}}{0.25 \text{ mg}}$

0.125 X = 0.25

X = 2 tablets (paras 2-5, 2-6, 2-16)

9. $\frac{20{,}000 \text{ units}}{1 \text{ ml}} = \frac{10{,}000 \text{ units}}{X \text{ ml}}$

20,000 X = 10,000

X = 0.5 ml (paras 2-5, 2-6, 2-18)

10. $\frac{0.4 \text{ mg}}{1 \text{ ml}} = \frac{0.6 \text{ mg}}{X \text{ ml}}$

0.4 X = 0.6

X = 1.5 ml (paras 2-5, 2-6, 2-18)

11. $\frac{10 \text{ mg}}{1 \text{ ml}} = \frac{4 \text{ mg}}{X \text{ ml}}$

10 X = 4

X = 0.4 ml (paras 2-5, 2-6, 2-18)

12. $\frac{50 \text{ mg}}{1 \text{ ml}} = \frac{35 \text{ mg}}{X \text{ ml}}$

50 X = 35

X = 0.7 ml (paras 2-5, 2-6, 2-18)

13. $\frac{10 \text{ mg}}{2 \text{ ml}} = \frac{8 \text{ mg}}{X \text{ ml}}$

10 X = 16

X = 1.6 ml (paras 2-5, 2-6, 2-18)

14. $\frac{1.5 \text{ ml}}{250 \text{ mg}} = \frac{X \text{ ml}}{350 \text{ mg}}$

250 X = 525

X = 2.1 ml

(paras 2-5, 2-6, 2-18)

15. $\frac{250 \text{ mg}}{1 \text{ mg}} = \frac{700 \text{ mg}}{X \text{ ml}}$

250 X = 700

X = 2.8 ml (paras 2-5, 2-6, 2-18)

16. $\frac{100 \text{ mg}}{2 \text{ ml}} = \frac{75 \text{ mg}}{X \text{ ml}}$

100 X = 150

X = 1.5 ml (paras 2-5, 2-6, 2-18)

17. $\frac{125 \text{ mg}}{0.5 \text{ ml}} = \frac{350 \text{ mg}}{\text{X ml}}$

125 X = 175

X = 1.4 ml (paras 2-5, 2-6, 2-18)

18. $\frac{1 \text{ unit}}{500 \text{ ml}} = \frac{3 \text{ units}}{\text{X ml}}$

X = 1500 ml

$\frac{1500 \text{ ml x } 10 \text{ gtts/ml}}{360}$

$\frac{15{,}000}{360}$ = 41.7 = 42 gtts/min (paras 2-5, 2-6, 2-7, 2-28)

19. $\frac{150 \text{ ml x } 15 \text{ gtts/ml}}{60}$

$\frac{2250}{60}$ = 37.5 = 38 gtts/min (paras 2-7, 2-26)

20. $\frac{100 \text{ ml x } 20 \text{ gtts/ml}}{30}$

$\frac{2000}{30}$ = 66.7 = 67 gtts/min (paras 2-7, 2-27)

21. $\frac{100 \text{ ml x } 15 \text{ gtts/min}}{60}$

$\frac{1500}{60}$ = 25 gtts/min (para 2-27)

22. $\frac{1500 \text{ ml x } 60 \text{ gtts/ml}}{1440 \text{ min}}$

$\frac{90{,}000}{1440}$ = 62.5 = 63 gtts/min (paras 2-7, 2-26)

23. $\frac{125 \text{ ml} \times 20 \text{ gtts/ml}}{60}$

$\frac{2500}{60} = 41.7 = 42$ gtts/min (paras 2-7, 2-16)

24. $\frac{25{,}000 \text{ units}}{500 \text{ ml}} = \frac{1500 \text{ units}}{X \text{ ml}}$

25,000 X = 750,000

X = 30 ml/hr

$\frac{30 \text{ ml} \times 60 \text{ gtts/ml}}{60 \text{ min}}$

$\frac{1800}{60} = 30$ gtts/min (paras 2-5, 2-6, 2-18)

25. a. 2.5 mg

b. $\frac{2.5 \text{ mg}}{1 \text{ tablet}} = \frac{5 \text{ mg}}{X \text{ tablets}}$

2.5X = 5

X = 2 tablets per dose

$\frac{2 \text{ tablets}}{1 \text{ dose}} = \frac{X \text{ tablets}}{3 \text{ doses}}$

X = 6 tablets per day

c. $\frac{200 \text{ mg}}{5 \text{ ml}} = \frac{X \text{ mg}}{1 \text{ ml}}$

5X = 200

X = 40 mg

d. $\frac{200 \text{ mg}}{5 \text{ ml}} = \frac{400 \text{ mg}}{X \text{ ml}}$ or $\frac{40 \text{ mg}}{1 \text{ ml}} = \frac{400 \text{ mg}}{X \text{ ml}}$

200 X = 2000   40 X = 400

X = 10 ml/dose   X = 10 ml/dose

$\frac{10 \text{ ml}}{1 \text{ dose}} = \frac{X \text{ ml}}{4 \text{ doses}}$

X = 40 ml/day

e. $\frac{40 \text{ ml}}{1 \text{ day}} = \frac{200 \text{ ml}}{X \text{ days}}$

40X = 200

X = 5 days

f. $\frac{40 \text{ mEq}}{30 \text{ ml}} = \frac{30 \text{ mEq}}{X \text{ ml}}$

40 X = 900

X = 22.5 ml

g. $\frac{15 \text{ ml (1 T)}}{4 \text{ oz}} = \frac{22.5 \text{ ml}}{X \text{ oz}}$

15 X = 90

X = 6 oz (paras 2-5, 2-6, 2-10, 2-11, 2-14, 2-16, 2-17, 2-31--2-35)

26. a. yes

$\frac{1 \text{ tsp}}{5 \text{ cc}} = \frac{1/2 \text{ tsp}}{X \text{ cc}}$

X = 2.5 cc

b. $\frac{0.8 \text{ ml}}{80 \text{ mg}} = \frac{2.5 \text{ ml}}{X \text{ mg}}$

$0.8\ X = 200$

$X = 250$ mg

c. If needed; if temp is 101 or greater.

d. 1400 + 4 = 1800 hrs

e. 5 ml

f. $\frac{2.2 \text{ lbs}}{1 \text{ kg}} = \frac{22 \text{ lbs}}{X \text{ kg}}$

$2.2X = 22$

$X = 10$ kg

$\frac{8 \text{ mg}}{1 \text{ kg}} = \frac{X \text{ mg}}{10 \text{ kg}}$

$X = 80$ mg trimethoprim/day

$\frac{80 \text{ mg}}{2 \text{ doses}} = \frac{X \text{ mg}}{1 \text{ dose}}$

$2X = 80$

$X = 40$ mg trimethoprim/dose

$\frac{40 \text{ mg}}{1 \text{ kg}} = \frac{X \text{ mg}}{10 \text{ kg}}$

$X = 400$ mg sulfamethoxazole/day

$\frac{400 \text{ mg}}{2 \text{ doses}} = \frac{X \text{ mg}}{1 \text{ dose}}$

$2X = 400$

$X = 200$ mg sulfamethoxazole/dose (paras 2-5, 2-6, 2-10, 2-14, 2-17, 2-31--2-35)

27. $\frac{1 \text{ tab}}{10 \text{ gr}} = \frac{X \text{ tabs}}{600 \text{ mg}}$

$\frac{60 \text{ mg}}{1 \text{ gr}} = \frac{600 \text{ mg}}{X \text{ gr}}$

60 X = 600

X = 10 gr

10 gr = 1 tab (paras 2-5, 2-6, 2-10, 2-16)

28. 1 oz = 2 tbsp (para 2-10)

29. $\frac{1 \text{ tab}}{500 \text{ mg}} = \frac{X \text{ tabs}}{2.0 \text{ gm}}$

$\frac{1 \text{ gm}}{1000 \text{ mg}} = \frac{2.0 \text{ gm}}{X \text{ mg}}$

X = 2000 mg

$\frac{1 \text{ tab}}{500 \text{ mg}} = \frac{X \text{ tabs}}{2000 \text{ mg}}$

500 X = 2000

X = 4 tabs (paras 2-5, 2-6, 2-10, 2-16)

30. $\frac{1 \text{ oz}}{30 \text{ ml}} = \frac{X \text{ oz}}{45 \text{ ml}}$

30 X = 45

X = 1 1/2 oz (paras 2-5, 2-6, 2-10, 2-17)

31. $\frac{1 \text{ tab}}{\text{gr } 1/64} = \frac{X \text{ tabs}}{\text{gr } 1/32}$

1/64 X = 1/32

X = 2 tabs (paras 2-5, 2-6, 2-16)

32. $\frac{1 \text{ tab}}{125 \text{ mg}} = \frac{X \text{ tabs}}{0.5 \text{ gm}}$

$\frac{1 \text{ gm}}{1000 \text{ mg}} = \frac{0.5 \text{ gm}}{X \text{ mg}}$

X = 500 mg

$\frac{1 \text{ tab}}{125 \text{ mg}} = \frac{X \text{ tabs}}{500 \text{ mg}}$

125 X = 500

X = 4 tabs (paras 2-5, 2-6, 2-10, 2-16)

33. $\frac{1 \text{ tab}}{0.125 \text{ mg}} = \frac{X \text{ tabs}}{250 \text{ mcg}}$

$\frac{1 \text{ mg}}{1000 \text{ mcg}} = \frac{X \text{ mg}}{250 \text{ mcg}}$

1000 X = 250

X = 0.25 mg

$\frac{1 \text{ tab}}{0.125 \text{ mg}} = \frac{X \text{ tabs}}{0.25 \text{ mg}}$

0.125 X = 0.25

X = 2 tabs (paras 2-5, 2-6, 2-10, 2-16)

34. $\frac{1 \text{ cap}}{\text{gr } 1/8} = \frac{X \text{ caps}}{30 \text{ mg}}$

$\frac{60 \text{ mg}}{1 \text{ gr}} = \frac{X \text{ mg}}{1/8 \text{ gr}}$

X = 7.5 mg

$\frac{1 \text{ cap}}{7.5 \text{ mg}} = \frac{X \text{ caps}}{30 \text{ mg}}$

7.5 X = 30

X = 4 caps (para 2-16)

35. a. $\frac{125 \text{ mg}}{5 \text{ ml}} = \frac{0.25 \text{ gm}}{X \text{ tsp}}$

b. $\frac{1 \text{ gm}}{1000 \text{ mg}} = \frac{0.25 \text{ gm}}{X \text{ mg}}$

X = 250 mg

c. $\frac{125 \text{ mg}}{1 \text{ tsp (5 ml)}} = \frac{250 \text{ mg}}{X \text{ tsp}}$

125 X = 250

X = 2 tsp (paras 2-5, 2-6, 2-10, 2-11, 2-17)

36. $\frac{1 \text{ tab}}{0.05 \text{ mg}} = \frac{X \text{ tabs}}{25 \text{ mcg}}$

$\frac{1 \text{ mg}}{1000 \text{ mcg}} = \frac{X \text{ mg}}{25 \text{ mcg}}$

1000 X = 25

X = .025 mg

$\frac{1 \text{ tab}}{0.05 \text{ mg}} = \frac{X \text{ tabs}}{.025 \text{ mg}}$

0.05 X = .025

X = 0.5 or 1/2 tab (paras 2-5, 2-6, 2-10, 2-16)

37. a. Sterile water or sodium chloride.

b. 1.4 ml.

c. $\frac{100 \text{ ml X } 60 \text{ gtts/ml}}{90}$

$\frac{6000}{90} = 66.7 = 67$ gtts/min

d. $\frac{325 \text{ mg}}{1 \text{ tab}} = \frac{X \text{ mg}}{2 \text{ tabs (1 dose)}}$

X = 650 mg/dose

e. $\frac{650 \text{ mg}}{1 \text{ dose}} = \frac{X \text{ mg}}{6 \text{ doses}}$

X = 3900 mg (paras 2-5, 2-6, 2-11, 2-28, 2-31--2-35)

38. a. $\frac{300 \text{ mg}}{2 \text{ ml}} = \frac{120 \text{ mg}}{X \text{ ml}}$

300 X = 240

X = 0.8 ml

b. $\frac{50 \text{ ml x } 60 \text{ gtts/ml}}{30}$

$\frac{3000}{30}$ = 100 gtts/min (paras 2-5, 2-6, 2-27)

39. $\frac{\text{gr } 1/150}{1 \text{ ml}} = \frac{0.3 \text{ mg}}{X \text{ ml}}$

$\frac{1 \text{ gr}}{60 \text{ mg}} = \frac{1/150 \text{ gr}}{X \text{ mg}}$

X = 0.4 mg

$\frac{0.4 \text{ mg}}{1 \text{ ml}} = \frac{0.3 \text{ mg}}{X \text{ ml}}$

0.4 X = 0.3

X = 0.75 = 0.8 ml (paras 2-5, 2-6, 2-7, 2-10, 2-18)

40. $\frac{250 \text{ units}}{500 \text{ ml}} = \frac{7 \text{ units}}{X \text{ ml}}$

250 X = 3500

X = 14 ml/hr

$\frac{14 \text{ ml x } 60 \text{ gtts/ml}}{60}$

$\frac{840}{60}$ = 14 gtts/min (paras 2-5, 2-6, 2-28)

41. $\frac{100 \text{ ml} \times 20 \text{ gtts/ml}}{30}$

$\frac{2000}{30} = 66.7 = 67$ gtts/min

(paras 2-7, 2-27)

42. a. $\frac{500 \text{ mg}}{2.7 \text{ ml}} = \frac{480 \text{ mg}}{X \text{ ml}}$

$500 X = 1286$

$X = 2.6$ ml

b. $\frac{25 \times 60 \text{ gtts/ml}}{30}$

$\frac{1500}{30} = 50$ gtts/min (paras 2-5, 2-6, 2-7, 2-27)

43. $\frac{100 \text{ units}}{1 \text{ ml}} = \frac{47 \text{ units}}{X \text{ ml}}$

$100 X = 47$

$X = 0.47$ ml (paras 2-5, 2-6, 2-18d)

44. $\frac{20{,}000 \text{ u}}{500 \text{ ml}} = \frac{700 \text{ u/hr}}{X \text{ ml/hr}}$

$20{,}000 X = 350{,}000$

$X = 17.5$ ml/hr

$\frac{17.5 \text{ ml} \times 60 \text{ gtts/ml}}{60}$

$\frac{1050}{60} = 17.5 = 18$ gtts/min (paras 2-5, 2-6, 2-18c)

45. $\frac{40{,}000 \text{ units}}{1 \text{ ml}} = \frac{11{,}000 \text{ units}}{X \text{ ml}}$

40,000 X = 11,000

X = 0.275 = 0.28 ml (paras 2-5, 2-6, 2-7, 2-18c)

46. $\frac{4 \text{ mg}}{1 \text{ ml}} = \frac{5 \text{ mg}}{X \text{ ml}}$

4 X = 5

X = 1.25 = 1.3 ml paras 2-5, 2-6, 2-7, 2-18)

47. $\frac{50 \text{ mg}}{1 \text{ ml}} = \frac{30 \text{ mg}}{X \text{ ml}}$

50 X = 30

X = 0.6 ml (paras 2-5, 2-6, 2-18)

48. $\frac{80 \text{ mg}}{15 \text{ ml}} = \frac{100 \text{ mg}}{X \text{ ml}}$

80 X = 1500

X = 18.75 = 18.8 ml (paras 2-5, 2-6, 2-7, 2-17)

49. $\frac{250 \text{ mg}}{5 \text{ ml}} = \frac{375 \text{ mg}}{X \text{ ml}}$

250 X = 1875

X = 7.5 ml (paras 2-5, 2-6, 2-17)

50. $\frac{125 \text{ ml} \times 15 \text{ gtts/ml}}{60}$

$\frac{1875}{60} = 31$ gtts/min (paras 2-7, 2-26)

End of Lesson 2

This page intentionally left blank.

Introduction to Practical Nursing

Subcourse MD0910

This page intentionally left blank.

U.S. ARMY MEDICAL DEPARTMENT CENTER AND SCHOOL
FORT SAM HOUSTON, TEXAS 78234-6100

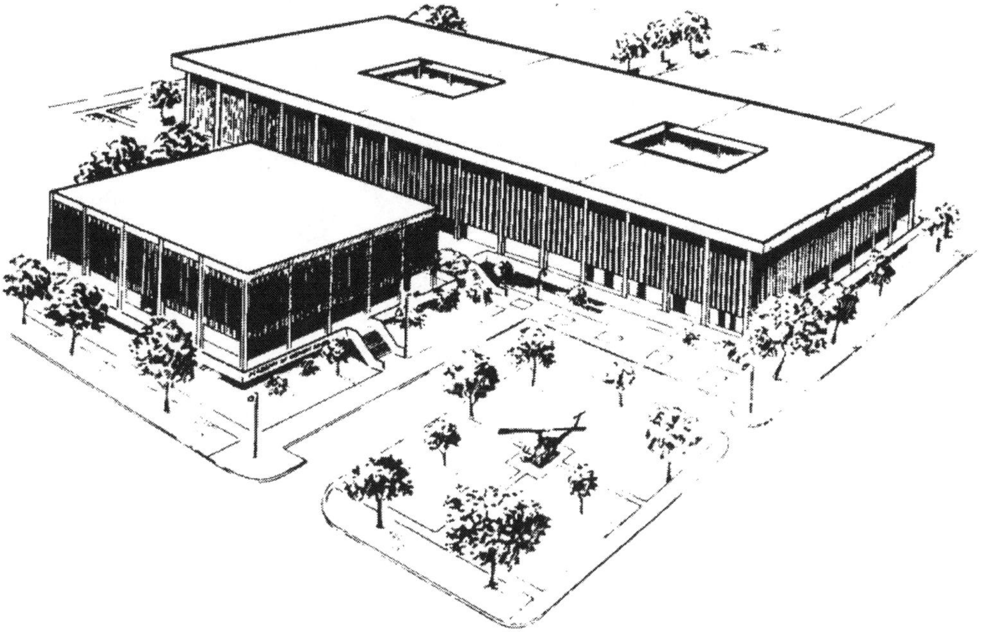

INTRODUCTION TO PRACTICAL NURSING

SUBCOURSE MD0910 EDITION 100

DEVELOPMENT

This subcourse is approved for resident and correspondence course instruction. It reflects the current thought of the Academy of Health Sciences and conforms to printed Department of the Army doctrine as closely as currently possible. Development and progress render such doctrine continuously subject to change.

The education specialist responsible for development of this edition was Mr. Joe McNaul, DSN 471-6346 or area code 210-221-6346, Academy of Health Sciences, ATTN: MCCS-HNP, Fort Sam Houston, Texas 78234-6100.

The organization responsible for the subject matter content of this edition is the Nursing Science Division, DSN 471-3086 or area code (210) 221-3086; Director, Phase I, M6 Branch, Academy of Health Sciences, ATTN: MCCS-HNP, Fort Sam Houston, Texas 78234-6100.

ADMINISTRATION

Students who desire credit hours for this correspondence subcourse must meet eligibility requirements and must enroll through the Nonresident Instruction Branch of the U.S. Army Medical Department Center and School (AMEDDC&S).

Application for enrollment should be made at the Internet website: http://www.atrrs.army.mil. You can access the course catalog in the upper right corner. Enter School Code 555 for medical correspondence courses. Copy down the course number and title. To apply for enrollment, return to the main ATRRS screen and scroll down the right side for ATRRS Channels. Click on SELF DEVELOPMENT to open the application and then follow the on screen instructions.

For comments or questions regarding enrollment, student records, or shipments, contact the Nonresident Instruction Branch at DSN 471-5877, commercial (210) 221-5877, toll-free 1-800-344-2380; fax: 210-221-4012 or DSN 471-4012, e-mail accp@amedd.army.mil, or write to:

NONRESIDENT INSTRUCTION BRANCH
AMEDDC&S
ATTN: MCCS-HSN
2105 11TH STREET SUITE 4191
FORT SAM HOUSTON TX 78234-5064

CLARIFICATION OF TERMINOLOGY

When used in this publication, words such as "he," "him," "his," and "men" 'are intended to include both the masculine and feminine genders, unless specifically stated otherwise or when obvious in context.

TABLE OF CONTENTS

CORRESPONDENCE COURSE OF
THE U.S. ARMY MEDICAL DEPARTMENT CENTER AND SCHOOL

SUBCOURSE MD0910

INTRODUCTION TO PRACTICAL NURSING

INTRODUCTION

The purpose of this subcourse is to introduce you to the ASI M6, Practical Nurse. The M6 practical nurse is an important link in the chain of health care providers within the Army Medical Department. The M6 serves in the dual roles of providing expert technical support to professional health care providers, while functioning as an enlisted military leader.

The M6 practical nurse is equivalent to the civilian occupation of licensed practical/vocational nurse. Because the Practical Nurse Course is approved by the Texas Board of Vocational Nurse Examiners, graduates of the course are eligible to apply for licensure examination and take the National Council Licensure Examination (NCLEX) for Practical Nurses. By simply maintaining licensure in the state of your choice, your ASI becomes a civilian occupation that will be available to you at the completion of your military career.

The NCLEX-PN is a one-day, three-hour, computer-based examination designed by the National Council of State Boards of Nursing to test the graduate's ability to practice practical nursing in a safe, effective manner. Licensure is required to maintain the ASI M6.

The M6 Practical Nurse Preparatory Correspondence Course is designed to be studied by the prospective M6. If you have not yet decided to apply for the resident M6 Course, this introductory subcourse will provide you with an overview of the duties, responsibilities, knowledge, and skills required of the practical nurse. With this information, you should be better prepared to decide whether practical nursing is for you. The M6 course is difficult and demanding. Maximum preparation is desirable for successful completion of the resident course. AMEDD personnel expecting to attend the 300-M6 Practical Nurse Course are encouraged to complete the M6 Practical Nurse Preparatory Correspondence Course in advance of resident training. The completion of the M6 correspondence course **does not** result in the awarding of the M6 ASI.

When you have passed all of the subcourses in the M6 correspondence course, a certificate of completion will be awarded to you. You should maintain a copy of this certificate and a copy will be placed in the your official 201 file. (Nonmilitary students should carry or mail a copy of the certificate to the local Directorate of Civilian Personnel for entry in their personnel file.)

The following list of suggested references is offered to assist you with your studies. These references should be available through the learning resource center and/or the library on your post. You will find them quite helpful as study and resource material during both your correspondence work and resident course work.

FM 21-11, First Aid for Soldiers.

FM 22-100, Army Leadership.

STP 21-1-SMCT Soldier's Manual of Common Tasks SL1.

Hole, J. Jr. Essentials of Human Anatomy &Physiology, 5th Ed. Dubuque, Iowa: Brown: 2000.

Kurzen, C. Contemporary Practical/Vocational Nursing, 3rd Ed. Philadelphia: Lippincott, 1997.

Burton, G. Microbiology for the Health Sciences, 4th Ed. Philadelphia: J.B. Lippincott, 1996.

Krause, A. Food, Nutrition & Diet Therapy, 9th Ed. W.B. Saunders, 1996.

Barry, P. Mental Health & Mental Illness, 7th Ed. Philadelphia: Lippincott, 1998.

Christensen, B. & Kockrow, E. Foundations of Nursing, 3rd Ed. St Louis: Mosby, 1999.

Christensen, B. & Kockrow, E. Adult Health Nursing, 3rd Ed. St Louis: Mosby, 1999.

Rosdahl, Caroline B. Textbook of Basic Nursing, 7th Ed. Philadelphia: Lippincott, 1999.

Scherer, J. Introduction to Medical Surgical Nursing, 7th Ed. Philadelphia: Lippincott, 1999.

Scherer, J. & Roach, S. Introductory Clinical Pharmacology, 6th Ed. Philadelphia: Lippincott, 2000.

Thompson, E.D. and Leifer, G. Introduction to Maternity and Pediatric Nursing, 3rd Ed. Philadelphia: WB Saunders Co., 1999.

Subcourse Components:

This subcourse consists of three lessons and an examination. The lessons are:

Lesson 1. The Practical Nurse in the AMEDD.

Lesson 2. The M6 Practical Nurse Course.

Lesson 3. Duties and Responsibilities of the M6 Practical Nurse

Credit Awarded:

Upon successful completion of this subcourse, you will be awarded 3 credit hours.

Procedures for Subcourse Completion:

You are encouraged to complete the subcourse lesson by lesson. When you have completed all of the lessons to your satisfaction, fill out the examination answer sheet and mail it to the U.S. Army Medical Department Center and School along with the Student Comment Sheet in the envelope provided. *Be sure that your name, rank, social security number, and return address are on all correspondence sent to the U.S Army Medical Department Center and School.* You will be notified by return mail of the examination results. Your grade on the exam will be your rating for the subcourse.

Study Suggestions:

Here are suggestions that may be helpful to you in completing this subcourse:

Read and study each lesson carefully.

Complete the subcourse lesson by lesson. After completing each lesson, work the exercises at the end of the lesson, marking your answers in this booklet.

After completing each set of lesson exercises, compare your answers with those on the solution sheet, which follows the exercises. If you have answered an exercise incorrectly, check the reference cited after the answer on the solution sheet to determine why your response was not the correct one.

As you successfully complete each lesson, go on to the next. When you have completed all of the lessons, complete the examination. Mark your answers in this booklet; then transfer your responses to the examination answer sheet using a #2 pencil.

Student Comment Sheet:

Be sure to provide us with your suggestions and criticisms by filling out the Student Comment Sheet (found at the back of this booklet) and returning it to us with your examination answer sheet. Please review this comment sheet before studying this subcourse.

LESSON ASSIGNMENT

LESSON 1 The Practical Nurse in the AMEDD.

LESSON ASSIGNMENT Paragraphs 1-1 through 1-17.

LESSON OBJECTIVES After completing this lesson, you should be able to:

1-1. Describe the mission of the AMEDD in peacetime and during mobilization.

1-2. State the four major functions of the AMEDD.

1-3. Define the health services support area concept.

1-4. Describe the levels of combat health support in the field.

1-5. List the major duties of the practical nurse in the AMEDD.

1-6. Describe the various roles of the M6 practical nurse in the AMEDD.

SUGGESTION After reading and studying the assignment, complete the exercises at the end of this lesson. These exercises will help you to achieve the lesson objectives.

LESSON 1

THE PRACTICAL NURSE IN THE AMEDD

Section I. REVIEW OF THE AMEDD

1-1. THE ARMY MEDICAL DEPARTMENT (AMEDD)

a. The personnel who comprise the Army Medical Department (AMEDD) are assigned to medical units and to positions that call for personnel with specialized health service training. The AMEDD consists of the following.

(1) The Office of The Surgeon General.

(2) The six officer corps.

(a) The Medical Corps (MC).

(b) The Army Nurse Corps (AN).

(c) The Dental Corps (DC).

(d) The Veterinary Corps (VC).

(e) The Medical Service Corps (MS).

(f) The Army Medical Specialist Corps (SP).

(3) Warrant Officers.

(4) Enlisted personnel.

(5) Civilian employees.

(6) AMEDD facilities, supplies, and equipment necessary for the mission.

b. The mission of the Army Medical Department is to maintain the health of the Army and conserve its fighting strength. Care is provided for eligible personnel in peacetime and, at the same time, preparations are made for health support of the Army in time of war, international conflict, or natural disaster. The four major functions of the AMEDD are:

(1) The selection of only the physically and mentally fit persons for military service.

(2) The prevention of unnecessary hazards to the health and efficiency of troops through a health and environment program.

(3) The medical treatment of those who become sick or injured and their prompt return to duty or other disposition as appropriate.

(4) The prompt evacuation of patients from the combat zone to medical treatment facilities designed to provide the type and extent of treatment required.

c. The AMEDD purpose is to provide the U.S. Army with the world's best trained, equipped, and supported leaders, soldiers, and civilians, ready to provide quality health service support in any environment across the operational continuum.

1-2. U.S. ARMY MEDICAL COMMAND

a. The U.S. Army Medical Department Command (MEDCOM) is a major Army command under the direction of Headquarters, Department of the Army. AMEDD personnel are found in all major Army commands (MACOM). MEDCOM's mission is to provide health services for the Army in the continental United States (CONUS) and other areas and organizations as directed by the Chief of Staff, U.S. Army. The MEDCOM has the additional mission of providing medical, dental, and veterinary education and training for AMEDD personnel and other personnel as directed.

b. The AMEDD provides health services to eligible personnel under the area support concept. The territory to which the AMEDD provides health services is divided into seven geographical areas of responsibility. Each of these has been designated as a health service region (HSR). Each HSR contains one U.S. Army Medical Center (MEDCEN). The health service regions are normally subdivided into two or more health service areas (HSA). A health service area is a geographical area for which a single medical treatment facility (MTF) has responsibility for providing health care services to authorized personnel within that area. For example, if a health service region contains a MEDCEN and three MEDDACs, this HSR would be divided into four health service areas. One HSA would have the MEDCEN as its primary MTF and each of the other HSAs would have one of the U.S. Army Medical Department Activities (MEDDAC) as its primary medical treatment facility.

c. A U.S. Army Medical Center (MEDCEN) is a specialized medical treatment and teaching facility that provides general and specialized medical and dental care and treatment. A U.S. Army Medical Department Activity (MEDDAC) is a fixed MTF with associated activities, all of which are responsible for providing health services.

d. Health services for areas not under the AMEDD are provided by AMEDD personnel within other MACOMs. For example, the 7th Medical Command in Heidelberg, Germany, is under the major Army command United States Army, Europe (USAREUR).

1-3. HEALTH SERVICE SUPPORT AREA CONCEPT

a. Under the Health Service Support Areas (HSSA) concept, the MEDCOM coordinates medical care in six regions of the United States with command authority in each region and subordinate commands for dental and veterinary services.

b. In November 1993, subordinate commands for the U.S. Dental Command (DENCOM) and Veterinary Command (VETCOM) were provisionally activated. Under the MEDCOM, Commanders of the Dental Service Support Areas (DSSA) integrate and coordinate dental care within their geographic areas of operation. The DSSA are seven regional organizations that parallel the Health Service Support Areas (HSSA) in the medical arena. The VETCOM controls seven Veterinary Service Support Areas (VSSA), whose boundaries may differ from the HSSA and DSSA because of Defense Department responsibilities.

c. Six medical centers have command and control over medical treatment facilities in their HSSA. These regional organizations are responsible for delivering health care in the AMEDD structure. The HSSAs are headquartered at Walter Reed, Eisenhower, Brooke, William Beaumont, Madigan, and Tripler Army Medical Centers.

1-4. COMBAT HEALTH SUPPORT IN THE FIELD

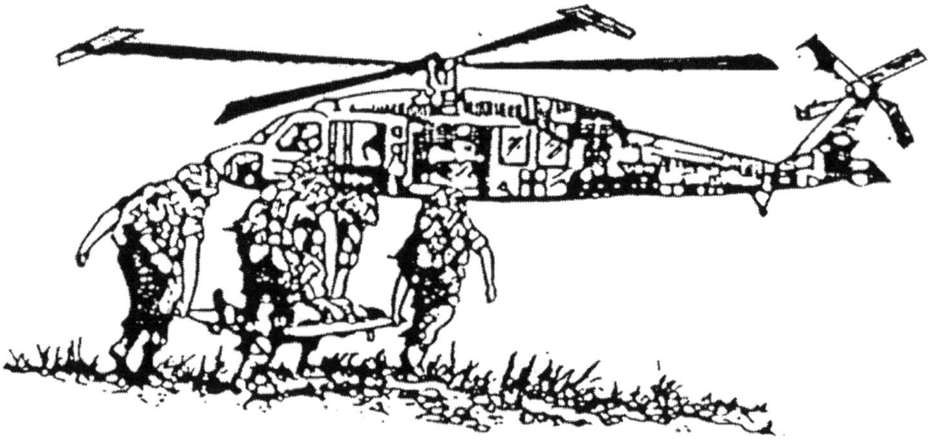

a. Combat health support (CHS) is provided for the Army in the field in war and peace by the utilization of a variety of medical modules and echelons of care. The medical system is functionally designed to prevent, collect, assess, treat, evacuate, and rehabilitate sick or injured soldiers. The combat health support system is designed to project, sustain, and protect the health of the soldier in war and operations other than war (OOTW). Consistent with strategic and tactical operations, CHS operates across all operational levels, from the forward line of own troops (FLOT) to the continental United States (CONUS) sustaining base. It is a system that provides continuous medical management throughout all echelons of care.

(1) The goals of the Army's CHS system in support of warfighting are to:

(a) Reduce the incidence of disease and nonbattle injuries (DNBI) through sound preventive medicine programs.

(b) Provide medical and surgical treatment for acute illnesses, injuries, or wounds.

(c) Evacuate patients through the echelons of care to the appropriate medical treatment facility (MTF) commensurate with requisite care.

(d) Maintain soldiers on duty or promptly return to duty (RTD) those who have recovered.

(e) Maintain a robust and aggressive science and technology base to enhance all capabilities related to health and the delivery of health care.

(2) These goals are the embodiment of the CHS battle field rules:

(a) Maintain medical presence with the soldier (be there).

(b) Maintain the health of the command.

(c) Save lives.

(d) Clear the battlefield.

(e) Provide state-of-the-art care.

(f) Ensure early return to duty.

b. Combat health support is arranged in levels or echelons of care. Each level of care reflects an increase in capability, yet the functions of each lower level of support are contained within the capabilities of all higher levels. The basic levels of health service support are the unit level, the division level, the corps level, the communication zone (COMMZ) level, and the CONUS support base.

c. The health service support system represents a continuum of care, beginning at the FLOT (forward line of own troops) and ending in the CONUS base. Each soldier is evacuated rearward only to that level of health service support having the medical treatment capabilities necessary to treat that patient's injuries. The objective of health service support in the field is to treat the soldier as far forward as possible and to return him to duty as soon as he is able.

d. Unit and division level medical care organizations are based on a modular design. In the future, modular components will even be employed at the corps and

COMMZ level. The system used at the division level and forward is comprised of six basic models as listed below.

(1) Combat medic. This module consists of one medic with a prescribed load of medical supplies and equipment. Combat medics are assigned to the medical platoon or section of the combat support battalions and are attached to the companies of the battalions as required.

(2) Treatment squad. The treatment squad consists of a primary care physician, a physician assistant (PA), and six medical specialists. The squad is trained and equipped to provide advanced trauma management (ATM) to the battlefield casualties. Advanced trauma management is physician or physician assistant directed care. It is designed to resuscitate and stabilize the patient for evacuation to the next echelon of medical care or to treat and return him to duty. Advanced trauma management provides maximum benefit if received within 60 minutes of injury. To maintain contact with the combat maneuver elements, each squad has two emergency treatment vehicles. Each squad can split into two treatment teams. These squads are organic to medical platoons or sections in maneuver battalions and designated combat support units. This module is the building block of the medical company.

(3) Ambulance squad. The ambulance squad module is comprised of four medical specialists and two ambulances. This squad operates in conjunction with the treatment squad. The squad provides patient evacuation throughout the operational continuum and care in route. Each ambulance carries a medical equipment set (MES) that includes intravenous fluids, oxygen, bandages, and splints, as well as other medical supplies and equipment to enable patient monitoring. In conjunction with the treatment squad, there is the capability to acquire a patient within 30 minutes of wounding, treat the patient, and coordinate for the rapid evacuation to the next level of care. Ambulance squads are organic to medical platoons and sections of maneuver battalions and squadrons, selected combat support units, divisional and nondivisional medical treatment companies, and ground ambulance companies of the medical evacuation battalion.

(4) Area support squad. This module is composed of a dental officer, a dental specialist, an x-ray specialist, a laboratory specialist, and associated medical equipment set (MES). The dentist is trained in advanced trauma management to augment the capabilities of the physician and/or physician assistant during periods of increased treatment requirements. The area support squad is organic to medical companies within the brigade support area, division support area, corps support area, or the COMMZ.

(5) Patient holding squad. This module is composed of practical nurses, medical specialists, and a medical equipment set (MES) specifically designed for the mission of the squad. Each squad is capable of providing limited medical support for minimal care patients who are expected to return to duty within 72 hours. Patient holding squads are assigned to a treatment platoon of the medical company.

(6) Forward surgical team. This module is staffed with two surgeons, two nurse anesthetists, a medical/surgical nurse, two operating room specialists, and two practical nurses. The forward surgical team is organized to provide early resuscitative surgery for seriously wounded or injured patients, to save life, and to preserve physical function. Early surgery is performed whenever a likely delay in the evacuation of a patient threatens life or the quality of recovery. This team collocates with the patient holding squad where postsurgical patients awaiting evacuation are held. The forward surgical team provides the required nursing care. Forward surgical teams are organic to the airborne and air assault divisions. All other surgical modules are called detachments and are not organic to these divisions. Forward surgical team members and their equipment can be transported by helicopter or air dropped, allowing for the provision of emergency surgical care.

e. Modular medical support characterizes Echelons I and II. The system standardizes medical subelements within these units. The modular design of the subelements enables the medical resource manager to rapidly tailor, augment, reinforce, or reconstitute the battlefield in areas of most critical need.

(1) The system is designed to provide emergency medical treatment and dental care, advanced trauma management, and routine sick call for soldiers of supported units. The modular medical support system is built around the six modules organic to division and nondivisional CHS units.

(2) It is oriented toward casualty assessment, collection, evacuation, treatment, and initial surgical resuscitation. When effectively employed, it provides assured flexibility, mobility, and patient care capabilities.

1-5. UNIT LEVEL (ECHELON I)

a. Unit level medical care is initial emergency medical treatment. Immediate far forward care consists of those lifesaving steps that do not require the knowledge and skill of a physician. Three different skill levels of personnel provide the care required in the far forward area.

(1) Self-aid/buddy-aid. Each soldier is trained in a variety of specific first aid procedures, with particular emphasis on the lifesaving tasks. This training enables the soldier or his buddy to apply immediate care in order to prevent or alleviate a life threatening situation.

(2) Combat lifesaver. The combat lifesaver is a non-medical member of a unit, selected by the commander, to receive additional training beyond the basic first aid procedures that are taught to all soldiers. The primary duty of the soldier does not change; additional duties as combat lifesaver are performed as the situation permits. The combat lifesaver assists the combat medic in providing immediate care for injuries. There should be at least one trained combat lifesaver per squad, crew, team, or

equivalent size unit. This training is normally provided by the medical personnel assigned or attached to the unit.

(3) Combat medic. The combat medic is the first individual in the combat health support chain who makes medically substantiated decisions based on military occupational specialty (MOS) specific medical training. The combat medic is trained to the emergency medical technician (EMT) level.

b. Additional unit level care is provided by the battalion aid station.

(1) Personnel and equipment. When required by the tactical situation, the battalion medical platoon has sufficient personnel and equipment for the temporary, simultaneous operation of two aid stations. When a single aid station is operating, the physician (medical platoon leader) supervises the treatment provided in the aid station and also performs emergency medical treatment therein. He is assisted by the physician assistant (PA) and other members of the aid station element. Included in this element are senior emergency medical aidman and medical aidmen, who assist in the treatment of patients, the conduct of sick call, and overall operation of the aid station.

(2) Location. The aid station is established as far forward in the battalion area of operation as the tactical situation permits, generally in the battalion support area. The location of the aid station may be farther forward in the attack than the defense.

1-6. DIVISION LEVEL (ECHELON II)

a. Division level medical support is designed as a modular medical support system that standardizes medical elements throughout the division. It is tactically mobile and responsive to the needs of the division. Division level medical care is rendered at the divisional and nondivisional clearing station.

b. Here the casualty is examined and his wounds and general status are evaluated to determine his priority for continued evacuation to the rear. Emergency care/resuscitation is continued and, if necessary, initial urgent surgery is performed.

c. Limited dental, laboratory, optometry, preventive medicine, and mental health services are also provided at this echelon, in addition to medical resupply of supported forces. These functions are typically performed by medical companies/troops organic to support battalions or divisions, support battalion of separate infantry brigades (SIB), support squadrons of armored cavalry regiments (ACR), and area support medical battalions. These Echelon II units are employed in the combat zone (brigade, division, and corps support areas) and the COMMZ.

1-7. CORPS LEVEL (ECHELON III) AND COMMZ LEVEL (ECHELON IV)

Corps and COMMZ level medical support is provided by units assigned to the corps medical group, medical brigade, or theater Army (TA) medical command. Area medical support is provided by units such as the area support medical battalion, dental battalions, veterinary service units, and preventive medicine units. Facilities are organized and equipped in modules that contain standardized medical equipment sets (MES) or medical material sets (MMS). The mission for the hospital system is two-fold. First, it is designed to maximize return to duty of patients. Second, it provides the necessary treatment to stabilize those patients not expected to return to duty for evacuation within the limits of the theater evacuation policy.

a. **Echelon III Corps Level Hospitals**. At Echelon III, patients are admitted to and treated in the combat support hospital (CSH), which is staffed and equipped to provide care for all categories of patients. Here, patients are treated and held within the parameters of the theater/corps evacuation policy. Patients are either returned to duty or evacuated to an Echelon IV hospital. The CSH is a 296-bed facility and is normally deployed in the corps area.

b. **Echelon IV COMMZ Level Hospitals**.

(1) At Echelon IV, the patients receive medical care in hospitals that are staffed and equipped to provide general and specialized medical care. There are two different hospitals employed at Echelon IV. One is employed to recondition and rehabilitate soldiers who can be returned to duty within theater policy guidelines. The other is employed to treat and stabilize patients destined to be evacuated to Echelon V (CONUS based hospitals).

(a) The general hospital (GH) is a 476-bed hospital that provides care to all classes of patients. The GH is the primary conduit for patients awaiting evacuation to CONUS.

(b) The field hospital (FH) is a 505-bed hospital that is staffed and equipped to treat all categories of patients. However, its principal mission is to treat and rehabilitate those patients who can return to duty within the stated theater evacuation policy.

(2) The medical treatment company receives, sorts, and provides resuscitation and stabilization of patients until evacuated and provides treatment for patients with minor illnesses or injuries. It may be employed to expand hospital capacities or as a holding facility of up to 1200 total cots for minimal care patients. It is 100 percent mobile and is allocated on the basis of one per division supported in the combat zone and one per two divisions supported in the COMMZ.

(3) This echelon characterizes the theater (operational) level combat health support system, which is oriented toward providing support to the forward deployed corps. Echelon IV contains all the services outlined for Echelon III to include theater

medical logistics management and medical laboratory assets. Support for contingency operations is normally initialized at this echelon.

1-8. CONUS SUPPORT BASE (ECHELON V)

a. Echelon V care is generally characterized by definitive care given to all categories of patients. It is provided by CONUS-based Department of Defense (DOD) tri-service hospitals and Department of Veterans Administration (DVA) hospitals. Patients evacuated from the theater of operations who are expected to return within 60 days are admitted to tri-service hospitals to the maximum extent possible. Patients requiring long term care are admitted to Veterans Administration hospitals and civilian hospitals participating in the National Disaster Medical System. During mobilization, the National Disaster Medical System may be activated. Under this system, patients overflowing DOD and DVA hospitals will be cared for in civilian hospitals. Strategic and operational planning and deployment of combat health support system assets also takes place at this level.

b. During peacetime, the bulk of CONUS hospital military personnel are organized into Table of Organization and Equipment (TOE) units which, upon mobilization, deploy to the theater of operations. Reserve Component organizations would then maintain the CONUS hospitals at current operational capacities. The capacities can be expanded through the use of individual mobilization augmentees, draftees, enlistments, and retired recalls. The CONUS peacetime health care structure is designed to provide for wartime readiness and to provide early-on medical assets to the theater of operations.

1-9. OTHER SUPPORT

a. Units that lack an organic medical capability are provided routine and emergency medical treatment on an area support basis. Within corps and echelons above corps (EAC), this service is provided by area support medical battalions, which are organized similar to divisional medical battalions. The battalion consists of medical companies that have a treatment platoon (area support squad, treatment squad, and patient holding squad) and an ambulance platoon. In addition to a normal battalion staff, the headquarters has optometry, preventive medicine, mental health, and medical logistics sections.

b. The ambulance exchange point (AXP) is an intermediate point of patient transfer. Ambulance exchange points are established when threats to air resources prevent evacuation by air from forward units. These points will be established to the rear of the battlefield air support (BAS). During deep operations, these points may be established to ensure that lines of communications of unit/ division/corps level resources are not overextended. The AXP is manned by the maneuver battalion medical platoon and medical company personnel.

1-10. COMMAND, CONTROL, COMMUNICATIONS, COMPUTERS, AND INTELLIGENCE (C^4I)

a. Command, control, communications, computers, and intelligence (C^4I) is the responsibility of medical organizations at all levels of command. Normally C^4I is handled by a medical command, medical brigade, or a medical group. The type of medical C^4I headquarters employed in an operational area is dependent on the size of the deployed force.

b. The medical C^4I headquarters is designed to implement Level II through Level IV combat health support operations across the operational continuum. Combat health support C^4I headquarters employ the principle of "first in--last out." The appropriate medical C^4I headquarters must arrive as lead elements with a deploying force to orchestrate the arrival of medical units into an operational area and they are among the last to leave.

c. The medical C^4I headquarters has sophisticated automation hardware and software as well as assured communications. Based on intelligence analysis, medical C^4I staff articulates priorities, synchronize operations, and ensure uninterrupted medical support to the medical units. Automation, communications, and command and control procedures must allow for interface among Army systems, among all levels of command, among other services, and (when feasible) among supported allied forces. Automated data processing systems aid in patient accountability, tracking the movement of patients/casualties across the battlefield, regulating patients into and out of theater hospitals, and management of health service logistics systems.

Section II. THE ROLE OF THE M6

1-11. HEALTH CARE TEAM

a. As a Department of the Army practical nurse, you will be one of the members of a group of people involved in the care of the patient--the health care team. Any person involved with the health and welfare of the patient is a member of the health care team. The needs of the patient will dictate who the primary team members will be. All of the following may be team members: the patient, the patient's family, the nursing staff, the physicians, the social workers, the physical therapists, the dieticians, the occupational therapists, the chaplains, and the administrative support staff.

b. Whether you find yourself working in a large MEDCEN or in a field unit, you are still a health care provider and a crucial member of the health care team.

1-12. PRACTICAL NURSING

Department of the Army practical nursing encompasses a wide range of nursing skills and military leadership responsibilities. The major duties of the practical nurse are to perform preventive, therapeutic, and emergency nursing care procedures; to manage other paraprofessional personnel; and to manage ward or unit operations. (These duties will be discussed in Lesson 3.) Specific duties performed and skills required will depend upon your rank, skill level, and current duty assignment. 91WM6s are the primary enlisted personnel performing nursing care duties at the various levels of health care. Therefore, the practical nurse must always be proficient in providing basic practical nursing care to a variety of patients during peacetime and during mobilization. Additionally, the practical nurse must always be able to function as an effective and efficient soldier, demonstrating proficiency in the common soldier tasks and exercising the principles of military leadership. The following paragraphs discuss the health care roles filled by the M6 practical nurse.

1-13. THE M6 PRACTICAL NURSE

The M6 practical nurse may work in a ward, unit, or clinic setting. The types of duties performed and skills required will depend upon the workplace and its immediate mission. Duties performed may be very specialized, as in a neonatal intensive care unit or thoracic surgery ward, or may be very broad, as on a multi-service medical-surgical ward. The practical nurse works as a staff member giving direct patient care under the supervision of a professional nurse while, at the same time, supervising subordinates. The M6 practical nurse is concerned not only with direct nursing care, but with health teaching; patient comfort and safety; clerical administration such as admissions, discharges, consultations and referrals; and the requisition and maintenance of supplies and equipment. At each higher grade and skill level, the M6 practical nurse assumes increased supervisory and managerial responsibilities. As administrative duties increase, time spent in direct patient care will consequently decrease. Rather than perform direct patient care, the senior practical nurse will supervise and instruct subordinates in patient care techniques.

1-14. THE M6 PRACTICAL NURSE AS MANAGER

Any M6 practical nurse may be utilized as a manager. Senior enlisted supervisors will delegate selected administrative, logistical, or supervisory tasks to designated subordinates so that the individual has the opportunity to learn, under supervision, tasks needed to master the next skill level. These "mini-management" experiences help to prepare the practical nurse for future duty positions.

a. Management experience prepares practical nurses to be Senior Clinical NCOs or Clinical NCOs. These positions are normally held by an E6, E7, or E8 who will manage that particular ward, unit, or section and supervise all paraprofessional personnel assigned to that area. This supervisory experience, in turn, will further prepare the soldier for positions of higher responsibility.

b. Some practical nurses in grades E8 and E9 are utilized as chief clinical NCOs while those in grades E7 and E8 may serve as assistant chief clinical NCO. These assignments involve supervising the entire staff of enlisted personnel within the medical facility's Department of Nursing. As the senior nursing NCO, the practical nurse has the responsibility for the operation of all areas of the hospital involved with providing some form of nursing care. Needless to say, much of this responsibility is shared by the clinical NCOs and NCOs within the department.

c. A great amount of authority is delegated to subordinate supervisors. It is up to each practical nurse supervisor to ensure that his subordinate supervisors and subordinate workers are performing to standards. You can see that each management experience assists in preparing the individual to manage larger and more complex areas and larger numbers of personnel. An E5 in charge of a small clinic with one or two personnel could eventually find himself as an E8 in the position of Chief Clinical NCO at a MEDCEN.

1-15. THE M6 PRACTICAL NURSE IN THE FIELD

Yes, M6 practical nurses are found in "field" units. You may be the "medic" that will accompany a platoon to combat or the "aidman" on a MEDEVAC helicopter.

a. M6 practical nurses are utilized in the field type hospitals just as in any other hospital. M6 practical nurses are needed to staff the wards and serve as clinical NCOs and section NCOs. There are positions for a chief clinical NCO and an assistant chief clinical NCO. As in a regular hospital, these positions are filled by practical nurses. Any field unit that has patient holding capabilities may utilize practical nurses.

b. When a field medical element is not operational, it will be engaged in various levels of training for mobilization. Mobilization training means readiness training. The unit as a collective group, the elements within the group, and the individuals within each element must all be thoroughly prepared for mobilization on short notice. Training to achieve this readiness involves all aspects of operations in any given unit. Individuals must be proficient in their MOS/ASI and common soldier tasks. Each work center, no matter what its function, must be able to perform as a cohesive element. All the individual work centers must be able to work with the other elements of the unit in order to accomplish the mission. If any element or any individual is unprepared, the integrity of the entire unit is compromised. Training, then, is accomplished on varying levels, from individual training to unit training. A very large part of being assigned to a field unit is being involved in the process of training for mobilization.

1-16. SPECIAL OPTIONS FOR THE M6 PRACTICAL NURSE

a. Upon completion of an approved faculty development or instructor training course of instruction, the M6 practical nurse will be awarded the special qualification identifier (SQI) of "H," which designates instructor qualification. Practical nurses are authorized to be utilized as instructors in a number of settings. As a service school instructor, the practical nurse may instruct soldiers in an MOS/ASI producing course utilizing the classroom, the hospital, and/or the field as educational settings. Examples are advanced individual training (AIT) for MOS 91W or ASI M6. M6 practical nurses are also utilized as enlisted instructors in the Nursing Education and Staff Development (NESD) section of Army hospitals. As a practical nurse assigned to NESD, you will be involved in preparing, presenting, and supervising various types of training. The larger the hospital, the more diversified the activities of NESD. In a small MEDDAC, for example, the entire NESD operation may be run by one M6. At a MEDCEN, however, NESD may be organized into many sections and staffed by a large number of AN officers and AMEDD enlisted personnel. Some of the functions of the NESD are to conduct in-service training, manage continuing education for nursing personnel, and provide cardiopulmonary resuscitation (CPR) certification training. Many MEDDACs and MEDCENs are sites for Phase II training for MOS producing courses such as 91D or ASI M6. NESD may be the coordinating liaison or managing office for these Phase II instruction sites and may be involved in the training process.

b. An additional skill identifier (ASI) available to the 91W is M3, Renal Dialysis Technician. Upon completion of the required training, the 91W is awarded the ASI of M3 and assigned to work as a member of a dialysis team or unit. All dialysis related duty positions are found in the MEDCENs.

c. For additional SQI or ASI options, refer to Army Regulation 611-201.

1-17. CONCLUSION

In this lesson, we have looked at the AMEDD and the role of the M6 practical nurse within the AMEDD. U.S. Army practical nurses are unique individuals with varied levels of training, education, and experience. Duty assignments take the M6 practical nurse from CONUS to overseas and from the MEDCEN to the field. The M6 practical nurse plays a part in providing health service support in all areas of the AMEDD.

Continue with Exercises

EXERCISES, LESSON 1

INSTRUCTIONS. Complete the statements in the following exercises. After you have completed all statements in the exercises, turn to "Solutions to Exercises" at the end of this lesson and check your answers.

1. The mission of the Army Medical Department is to ________________________

   ____.

2. During peace time, preparations are made for ___________________________

   ____.

3. The four major functions of the AMEDD are:

   ____.
   ____.
   ____.
   ____.

4. Patients evacuated from the theater of operations and expected to return within 60 days are admitted to _______________________hospitals. Patients requiring long term care are admitted to ____________________________hospitals and civilian hospitals participating in the National Disaster Medical System.

5. Combat health support (CHS) is arranged in ___________________________ of care.

6. Unit level medical care is ____________________________________.

7. At ___________________ level, the casualty is examined, his wounds and general

   status are evaluated to determine his priority for continued evacuation to the rear, emergency care/resuscitation is continued, and urgent surgery is performed if necessary.

8. The CSH is a ________________________ level hospital.

9. The GH and FH are _______________________ level hospitals.

10. A major duty of the M6 practical nurse is to perform _____________________, ________________________, and ________________________ nursing care procedures.

11. Duties of the M6 practical nurse also involve management of ________________ ______________________________ and ______________________________.

12. At each higher grade and skill level, the M6 practical nurse assumes more ____ and spends less time in ____ .

13. In addition to being proficient in providing practical nursing care, the M6 must demonstrate proficiency in ____ and exercising the ____.

14. Two areas of specialization available to the M6 practical nurse are ___________________________ and ___________________________________ .

Check Your Answers on Next Page

SOLUTIONS TO EXERCISES, LESSON 1

1. Maintain the health of the Army and conserve its fighting strength. (para 1-1b)

2. Health support of the Army in time of war, international conflict, or natural disaster. (para 1-1b)

3. Selection of fit personnel for military service.
   Prevention of unnecessary health hazards.
   Medical treatment of the sick and injured.
   Evacuation of patients. (paras 1-1b(1), (2), (3), (4))

4. DOD tri-service hospitals; Veterans Administration hospitals. (para 1-8a)

5. Levels or echelons. (para 1-4b)

6. Initial emergency medical treatment. (para 1-5a)

7. Division. (para 1-6b)

8. Corps. (para 1-7a)

9. COMMZ. (paras 1-7b(1)(a), (b))

10. Preventive; therapeutic; emergency. (para 1-12)

11. Other paraprofessional personnel; ward or unit operations. (para 1-12)

12. Supervisory and managerial responsibility; direct patient care. (para 1-13)

13. Common soldier tasks; principles of military leadership. (para 1-12)

14. Instructor; dialysis technician. (paras 1-16a, b)

END OF LESSON 1

LESSON ASSIGNMENT

LESSON 2 The M6 Practical Nurse Course.

LESSON ASSIGNMENT Paragraphs 2-1 through 2-7.

LESSON OBJECTIVES After completing this lesson, you should be able to:

2-1. State the purpose of the M6 Practical Nurse Course.

2-2. State the objectives of the M6 Practical Nurse Course.

2-3. Describe the content of the M6 Practical Nurse Course.

SUGGESTION After reading and studying the assignment, complete the exercises at the end of this lesson. These exercises will help you to achieve the lesson objectives.

LESSON 2

THE M6 PRACTICAL NURSE COURSE

2-1. COURSE PURPOSE

The purpose of the Practical Nurse Course is to prepare qualified Army Medical Department enlisted personnel to provide basic practical nursing care in a variety of settings during peacetime and mobilization. Students are expected to achieve entry-level practical nursing competencies for medical-surgical nursing, obstetrics, newborn, and pediatric nursing. Students are also introduced to the role and functions of the Department of the Army practical nurse as a soldier and noncommissioned officer.

2-2. TERMINAL LEARNING COURSE OBJECTIVES

Upon completion of the Practical Nurse Course, the soldier will have been trained in a variety of skills in many different subject areas. This learning experience can be summed up in several terminal learning course objectives that the soldier will meet upon completion of the course. The Practical Nurse Course graduate will do the following.

a. **Phase I**.

(1) Identify principles of basic-level anatomy, physiology, microbiology, and nutrition.

(2) Perform basic-level pharmacological calculations.

b. **Phase II**.

(1) Administer safe and effective beginning-level practical nursing care in a variety of health care settings during peacetime and war.

(2) Demonstrate the ability to integrate the knowledge of drug therapy into nursing practice.

(3) Demonstrate effective oral and written communication skills in the health care setting.

(4) Display the ability to function effectively as a team member and team leader.

(5) Identify the basic principles of field nursing.

2-3. TRAINING SEQUENCE

The Practical Nurse Course is a 52-week training program conducted in two phases. Phase I is 6 weeks in length and is conducted at the U.S. Army Academy of Health Sciences (AHS), Fort Sam Houston, Texas,. Phase II is 46 weeks in length and is conducted at one of five designated medical treatment facilities in the continental United States (CONUS). Phase II sites are:

a Brooke Army Medical Center, Fort Sam Houston, Texas.

b. Dwight D. Eisenhower Army Medical Center, Fort Gordon, Georgia.

c. Walter Reed Army Medical Center, Washington, DC.

d. Madigan Army Medical Center, Fort Lewis, Washington.

e. William Beaumont Army Medical Center, Fort Bliss, Texas.

2-4. CURRICULUM

a. **Phase I.**

(1) Orientation to the practical nurse course. During orientation, an assessment of the student's academic knowledge will be completed. Academic confidence training and instruction in techniques of effective learning is given in order to enhance learning potential. An overview of practical nursing discusses organizations and publications for practical nurses and the history and trends of practical nursing. The standards of nursing practice and the duties and responsibilities of the practical nurse are discussed with the role of the practical nurse as a member of the health care team. Some of the many career opportunities for practical nurses are also presented to the student.

(2) Basic sciences for practical nurses. An introduction to the basic sciences for practical nurses is presented. Topics included are nursing and medical terminology, nutrition, anatomy and physiology, microbiology, pharmacology, and pharmacological mathematics.

b. **Phase II.**

(1) Medical-surgical nursing I. Basic practical nursing skills are learned in an integrated classroom and clinical experience approach. Basic nursing competencies are practiced on medical and surgical nursing units, to include the care of geriatric and pediatric patients.

(2) Medical-surgical nursing II. Basic medical-surgical nursing skills and knowledge are expanded with classroom and clinical instruction in the nursing care of a patient with problems in various body systems, to include musculoskeletal, blood and blood forming, cardiovascular, respiratory, gastrointestinal, nervous, and endocrine systems.

(3) Medical-surgical nursing III. Students receive theoretical instruction and clinical experience in the delivery of practical nursing care to adult patients with cancer, reproductive disorders, and mental illness. Nursing care related to obstetrics is included.

(4) Field nursing. Instruction and performance oriented training in the administration of emergency care and first aid to combat casualties is presented in classroom and field settings. Training is given in the protection of self and subordinates when operating in a nuclear-biological-chemical contaminated environment.

(5) State Board Examination preparation and outprocessing. A review of major content areas, administration of achievement tests, and group study prepares the student for the Practical Nurse Licensure Examination. During this module, outprocessing is accomplished and the students are assisted with permanent change of station (PCS) to their follow-on assignment.

2-5. DIDACTIC ACHIEVEMENT EVALUATION

The student's didactic (theory) achievement will be measured by the administration of a series of written examinations in the major didactic subject areas. Each examination question is multiple-choice in nature and is keyed to the lesson plan objectives.

2-6. CLINICAL ACHIEVEMENT EVALUATION

The student's achievement in clinical performance training will be graded pass/fail, based upon the performance of a series of tasks related to the different clinical subject areas. At the beginning of each clinical rotation, the student will receive a list of objectives for that particular clinical area. The student must successfully accomplish those objectives during the time allotted for that clinical rotation. The clinical areas include the following:

a. Medical-surgical ward.

b. Intensive care unit.

c. Recovery room.

d. Pediatrics.

e. Obstetrics.

f. Newborn nursery.

g. Clinics.

2-7. OTHER REQUIREMENTS

In addition to passing the clinical and didactic portions of the Practical Nurse Course, the student is required to meet height and weight standards in accordance with regulation. A diagnostic Army Physical Fitness Test (APFT) will be conducted during Phase I. The APFT for record will be conducted near the end of Phase II. Students who fail to pass the APFT for record will not graduate and will not receive a diploma.

Continue with Exercises

EXERCISES, LESSON 2

INSTRUCTIONS. Complete the statements in the following exercises. After you have completed all statements in the exercises, turn to "Solutions to Exercises" at the end of this lesson and check your answers.

1. One purpose of the Practical Nurse Course is to train personnel to provide basic practical nursing care during________________________ and ________________________________.

2. Another purpose of the Practical Nurse Course is to introduce personnel to the role and functions of the U.S. Army practical nurse as __________________________ and ____.

3. A Practical Nurse Course graduate will be able to identify principles of basic-level ___________________________, __________________________________, ___________________________, and _______________________________.

4. The Practical Nurse Course graduate will be able to administer beginning-level practical nursing care during ________________________ and ______________.

5. The Practical Nurse Course graduate will be able to function effectively as a team ________________________ and a team _____________________________.

6. The Practical Nurse Course is a 52-week program conducted in _______ phases.

7. During the clinical phase of training in the Practical Nurse Course, students receive a list of ______________________________ to accomplish for each clinical area.

8. To graduate from the Practical Nurse Course, the soldier must meet ________________________ and ________________________ standards and pass the ____.

Check Your Answers on Next Page

SOLUTIONS TO EXERCISES, LESSON 2

1. Peacetime; mobilization. (para 2-1)

2. Soldier; noncommissioned officer. (para 2-1)

3. Anatomy; physiology; microbiology; nutrition. (para 2-2a(1))

4. Peacetime; war. (para 2-2b(1))

5. Member; leader. (para 2-2b(4))

6. Two. (para 2-3)

7. Objectives. (para 2-6)

8. Height; weight; Army Physical Fitness Test (APFT). (para 2-7)

END OF LESSON 2

LESSON ASSIGNMENT

LESSON 3 Duties and Responsibilities of the M6 Practical Nurse.

LESSON ASSIGNMENT Paragraphs 3-1 through 3-13.

LESSON OBJECTIVES After completing this lesson, you should be able to:

3-1. Identify the clinical duties and responsibilities of the M6 practical nurse.

3-2. Identify the managerial duties and responsibilities of the M6 practical nurse.

SUGGESTION After completing the assignment, complete the exercises at the end of this lesson. These exercises will help you to achieve the lesson objectives.

LESSON 3

DUTIES AND RESPONSIBILITIES OF THE M6 PRACTICAL NURSE

Section I. CLINICAL DUTIES AND RESPONSIBILITIES OF THE M6 PRACTICAL NURSE

3-1. INTRODUCTION

The M6 practical nurse performs or supervises preventive, therapeutic, and emergency nursing care procedures under the supervision of a physician, nurse, or senior NCO. The recipients of this care include infants, children, adolescents, active duty soldiers, retirees, and civilian emergencies. All have different health care needs, and the practical nurse must be able to provide the nursing care related to those needs. Flexibility is a necessity when expected to provide care to all these categories of patients. Additionally, the practical nurse must be able to adapt that clinical ability to various settings and situations, including the field environment. The first step in providing health care is to determine the needs of the patient. All the nursing care needs of the patient may be determined and fulfilled by a logical application of four easy steps--assessment, planning, implementation, and evaluation.

3-2. ASSESSMENT

a. In order to provide nursing care, one must first determine the needs of the patient. Patient needs vary in relation to the illness or injury, the age and overall physical condition of the patient, the support or nonsupport of the patient's family and friends, the mental status of the patient, and the length of time expected for recovery. These are the most significant of the many variables involved. All the information and medical data obtained will be applied to a general assessment of the patient's needs. The practical nurse supports the professional nursing staff in the assessment of nursing care needs by:

(1) Using basic communication skills in the patient care setting, interacting with the patient and his family to obtain subjective information relative to the patient's condition.

(2) Obtaining objective data from the patient through observation and goal-directed interviews.

(3) Participating in the identification of physical, emotional, spiritual, cultural, and learning needs of the patient through data collection.

(4) Determining the significance of the data collected in relation to the patient's pathophysiology.

b. Once the specific needs of the patient have been identified, the health care team members go to the next step, which is the planning phase.

3-3. PLANNING

a. Once the needs of the patient have been identified, several questions must be asked by the health care team in order to develop the nursing care plan. A plan of care is goal-oriented, with short-term and long-term goals identified. When you have identified the needs of the patient in the assessment phase, you also begin to determine what the results of fulfilling those needs should be. Do you expect results on a short- or long-term basis? How, specifically, will those goals be achieved? What action will be taken, and by whom? What shall be done first, second, last, and so on? The practical nurse supports the professional nursing staff in the planning of nursing care by:

(1) Assisting the professional nurses in determining the nursing care priorities and planning the nursing care to be provided.

(2) Working with other team members to develop a written plan of care.

(3) Participating in the development of long-term and/or preventive health plans with the patient and his family.

b. After the patient's needs have been identified and the plan of care has been developed, the process of implementation begins.

3-4. IMPLEMENTATION

a. In order to participate in the implementation of the planned nursing care, the M6 practical nurse must be clinically proficient and capable of providing and/or supervising nursing care. This care includes basic nursing care procedures such as obtaining and interpreting vital signs, collecting blood specimens, and changing wound dressings. Nursing care also includes activities involved with patient comfort and safety such as bathing the patient, administering range-of-motion exercises, and application of restraints to a disoriented patient. Also within the scope of practical nursing duties is the administration of medications and intravenous therapy. The practical nurse must also be able to reinforce the teaching done by the professional staff. To achieve patient awareness and cooperation, it is necessary to explain the "how" and "why" of nursing care procedures. This is especially important if the patient will have continuing treatments, medications, or special instructions at home with little or no supervision from the health care team. With this clinical nursing proficiency, the practical nurse supports the professional nursing staff in the implementation of the planned nursing care by:

(1) Applying a working knowledge of patients' rights and protecting the rights and privacy of the patient and his family.

(2) Safely performing or supervising nursing care in the form of therapeutic and preventive procedures that have been specifically planned for each individual patient.

(3) Observing the patient and reporting significant findings to the health care team members as appropriate.

(4) Contributing to the development and reinforcement of health care teaching plans for patients and their family members.

(5) Maintaining current knowledge, skills, and certification necessary to provide quality care.

b. Providing appropriate nursing care to the patient is not the end of the M6 practical nurse's responsibility. The care being given must continually be evaluated for effectiveness.

3-5. EVALUATION

a. It is necessary to determine whether the care provided is appropriate and effective. Are the long- and short-term goals being achieved? What is the patient's physiological and psychological status now, in comparison to earlier? Would some other course of action be more beneficial or more significant? The nursing care plan must be continually evaluated and updated in response to the changes in the patient. If not, something significant may be overlooked and the course of recovery for the patient may be delayed. The practical nurse coordinates with and assists the professional nursing staff in the evaluation of nursing care by:

(1) Contributing to the identification of the strengths and weaknesses in the plan of nursing care.

(2) Communicating with the patient and his family to maintain awareness of the patient's feelings and condition.

(3) Observing the patient and documenting the information obtained through observation and communication.

(4) Seeking assistance in improving <u>his</u> <u>own</u> personal weaknesses if any are identified in the course of patient care.

b. As the nursing plan of care is evaluated, it will become necessary to periodically reassess the patient's needs and formulate a new plan to be implemented. This four step method of assessing, planning, implementing, and evaluating is a circular process of continued nursing care (see figure 3-1). This process can be utilized for developing all types of nursing care. This circular process is illustrated in the following situation.

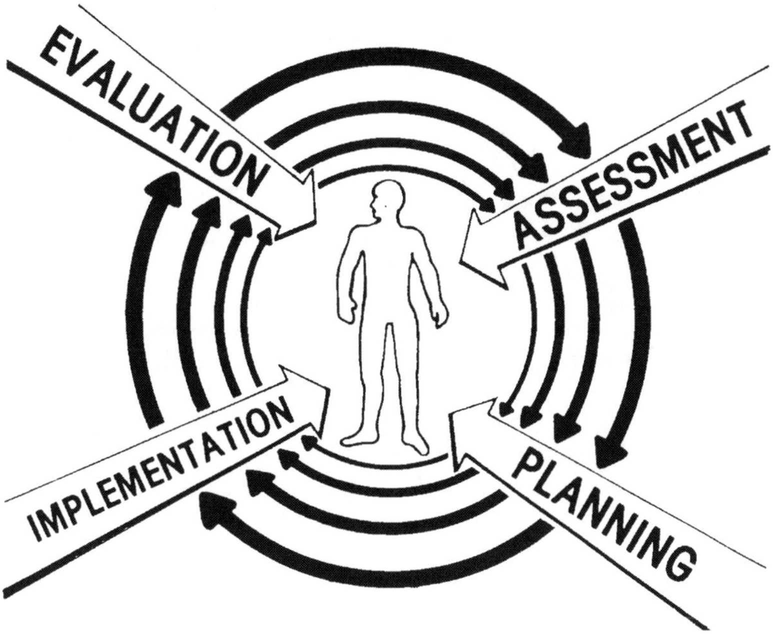

Figure 3-1. Circular process of nursing care.

3-6. ILLUSTRATION

a. You are a M6 practical nurse assigned to a surgical ward. It is 1630 hours, and the Emergency Department calls to inform the registered nurse (RN) in charge that the ward will be receiving an admission. Sergeant Jones, age 30, is admitted to the ward a short time later. His diagnosis is traumatic amputation and avulsion of a portion of the right foot. The injury occurred when Sergeant Jones accidentally entangled his foot in the blades of his power mower. You assist the RN in assessing Sergeant Jones. You find that he appears generally healthy and well nourished. He is alert and oriented, and his vital signs, although slightly abnormal, are stable. His skin is cool and clammy, his face pale. He has an intravenous infusion (IV) that is infusing well. The surgeon on duty removes the bulky dressing in order to evaluate the injury. You observe that the 4th and 5th toes are missing and that a portion of the lateral foot has been avulsed. The wound is slowly oozing blood. The surgeon decides to take Sergeant Jones to the operating room (OR) as soon as possible. He discusses the preparations with the RN in charge. As you are obtaining the preoperative laboratory specimens from Sergeant Jones, he tells you that he is extremely concerned about the welfare of his two small children, now waiting in the cafeteria with a neighbor. Sergeant Jones explains that his wife is on temporary duty (TDY) elsewhere and there is no one at home to care for the children while he is hospitalized. You relay this information to the RN, who is completing the assessment of Sergeant Jones. Based upon the assessment, the following needs have been identified. Sergeant Jones is stable, but must be closely observed for shock. Surgical repair of the foot is necessary and Sergeant Jones must be prepared for surgery. There is also the need to alleviate his anxiety over the welfare of his children.

b. The nursing plan is to prepare Sergeant Jones for surgery, scheduled for one hour later. You will monitor him closely since a change in vital signs could indicate a change in his stable condition. While the RN begins the pre-operative arrangements for Sergeant Jones, you will call social services to arrange for someone to help Sergeant Jones with childcare. These are Sergeant Jones' immediate needs. Several projected needs have also been identified. As the wound is considered "dirty," there is an additional danger of infection for Sergeant Jones. The RN decides that it would be best to isolate Sergeant Jones in a private room post-operatively, and you begin to make the necessary preparations for the room. Additionally, Sergeant Jones will need the services of other activities. Physical therapy will be consulted for post-surgical rehabilitation. Since Sergeant Jones will most likely suffer a sense of loss and depression caused by the disfigurement of his foot, mental health services will be consulted.

c. The ward staff now begins to implement the plan. The surgical paperwork is prepared and placed in Sergeant Jones' chart. The RN accompanies the surgeon to Sergeant Jones' room to witness the surgical counseling and signing of the operative permit. Sergeant Jones' vital signs are taken every 15 minutes in order to monitor his status. Since the RN had assigned you the duty of passing medications for that shift, you prepare and administer the pre-op medication ordered by the physician. Social work services has sent a representative to the ward to assist Sergeant Jones and child care arrangements are made. A patient administration clerk is notifying Sergeant Jones' unit of his admission and will request that a representative of the unit come in the hospital to visit Sergeant Jones and assist him with his personal matters.

d. The staff evaluates the plan 45 minutes later and finds that Sergeant Jones' condition is stable and he is ready for surgery. The appropriate paperwork is completed and placed in the patient's chart. Social work services have arranged for Sergeant Jones' neighbor to care for the children until his wife can be notified and return from TDY. A private room has been prepared for Sergeant Jones to occupy following surgery. Pre-op blood and urine specimens have been sent to the lab. X-rays have been obtained from the radiology section and are ready to be sent to the OR with Sergeant Jones. The RN has completed pre-op counseling and teaching and you have taken Sergeant Jones through his first coughing and deep breathing exercises. Based upon this evaluation, it is determined that all of the initial short-term nursing care goals have been accomplished. As he is transported to the operating room, you are already preparing for Sergeant Jones' return, when a re-assessment must be done and a new plan implemented.

3-7. SUMMARY

a. You can see that the clinical duties and responsibilities of the practical nurse involve much more than simply performing patient care tasks. In addition to having performance proficiency in nursing care tasks, the practical nurse must also maintain a strong knowledge base from which to work. The practical nurse must be a communicator, an observer, an interviewer, and a teacher. The M6 practical nurse must be able to interpret data, prioritize needs, and act appropriately to assist in the implementation of a plan of nursing care. Some patient needs may require the M6 practical nurse to think and act quickly to save life or limb, while other needs may require projecting ahead to the future. Most importantly, the practical nurse must be a team worker.

b. All these things are part of clinical practical nursing. The majority of the MOS related tasks performed by the practical nurse are clinical in nature; that is, they involve providing patient care. As a soldier advances to the next skill level, he assumes the responsibility for proficiency in more tasks. For the M6 practical nurse, the higher skill levels include not only more advanced nursing care, but managerial tasks as well. These tasks will be discussed in the next section of this lesson.

Section II. MANAGERIAL DUTIES AND RESPONSIBILITIES OF THE M6 PRACTICAL NURSE

3-8. INTRODUCTION

In addition to clinical proficiency and soldier skills, the practical nurse must learn to be an effective manager and leader (see figure 3-2). As rank increases, the M6 must maintain additional managerial and supervisory expertise. Clinical areas must be well managed in order to provide consistent quality care. Supplies and equipment must be maintained, and paperwork must flow smoothly. The needs of the patients and staff must be dealt with in a fair and professional manner. As with clinical skills, these managerial skills must be adaptable to different areas of assignment. Practical nurse management responsibilities can be categorized into three basic areas of concern: managing supplies and equipment, managing work center operations, and managing personnel.

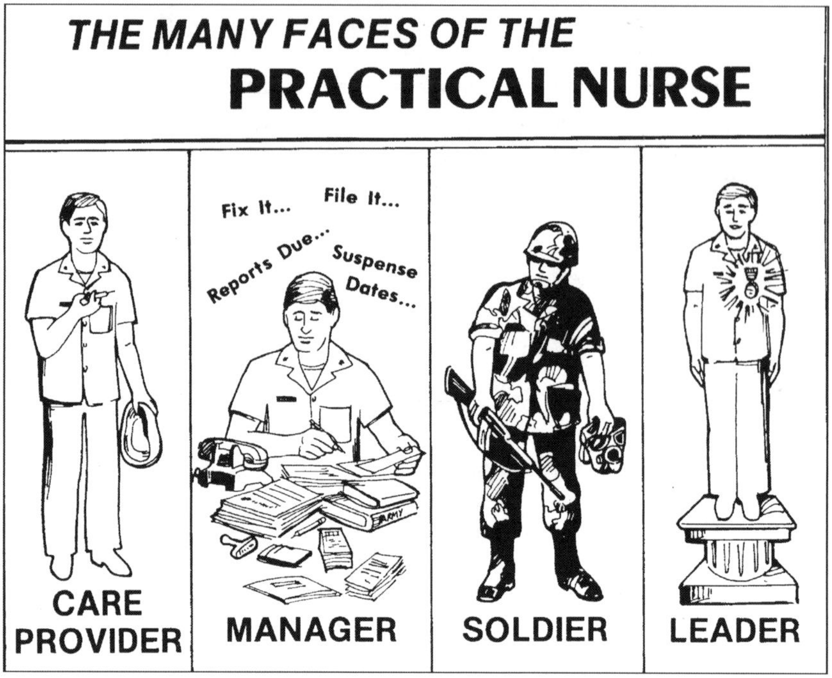

3-9. MANAGING SUPPLIES AND EQUIPMENT

a. Managing supplies and equipment involves much more than keeping the storage area neat. The first priority in supply and equipment management is knowing how to procure the things that are needed. The procurement process involves several steps. First, requirements must be established. The practical nurse manager must maintain ward, clinic, or area readiness by knowing what supplies and equipment are needed for daily operations (to accomplish the mission). The next step is to requisition the supplies and equipment through the proper channels. In order to do this, the manager must have a working knowledge of the basics of the supply system. This does not mean you must be a logistics expert, but you do need to know where to look for information and whom to see for assistance. When the requested items arrive in your work place, they must be properly received, inspected, and stored. Additionally, supplies and equipment must be properly safeguarded against damage and loss, periodically inventoried and inspected, and properly issued for use. The practical nurse manager is responsible for the readiness of his or her area of responsibility.

b. Another part of supply and equipment management is maintaining the associated paperwork and records. Hand receipts must be kept up to date, budgets controlled, and supply documents noted and filed. Equipment found to be unserviceable must be turned in or sent for repair. As the manager, the practical nurse is responsible for accountability of supplies and equipment, whether used, disposed of, or sent for repair.

c. Maintenance and serviceability of equipment are also management responsibilities. Equipment must be checked for proper function, inspected for damage or leaks, calibrated, and tested on a regular basis. Local policy dictates what is to be done, but it is the responsibility of the enlisted manager to make sure that it does get done at the proper time and by the appropriate personnel. Much supply and equipment maintenance is done on the "user" level and, again, it is the responsibility of the enlisted manager to be certain that the individuals using the equipment are familiar with the correct procedures for its operation and maintenance.

3-10. MANAGING WORK CENTER OPERATIONS

Support of health care operations involves management of the work center itself, in day-to-day operations and in long range planning strategies. Readiness of personnel and equipment must be maintained for efficient operations. To sustain readiness, a paraprofessional in-service program must be developed and implemented. Individual progress and abilities of each subordinate must be tracked and documented. Time schedules and task assignment rosters must be prepared to support daily operations in the work place. The work center itself must be set up and maintained in a manner that allows for efficient operations. A ward, unit, or section SOP must be implemented and enforced in order to provide guidance and standardization for procedures. Periodic inspections must be conducted to ensure safety and cleanliness. The enlisted managers must be familiar with all aspects of operations in their section and act as "troubleshooters" when observing daily activities and operations.

3-11. MANAGING PERSONNEL

a. Of all the management skills required, the ability to effectively manage personnel is the most crucial and most difficult. When managing personnel, the M6 practical nurse is concerned with daily appearance and military bearing, attitude, job performance, and training needs. The manager must also be informed about the soldier's off-duty activities and behavior. Additionally, each soldier's first-line supervisor is responsible for overseeing the development of that individual into an effective and efficient soldier and future NCO. The practical nurse manager must be aware of the educational needs, performance capabilities, and personal goals of each subordinate worker, whether military or civilian. Taking the time and initiative to know your personnel as individuals will make managing them easier for you and communicating with you easier for them.

b. The following categories identify the responsibilities of the enlisted manager in the scope of personnel management. Listed under each area are only a few examples of the tasks performed by the practical nurse manager.

(1) <u>Personal and professional development of the soldier</u>.

(a) Recommend promotions, awards, and punitive actions.

(b) Counsel soldiers in their strengths and weaknesses and how each affects their duty performance.

(c) Ensure soldiers are utilized in their MOS.

(d) Ensure that required technical publications are available and utilized.

(e) Ensure that deserving soldiers attend appropriate service schools.

(f) Conduct professional development training.

(2) Individual training of the soldier.

(a) Educate soldiers in history and traditions of the service, military courtesy, drill and ceremonies, standards of conduct, personal hygiene, and standards for military bearing and appearance.

(b) Train enlisted personnel as effective team members.

(c) Train individual soldiers in their MOS/ASI skills.

(d) Train soldiers for survival on the battlefield.

(e) Train soldiers in common training tasks (CTT) and for self development tests (SDT).

(3) Accountability for squad/section/team.

(a) Know what soldiers are doing during duty hours.

(b) Know where all soldiers live and how to locate them.

(c) Know why soldiers are going to sick call or other appointments, how they are treated, and what the results are.

(d) Use squad/section/team as a unit to accomplish goals/objectives/mission.

(4) Military appearance and physical condition of the soldier.

(a) Make on-the-spot corrections for deficiencies in military appearance.

(b) Conduct physical training and enforce physical fitness standards.

(c) Assist personnel with physical training problems.

(d) Enforce and appearance standards.

(e) Train soldiers how to properly maintain and wear uniforms and equipment.

(5) Physical and mental well-being of the soldier and the family.

(a) Know where and how soldiers live.

(b) Know soldiers' family situations and provide assistance if needed.

(c) Inform soldiers of services available to them and their families through the military.

(d) Visit soldier support activities and ensure that they are acting in the best interest of the soldiers.

(e) Visit soldiers and family members who are sick and provide needed assistance.

(f) Refer soldiers for medical assistance when necessary.

(6) Supervision, control, and discipline.

(a) Conduct counseling and maintain counseling records.

(b) Support actions of subordinate NCO leaders.

(c) Educate personnel on the Uniformed Code of Military Justice (UCMJ).

(d) Recommend punitive action through appropriate channels.

(e) Conduct remedial training when required.

(f) Use the chain of command and appropriate supporting channels.

(g) Listen and respond to soldiers' suggestions and complaints.

(h) Support and explain reasons for current policies to the soldiers.

(i) Instill the feeling of unit pride, integrity, and loyalty.

(j) Supervise the execution of established policy.

(7) Maintain established standards of professionalism and performance.

(a) Conduct special training to resolve areas of training weakness.

(b) Train subordinates to meet, and then exceed, standards.

(c) Provide up-to-date information for all levels of training (CTT/SDT).

(d) Set the example, so that subordinates can see the professional NCO in action.

(8) Demonstrate proficiency in and teach leadership traits.

(a) Professional ethics.

(b) Technical competence.

(c) Tactical competence.

(d) Communicating.

(e) Supervising.

(f) Counseling.

(g) Management ability.

(h) Planning ability.

(b) Decision-making ability.

(b) Soldier-team development ability.

3-12. SUMMARY

In the role of enlisted leader, the M6 practical nurse manager must remember that he is responsible for the development of subordinate personnel. Therefore, when teaching, strive to teach excellence. When leading, lead by example. Only by demonstrating personal and professional excellence can the practical nurse manager motivate subordinates to develop competence, commitment, and integrity. The practical nurse must demonstrate both candor and tact when dealing with people. The practical nurse must be decisive, having the knowledge, initiative, and self-confidence to perform in a professional manner. The practical nurse must maintain enthusiasm and humor in the face of even the most unpleasant or demoralizing situations. By maintaining professional bearing and demonstrating these qualities, the practical nurse manager will influence other soldiers to do the same.

3-13. CLOSING

This subcourse has introduced you to the many aspects of U.S. Army practical nursing. In order to be a competent M6 practical nurse, you must first have an understanding of the mission of the Army Medical Department and your role in helping to accomplish that mission. You must also be aware of, and proficient in, your duties and responsibilities, not only as a practical nurse, but also as a soldier in the United States Army. Only then will you be able to fulfill the challenging role of a U.S. Army practical nurse.

Continue with Exercises

EXERCISES, LESSON 3

INSTRUCTIONS. Complete the statements in the following exercises. After you have completed all statements in the exercises, turn to "Solutions to Exercises" at the end of this lesson and check your answers.

1. The practical nurse performs or supervises ______________________________, ____________________, and ________________________ nursing care procedures.

2. The first step in providing health care is to ______________________________.

3. A plan of care is ______________________ -oriented, with both long- and short-term ____.

4. The practical nurse supports the implementation of the planned nursing care by contributing to the development and reinforcement of ____ plans.

5. The practical nurse assists with the evaluation of nursing care by _______________ the patient and ____________________________________ information.

6. Nursing care is a continuous, ____ process of ______________________ , ______________________ ______________________, and ______________________ .

7. The ____ must be evaluated and updated in response to changes in the patient.

8. During evaluation, the nursing staff must determine whether the care provided is ________________________________ and ________________________________.

9. Management responsibilities can be categorized into the three basic areas of managing ______________________, ____________________________________ , and ____.

10. In addition to clinical proficiency and soldier skills, the practical nurse must learn to be an effective ________________________ and ________________________.

Turn Page for Self-Test

SOLUTIONS TO EXERCISES, LESSON 3

1. Preventive; therapeutic; emergency. (para 3-1)
2. Determine the needs of (assess) the patient. (paras 3-1, 3-2a).
3. Goal; goals. (para 3-3a)
4. Health care teaching. (para 3-4a(4))
5. Observing; documenting. (para 3-5a(3))
6. Circular; assessing; planning; implementing; evaluating. (para 3-5b; fig. 3-1)
7. Nursing care plan. (para 3-5a)
8. Appropriate; effective. (para 3-5a)
9. Personnel; supplies and equipment; work center operations. (para 3-8)
10. Manager; leader. (para 3-8)

END OF LESSON 3

COMMENT SHEET

SUBCOURSE MD0910 INTRODUCTION TO PRACTICAL NURSING EDITION 100

Your comments about this subcourse are valuable and aid the writers in refining the subcourse and making it more usable. Please enter your comments in the space provided. ENCLOSE THIS FORM (OR A COPY) WITH YOUR ANSWER SHEET **ONLY** IF YOU HAVE COMMENTS ABOUT THIS SUBCOURSE..

FOR A WRITTEN REPLY, WRITE A SEPARATE LETTER AND INCLUDE SOCIAL SECURITY NUMBER, RETURN ADDRESS (and e-mail address, if possible), SUBCOURSE NUMBER AND EDITION, AND PARAGRAPH/EXERCISE/EXAMINATION ITEM NUMBER.

PLEASE COMPLETE THE FOLLOWING ITEMS:

(Use the reverse side of this sheet, if necessary.)

1. List any terms that were not defined properly.

____
____
____
____

2. List any errors.

paragraph error correction

____
____
____
____
____
____
____
____

3. List any suggestions you have to improve this subcourse.

____
____
____
____

4. Student Information (optional)

Name/Rank ____________________
SSN ____________________
Address ____________________
____
E-mail Address ____________________
Telephone number (DSN) ____________________
MOS/AOC ____________________

PRIVACY ACT STATEMENT (AUTHORITY: 10USC3012(B) AND (G))

PURPOSE: To provide Army Correspondence Course Program students a means to submit inquiries and comments.

USES: To locate and make necessary change to student records.

DISCLOSURE: **VOLUNTARY.** Failure to submit SSN will prevent subcourse authors at service school from accessing student records and responding to inquiries requiring such follow-ups.

U.S. ARMY MEDICAL DEPARTMENT CENTER AND SCHOOL Fort Sam Houston, Texas 78234-6130

Drug Dosage and Therapy

Subcourse MD0913

This page intentionally left blank.

U.S. ARMY MEDICAL DEPARTMENT CENTER AND SCHOOL
FORT SAM HOUSTON, TEXAS 78234-6100

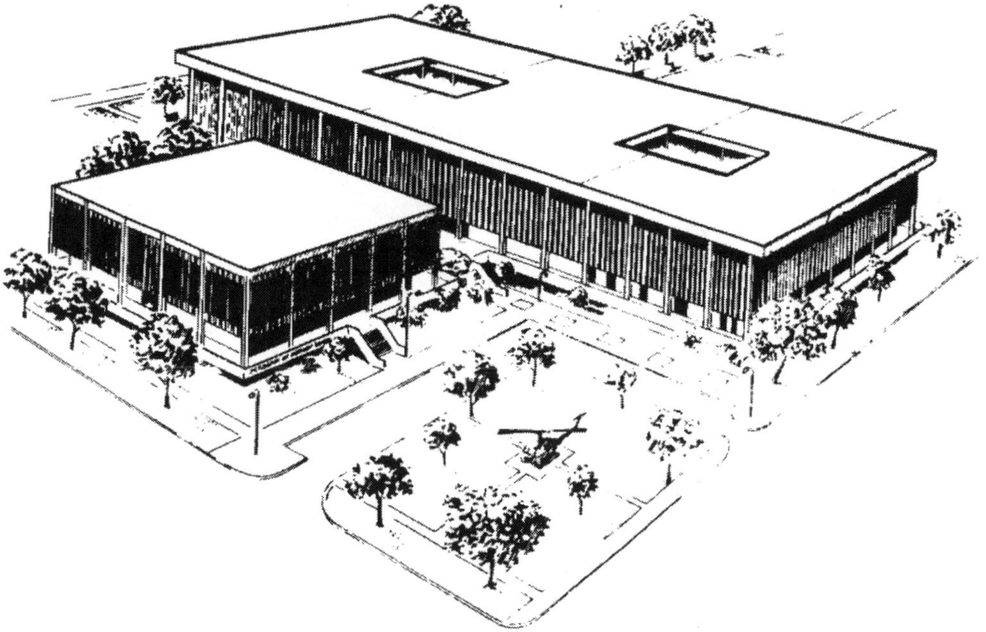

DRUG DOSAGE AND THERAPY

SUBCOURSE MD0913

EDITION 100

DEVELOPMENT

This subcourse is approved for resident and correspondence course instruction. It reflects the current thought of the U.S. Army Medical Department Center and School and conforms to printed Department of the Army doctrine as closely as currently possible. Development and progress render such doctrine continuously subject to change.

Content accuracy of this edition was the responsibility of the Pharmacy Branch, Medicine and Surgery Division; DSN 471-8420 or area code 512-221-8420; Commander, U.S. Army Medical Department Center and School, ATTN: HSHA-MM, Fort Sam Houston, Texas 78234-6100.

ADMINISTRATION

Students who desire credit hours for this correspondence subcourse must meet eligibility requirements and must enroll through the Nonresident Instruction Branch of the U.S. Army Medical Department Center and School (AMEDDC&S).

Application for enrollment should be made at the Internet website: http://www.atrrs.army.mil. You can access the course catalog in the upper right corner. Enter School Code 555 for medical correspondence courses. Copy down the course number and title. To apply for enrollment, return to the main ATRRS screen and scroll down the right side for ATRRS Channels. Click on SELF DEVELOPMENT to open the application and then follow the on screen instructions.

For comments or questions regarding enrollment, student records, or shipments, contact the Nonresident Instruction Branch at DSN 471-5877, commercial (210) 221-5877, toll-free 1-800-344-2380; fax: 210-221-4012 or DSN 471-4012, e-mail accp@amedd.army.mil, or write to:

NONRESIDENT INSTRUCTION BRANCH
AMEDDC&S
ATTN: MCCS-HSN
2105 11TH STREET SUITE 4191
FORT SAM HOUSTON TX 78234-5064

CLARIFICATION OF TERMINOLOGY

When used in this publication, words such as "he," "him," "his," and "men" 'are intended to include both the masculine and feminine genders, unless specifically stated otherwise or when obvious in context.

USE OF PROPRIETARY NAMES

The initial letters of the names of some products are capitalized in this subcourse. Such names are proprietary names, that is, brand names or trademarks. Proprietary names have been used in this subcourse only to make it a more effective learning aid. The use of any name, proprietary or otherwise, should not be interpreted as endorsement, deprecation, or criticism of a product. Nor should such use be considered to interpret the validity of proprietary rights in a name, whether it is registered or not.

TABLE OF CONTENTS

CORRESPONDENCE COURSE OF THE U.S. ARMY MEDICAL DEPARTMENT CENTER AND SCHOOL

SUBCOURSE MD0913

DRUG DOSAGE AND THERAPY

INTRODUCTION

The administration of drugs is one of the most important and exacting duties performed in caring for sick and injured patients. The appropriate drug given in the correct dosage will very often hasten a patient's recovery. On the other hand, an inappropriate drug or dosage may worsen a patient's condition or even result in his death.

The enlisted person charged with the administration of drugs is therefore faced with a grave responsibility, whether medical supervision is immediately available or not.

The purpose of this subcourse is to familiarize you with basic drugs that are standard for the U.S. Army. Discussion includes the actions, clinical uses, administration, untoward effects, cautions, and contraindications in the use of these drugs, as well as their forms of issue.

Subcourse Components:

This subcourse consists of six lessons:

Lesson 1. Dosage Calculations.

Lesson 2. Basic Pharmacology; Antiseptics, and Disinfectants; Other Topical Drugs; Gastrointestinal Agents; Respiratory Drugs; Local Anesthetics.

Lesson 3. Central Nervous System Drugs.

Lesson 4. Autonomic and Cardiovascular Drugs.

Lesson 5. Drugs Used to Prevent and Treat Infection I.

Lesson 6. Drugs Used to Prevent and Treat Infection II.

Credit Awarded:

Upon successful completion of this subcourse, you will be awarded 16 credit hours.

LESSON ASSIGNMENT

LESSON 1 Dosage Calculations

LESSON ASSIGNMENT Paragraphs 1-1 through 1-25

LESSON OBJECTIVES After completing this lesson, you should be able to:

1-1 Interpret drug orders.

1-2 Convert units within the metric system.

1-3 Convert units between the apothecary and metric systems.

1-4 Given the strength of a drug, calculate and measure an injection dose.

1-5 Given an antibiotic or other drug in dry powder form, dilute the vial with an appropriate diluent and calculate the necessary volume dose.

1-6 Calculate pediatric doses, given the body weight and either the dose per unit of body weight or the dose per unit of surface area.

SUGGESTIONS If you need to review basic mathematics, it is recommended that you enroll in Subcourse MD0900, Basic Mathematics.

After studying this assignment, complete the exercises at the end of this lesson. These exercises will help you to achieve the lesson objectives.

LESSON 1

DOSAGE CALCULATIONS

Section I. INTERPRETING MEDICAL ORDERS

1-1. COMMON MEDICAL ABBREVIATIONS

To calculate doses and administer drugs, you must be familiar with those abbreviations commonly used in medicine, especially those found in prescriptions and clients' charts. Table 1-1 is a list of common Latin terms and abbreviations used in medicine. Tables 1-2 and 1-3 are summaries of common abbreviations used to indicate times of administration, routes of administration, and dosage forms. Tables 1-4 and 1-5 give symbols or abbreviations for different units of measure.

1-2. ROMAN NUMERALS

Roman numerals are used in writing prescriptions. They are used to specify the amounts of ingredients when the apothecary system is being used. They are used to specify the number of units (capsules, tablets, powders, suppositories, and so forth) to be dispensed; for example, "Dispxxiv." And lastly, they are used in the signa or directions to the client. You should, therefore, be thoroughly familiar with the system of Roman numerals used in pharmacy. The basic symbols or numerals are:

ss, $\overline{ss}$	1/2
I	1
V	5
X	10
L	50
C	100
D	500
M	1000

These basic numerals may be combined to represent any number, and there are definite rules for the manner in which they are combined. Upper-case or lower-case letters may be used for Roman numerals. Prescribers usually prefer uppercase letters, but they dot the "I" for the sake of clarity. The rules for Roman numerals are as follows:

a. **Fractions**. Except for "ss" meaning one-half (1/2), all other fractions are represented by Arabic numerals (1/4, 3/8, 1/120, and so forth). (Note: The "ss" may be written with or without a bar--ss or $\overline{ss}$.)

b. **Repeating Numerals**. Numerals may be repeated. When they are, the value of the number is repeated. Thus, iii or III is 3 (1+1+1), XXX is 30 (10+10+10), and CCC is 300 (100+100+100). Any numeral that would be the same as another when

TERM OR PHRASE	ABBREVIATION	MEANING
ad		to, up to
ad libitum	ad lib	freely, at pleasure
ana	āā	of each
ante	a.	before
ante cibum	a.c.	before meals
bene	ben.	well, good
bis		twice
bis in die	b.i.d.	twice a day
capiat	Cap.	let the client take
capsula	caps.	capsule
cum	$\bar{c}$	with
dentur tales doses	D.T.D., d.t.d.	give of such doses
dispensa	Disp.	dispense
et		and
ex modo praescripto	e.m.p.	after the manner prescribed (as directed)
fac, fiat, fiant	ft.	make, let it be made
granum	gr.	grain
gutta, guttae	gt., gtt.	Drop, drops
hora	hor., h.	hour
hora somni	hor. som., h.s.	at the hour of sleep
injectio	inj.	injection
inter		between
lotio	lot.	lotion
non repetatur	non rep., non repetat.	do not repeat

Table 1-1. Common Latin terms and abbreviations (continued).

TERM OR PHRASE	ABBREVIATION	MEANING
octarius	O.	pint
oculus dexter	O.D.	right eye
oculus sinister	o.s., O.S.	left eye
oculi unitas	O.U.	both eyes
omni hora	Omn. hor.	every hour
per		through, by means of
per os	P.O.	by mouth
placebo		I will satisfy
post cibum	post cib., p.c.	after meals
pro re nata	p.r.n.	as needed, as circumstances require
pulvis	pulv.	powder
quantum satis	q.s.	a sufficient quantity
quantum satis ad	q.s. ad	a sufficient quantity to make
quaque	q.	every
quaque die	q.d.	every day
quaque hora	q.h.	every hour
quater in die	q.i.d.	four times a day
recipe	Rx	take thou
semi, semis	ss	a half
signa	sig.	write, label
sine	$\bar{s}$	without
solve, solvere, solutus	solv.	dissolve
statim	stat	immediately
tabella	tab.	tablet
ter	t.	three
ter in die	t.i.d., tid	three times daily
unguentum	ung.	an ointment
ut dictum	Ut dict.	as directed

Table 1-1. Common Latin names and abbreviations (concluded).

ABBREVIATION	MEANING	ABBREVIATION	MEANING
a.c.	before meals	q.h.	every hour
b.i.d., bid	twice a day	q.i.d., qid	four times a day
h.s.	at bedtime	q.3h., q3h	every 3 hours
non rep	do not repeat	q.6h., q6h	every 6 hours
p.c.	after meals	stat.	Immediately
p.r.n.	as needed	t.i.d., tid	three times a day

Table 1-2. Times of administration.

ABBREVIATION	MEANING	ABBREVIATION	MEANING
I.M., IM	intramuscularly	s.c., s.q.	subcutaneously
I.V., IV	intravenously	P.O.	by mouth
O.D.	right eye	caps.	capsule
o.s., O.S.	left eye	liq.	liquid, solution
O.U.	both eyes	tab.	tablet

Table 1-3. Routes of administration and dosage forms.

WEIGHT		VOLUME	
milligram	mg.	milliliter	ml.
gram	g., Gm.	cubic centimeter	cc.
kilogram	kg., Kg.	liter	l., L.

Table 1-4. Metric system abbreviations.

WEIGHT		VOLUME	
grain	gr.	fluid dram	f ʒ
dram	ʒ	fluid ounce	fl. oz., f ℥
ounce	oz., ℥	pint	O., pt.
		quart	qt.
		gallon	C., gal.

NOTE: The fluid dram and the fluid ounce are often abbreviated without the "f" being used. It can be assumed that when the dram symbol is used with a liquid, the fluid dram is intended.

Table 1-5. Apothecary system abbreviations.

repeated is NOT repeated. For example, VV is NOT used for 10 (5+5) because X is 10 and LL is NOT used for 100 (50+50) because C = 100).

c. **Smaller Numerals Before Larger**. When a smaller numeral placed before a larger one, the smaller value is subtracted from the larger one. Only one number can be subtracted in this way. Thus, IV (5 - 1) = 4; IX (10 - 1) = 9; and XC (100 - 10) = 90 are correct, but 3 is never written IIV.

d. **Smaller Numerals After Larger**. A smaller numeral placed after a larger one is added to the larger number. For example, VIII = (5+3) = 8 ; XIII = (10+3) = 13; CLX = (100+50+10) = 160.

e. **Smaller Numeral Between Two Larger**. A smaller numeral between two larger ones is ALWAYS subtracted from the larger numeral which follows it as CXL (100 + [50-10]) = 140; MCMLXXVI (1000 + [1000-100] + 50 + 10 + 10 + 5 + 1) = 1976.

f. **The Use of "j."** As a precaution against error, the last "i" may be replaced by a "j." When this method is used, 3 would be written as iij.

g. **Table of Roman Numerals**. Table 1-6 shows examples of Roman numerals and their equivalents.

ss	=	1/2	x	=	10	xx	=	20	li	=	51
i	=	1	xi	=	11	xxi	=	21	lix	=	59
ii	=	2	xii	=	12	xxii	=	22	lx	=	60
iii	=	3	xiii	=	13	xxiii	=	23	lxx	=	70
iv	=	4	xiv	=	14	xxiv	=	24	lxxx	=	80
v	=	5	xv	=	15	xxv	=	25	xc	=	90
vi	=	6	xvi	=	16	xxvi	=	26	c	=	100
vii	=	7	xvii	=	17	xxvii	=	27	ci	=	101
vii	=	8	xviii	=	18	xxviii	=	28	cxxi	=	121
ix	=	9	xix	=	19	xxix	=	29	d	=	500
									m	=	1000

Table 1-6. Examples of Roman numerals.

h. **Number After Modified Noun**. When a number expressed in Roman numerals is used to modify a noun, the number follows the noun. The noun is likely to be a unit of the apothecary system or a unit of dosage. For example, "gr ii" would be interpreted as "two grains" and "caps i" would mean "one capsule."

1-3. INTERPRETATION OF ORDERS FOR DRUGS

Prescribers use abbreviations extensively in writing orders for drugs. The enlisted soldier must be able to read such orders accurately. Examples of some orders for drugs and the interpretations are given below.

a. **Example 1**.

Order:	Tab ii stat, then tab i bid
Interpretation:	2 tablets at once, then 1 tablet twice a day.

b. **Example 2**.

Order:	Tsp i pc & hs
Interpretation:	1 teaspoonful after meals and at bedtime.

c. **Example 3**.

Order:	2 ml IM stat & q12h
Interpretation:	2 ml intramuscularly at once and every 12 hours.

d. **Example 4**.

Order:	Tab iv stat, then tab ii q4h
Interpretation:	4 tablets at once, then 2 tablets every 4 hours.

Section II. RATIO AND PROPORTION

1-4. BASIC MATHEMATICS

For a review of basic mathematics, you can enroll in Subcourse MD0900, Basic Mathematics, or Subcourse MED904, Pharmacology Math for the Practical Nurse. Subcourse MD0900 covers fundamental operations and practical problems in fractions, mixed numbers, decimals, percents, ratios, proportions, and square roots. Subcourse MD0904 covers basic arithmetic, fractions, decimals, percentages, ratio and proportion, and math required for pharmaceutical calculations.

1-5. IMPORTANCE OF RATIO AND PROPORTION

The principles of ratio and proportion are tools with which the student can solve many, if not all, dosage calculations. A firm understanding of these basics will enable the student to deal with later sections in which common dose problems are solved by applying simple ratio and proportion techniques.

1-6. RATIOS

a. A ratio is the relation between like numbers or values, or a way to express a fractional part of a whole. Ratios may be written:

As a fraction: $\frac{2}{3}$

As a division: $2 \div 3$

With the ratio or colon sign: 2:3

Using "per": 50 miles per hour (50mi/hr)

b. The strength or concentration of various drugs can be expressed as a ratio. First, read the label of the drug and find the strength or concentration. Express this strength as a ratio in fractional form, as in the following examples.

(1) Tolnaftate solution, 10 mg per ml = $\frac{10 \text{ mg}}{1 \text{ ml}}$

(2) Guinine injection, 0.3 gm per ml = $\frac{0.3 \text{ gm}}{1 \text{ ml}}$

(3) Kanamycin injection, 1.0 gm/3 ml = $\frac{1.0 \text{ gm}}{3 \text{ ml}}$

(4) Isoproterenol inhalation, 1:200 = $\frac{1}{200}$

(5) Epinephrine injection, 1:1000 = $\frac{1}{1000}$

(6) Phenoxymethyl penicillin tablets 200,000 units = $\frac{200{,}000 \text{ units}}{1 \text{ tablet}}$

Sulfisoxazole tablets, 0.5 gm = $\frac{0.5 \text{ gm}}{1 \text{ tablet}}$

1-7. PROPORTIONS

A proportion consists of two equal ratios and is essentially a statement of equality between two ratios. For example:

$$\frac{2}{5} = \frac{4}{10}$$

The value of the ratio on the right must always equal the value of the ratio on the left. A proportion may be written with the double colon, or proportion sign (::), or with the sign of equality (=).

2:5 :: 4:10 or $\frac{2}{5} = \frac{4}{10}$

a. **Parts of a Proportion**. In a proportion, there are four numbers. The two middle numbers are known as MEANS and the two end numbers are known as EXTREMES.

(1) Example: You find a 10-ml vial of Aminophylline in supply labeled "25 mg per ml." Thus, there are 250 mg of drug in this 10-ml vial.

(extreme)	25 mg	=	250 mg	(mean)
(mean)	1 ml		10 ml	(extreme)

(2) Notice that when you multiply the two extremes and the two means, the products are equal. For example: 25 x 10 = 250 x 1.

Multiply the extremes: $25 \times 10 = 250$
Multiply the means: $1 \times 250 = 250$

RULE: In a proportion, the product of the means is always equal to the product of the extremes.

b. **Solving Problems with Proportions**. Using the above rule of proportion and knowing the value of three parts of a proportion, then the fourth unknown part, call it "X," can be found. When confronted with a calculation, use the following steps to solve for X.

(1) Step 1. State problem in "if-then" form.

(2) Step 2. Convert the problem to an equation.

(a) Known information (labeled strength, and so forth) should be your IF ratio.

(b) The unknown ratio including X will be your THEN ratio.

(c) Put like units on the same side of each ratio. (For example, if the left side of the equation is expressed in mg/ml, then the right side must also be expressed in mg/ml).

(3) Step 3. Cross multiply means and extremes.

(4) Step 4. Solve for X.

c. **Example 1**. You have a 10-ml vial of aminophylline labeled "25 mg per ml". How many milliliters must be injected to administer a dose of 125 mg?

(1) Step 1. If there are 25 mg of drug per 1 ml, then there are 125 mg of drug per X ml.

(2) Step 2. IF $\frac{25 \text{ mg}}{1 \text{ ml}}$ THEN = $\frac{125 \text{ mg}}{X \text{ ml}}$

(3) Step 3. $25 \times X = 125 \times 1$

(4) Step 4. $25X = 125$

(5) Solve for X.

$$\frac{\cancel{25}X}{\cancel{25}} = \frac{125}{25}$$

X = 5 ml (answer) [125 divided by 25 is 5]

d. **Example 2**. How many milliliters must be injected from an ampule of Prochlorperazine labeled "10 mg/2 ml" in order to administer a dose of 7.5 mg?

(1) Step 1. If there are 10 mg of drug per 2 ml, then there are 7.5 mg of drug per X ml.

(2) Step 2. IF $\frac{10 \text{ mg}}{2 \text{ ml}}$ THEN = $\frac{7.5 \text{ mg}}{X \text{ ml}}$

(3) Step 3. $10 \times X = 2 \times 7.5$

(4) Step 4. $10X = 15$

(5) Solve for X.

$$\frac{\cancel{10}X}{\cancel{10}} = \frac{15}{10}$$

X = 1.5 ml (answer) [15 divided by 10 is 1.5]

Section III. THE METRIC SYSTEM

1-8. ADVANTAGES OVER OTHER SYSTEMS

a. Every weight and measure in the metric system bears a simple relation to the initial unit, the meter.

b. Every unit is multiplied or divided by the same number (that is, 10) to obtain the next higher or lower denomination, and an increase or decrease is expressed by moving the decimal point either to the right or to the left.

c. Its almost universal adoption makes it an international system.

1-9. VALUES OF PREFIXES

a. The three basic units of the metric system are the meter, the gram, and the liter. The names of the other units are formed by adding a prefix to one of these basic units. Each prefix has a corresponding numerical value. These are listed below.

Prefix		Value
micro (mc, μ)	=	$\frac{1}{1,000,000}$
milli (m)	=	$\frac{1}{1000}$
centi (c)	=	$\frac{1}{100}$
deci (d)	=	$\frac{1}{10}$
deka (dk)	=	10
hecto (h)	=	100
kilo (k)	=	1000

Basic Units
meter (m)
gram (gm)
liter (l)

b. For example, a milliliter (ml) is equal to $\frac{1}{1000}$ of a liter (l). A kilogram (kg) is equal to 1000 grams (g).

1-10. COMMONLY USED RELATIONSHIPS

a. **Length**. Three of the most commonly used length relationships in the metric system are:

1 kilometer (km)	=	1000 meters (m)
1 meter (m)	=	100 centimeters (cm) = 1000 millimeters (mm)
1 centimeter (cm)	=	10 millimeters (mm)

b. **Weight**. Two of the most commonly used weight relationships in the metric system are:

1 kilogram (kg)	=	1000 grams (gm)
1 gram (gm)	=	1000 milligrams (mg)

NOTE: We occasionally need the following relationship:

$$1 \text{ microgram (mcg)} = \frac{1}{1000} \text{ milligram (mg)}$$

c. **Volume**. Three of the most commonly used volume relationships in the metric system are:

1 liter (l)	=	1000 milliliters (ml)
1 liter (l)	=	1000 cubic centimeters (cc)
1 milliliter (ml)	=	1 cubic centimeter (cc)

NOTE: 1 milliliter of water weighs 1 gram

1-11. CONVERSION WITHIN THE METRIC SYSTEM

To convert a quantity in the metric system to a larger unit, we divide or move the decimal point to the left. To convert to a smaller unit, we multiply or move the decimal point to the right. Alternatively, we can use ratio and proportion as illustrated in the following examples:

a. **Example 1**: Convert 0.3 mg to grams. (There are 1000 mg in 1 gram.)

$$\text{IF } \frac{1000 \text{ mg}}{1 \text{ gm}} \text{ THEN } = \frac{0.3 \text{ mg}}{X \text{ gm}}$$

$$1000 \times X = 0.3 \times 1$$

$$\frac{\not{1000}X}{\not{1000}} = \frac{0.3}{1000}$$

$$X = 0.0003 \text{ gm (answer)}$$

b. **Example 2**: Express 30 liters in terms of milliliters. (There are 1000 ml in 1 liter.)

$$\text{IF } \frac{1000 \text{ ml}}{1 \text{ liter}} \text{ THEN } = \frac{X \text{ ml}}{30 \text{ liters}}.$$

$$1 \times X = 1000 \times 30 \text{ liters}$$

$$X = 30{,}000 \text{ ml (answer)}$$

Section IV. THE APOTHECARY SYSTEM

1-12. INTRODUCTION

Several systems of weight and measure are used currently in the United States. This is an unfortunate situation in the medical field, but until the metric system is universally adopted in this country, you must remain flexible and familiar with some of the commonly encountered units from other systems of measurement. Ultimately, all calculations will be performed in the metric system. The metric system is the official system for use in the U.S. Army. Conversion factors or equivalents are discussed and presented later in this lesson to enable you to convert quickly and accurately from other systems to the metric system. GIVEN A CALCULATION INVOLVING UNITS IN ANOTHER SYSTEM OF MEASURE, CONVERT TO AND WORK WITHIN THE METRIC SYSTEM.

1-13 APOTHECARY WEIGHT

Several years ago, the apothecary system of measure was widely used in calculations pertaining to the administration of medications. Recently, the apothecary system has been used less and less in favor of the metric system. One unit in the apothecary system (see Table 1-7) is still seen on some drug labels. As you see from Table 1-7, the abbreviation for grain is gr.

Apothecary	Abbreviation
grain	gr.

Table 1-7. A commonly encountered apothecary weight unit.

1-14. APOTHECARY VOLUME

The gallon, quart, pint, and fluid ounce of the apothecary system are the familiar units used in the United States to measure liquids such as milk, gasoline, and soft drinks. Table 1-8 provides some useful information on commonly encountered apothecary volume units.

1 gallon (C. or gal.)	=	4 quarts	=	8 pints
1 quart (qt.)	=	2 pints	=	32 fluid ounces
1 pint (pt.)	=	16 fluid ounces (fl. oz. or f℥)		

Table 1-8. Commonly encountered apothecary volume units.

Section V. CONVERSIONS

1-15. CONVERSION BETWEEN SYSTEMS

a. To convert quantities from one system of measurement to another, a familiar tool, ratio and proportion, can be used. Table 1-9 contains some useful approximate conversion factors. Remember, the conversion factors are approximate. When the exact conversion factors are required (that is, when prescriptions are compounded), pharmaceutical texts or references should be consulted.

	Weight	
2.2 pounds	=	1 kilogram (kg.)
1 grain (gr.)	=	60 milligrams (mg.)
	Fluid Measure	
1 fluid ounce (fl. oz., f℥)	=	30 milliliters
1 pint	=	473 milliliters

Table 1-9. Approximate conversion factors.

b. The process of converting from one system to another can be done with ease if three steps are followed:

(1) Write the conversion factor as your **IF** ratio.

(2) Write the unknown factor as your **THEN** ratio.

(3) Solve for the unknown as in any ratio and proportion problem.

c. Let's apply these principles in performing some conversions from other systems to the metric system.

(1) Weight. Express 5 grains as milligrams.

(a) Step 1. Write the conversion factor as your **IF** ratio:

$$\text{IF} \quad \frac{1 \text{ gr}}{60 \text{ mg}}$$

(b) Step 2. Write the unknown factor as your **THEN** ratio:

$$\text{THEN} \quad \frac{5 \text{ gr}}{X \text{ mg}}$$

(c) Step 3. Solve for the unknown as in any other ratio and proportion problem.

$$\text{IF} \quad \frac{1\text{gr}}{60 \text{ mg}} = \text{THEN} \quad \frac{5 \text{ gr}}{X \text{ mg}}$$

$$1 \times X = 5 \times 60$$

$$X = 300 \text{ mg (answer)}$$

(2) Volume. Express 4 fluid ounces as milliliters.

(a) Step 1. Write the conversion factor as your **IF** ratio:

$$\text{IF} \quad \frac{1 \text{ fl oz}}{30 \text{ ml}}$$

(b) Step 2. Write the unknown factor as your **THEN** ratio:

$$\text{THEN} \quad \frac{4 \text{ fl oz}}{X \text{ ml}}$$

(c) Step 3. Solve for the unknown.

$$\text{IF} \quad \frac{1 \text{ fl oz}}{30 \text{ ml}} \quad \text{THEN} = \quad \frac{4 \text{ fl oz}}{X \text{ ml}}$$

$$1 \times X = 4 \times 30$$

$$X = 120 \text{ ml (answer)}$$

1-16. APPROXIMATE HOUSEHOLD EQUIVALENTS

a. It is often necessary to express the dose of a fluid medication in common household unit for self-administration by the client. Ratio and proportion principles can be used to perform these conversions.

HOUSEHOLD MEASURE	APOTHECARY MEASURE	METRIC MEASURE
2 Tablespoonsful	1 fluid ounce (fl.oz., f℥)	30 milliliters (ml.)
1 Tablespoonful (tbsp.)	1/2 fluid ounce (fl. oz. $\overline{ss}$, f℥ $\overline{ss}$)	15 milliliters (ml.)
1 teaspoonful (tsp.)	1 fluid dram (fʒ)	5 milliliters (ml.)
1/2 teaspoonful	1/2 fluid dram (fʒ $\overline{ss}$)	2.5 milliliters (ml.)

Table 1-10. Approximate household equivalents.

b. Solve the following problem: A client is to receive 30 milliliters of a particular antacid preparation. Express this volume in tablespoons.

(1) Step 1. Write the conversion factor as your **IF** ratio:

$$\text{IF} \quad \frac{15 \text{ ml}}{1 \text{ Tbsp}}$$

(2) Step 2. Write the unknown factor as your **THEN** ratio:

$$\text{THEN} \quad \frac{30 \text{ ml}}{X \text{ Tbsp}}$$

(3) Step 3. Solve for the unknown as in any ratio and proportion problem.

$$\text{IF} \quad \frac{15 \text{ ml}}{1 \text{ Tbsp}} \quad \text{THEN} = \quad \frac{30 \text{ ml}}{X \text{ Tbsp}}$$

$$15 \times X = 1 \times 30$$

$$\frac{\cancel{15}X}{\cancel{15}} = \frac{30}{15}$$

$$X = 2 \text{ Tbsp (answer)}$$

Section VI. PERCENTAGE SOLUTIONS

1-17. EXPLANATION

a. **Variable Meaning of Percentage.**

(1) The word percentage can have different meanings under different circumstances. In solution, we are dealing with solids that are weighed and liquids that can be weighed or measured; thus, it is necessary to define the expression of age concentration of solutions. There are three different percentage solutions.

(a) Percentage weight in weight (w/w)--expresses the number of grams of solute in 100 ml of solution.

(b) Percentage weight in volume (w/v)--expresses the number of grams of solute in 100 ml of solution, regardless of whether water or another liquid is used as the solvent. Table 1-11 is helpful in preparing weight-in-volume solutions.

(c) Percentage volume in volume (v/v)--expresses the number of milliliters of solute in 100 ml of solution.

(2) The strength of a certain solution expressed in one of the ways is likely to be different from the strength expressed another way. It is therefore important to know whether a particular desired percentage strength for a prescription is w/w, w/v, or v/v. Some helpful rules are given below.

b. **Rules for Percentage Solutions.**

(1) Unless specifically stipulated otherwise, the following rules hold true for percentage solutions.

(a) Mixtures of solids are weight in weight (w/w).

(b) Solids in liquids are weight in volume (w/v).

(c) Liquids in liquids are volume in volume (v/v).

(d) Gases in liquids are weight in volume (w/v).

(2) For example, to make a 10 percent solution, dissolve 10 gm of a solid or 10 ml of a liquid in the amount of solvent necessary to make 100 ml of finished solution.

c. **Ratio Strengths**. Often the strength of a preparation, particularly the strength of a weak solution, may be expressed in terms of a ratio. Ratio strengths are also volume in volume (v/v), weight in weight (w/w), or weight in volume (w/v).

QUANTITY TO BE PREPARED								
%W/V	5 ml	10 ml	15 ml	30 ml	60 ml	120 ml	180 ml	240 ml
1/4 %	0.0125	0.025	0.0375	0.075	0.15	0.3	0.45	0.6
½ %	0.025	0.05	0.075	0.15	0.3	0.6	0.9	1.2
1 %	0.05	0.1	0.15	0.3	0.6	1.2	1.8	2.4
2 %	0.1	0.2	0.3	0.6	1.2	2.4	3.6	4.8
3 %	0.15	0.3	0.45	0.9	1.8	3.6	5.4	7.2
4 %	0.2	0.4	0.6	1.2	2.4	4.8	7.2	9.6
5 %	0.25	0.5	0.75	1.5	3.0	6.0	9.0	12.0
10 %	0.5	1.0	1.5	3.0	6.0	12.0	18.0	24.0
15 %	0.75	1.5	2.25	4.5	9.0	18.0	27.0	36.0
20 %	1.0	2.0	3.0	6.0	12.0	24.0	36.0	48.0
25 %	1.25	2.5	3.75	7.5	5.0	30.0	45.0	60.0
50 %	2.5	5.0	7.5	15.0	30.0	60.0	90.0	120.0

NOTE: The table above may be used to find the weight of solute in GRAMS required to prepare the indicated volume of solution with the desired percentage strength.

Table 1-11. Percentage solutions (w/v) in the metric system.

1-18. FIELD DILUTION OF ISOPROPYL ALCOHOL

Isopropyl alcohol is widely used in a 70 percent concentration as an antiseptic-disinfectant. Since its effective range of activity is 70 percent to 90 percent, great accuracy is not required in the dilution of stock 99 percent isopropyl alcohol. The field method is to:

a. Fill container (pt, qt, or gal) approximately three-fourths full with 99 percent isopropyl alcohol.

b. Using distilled water, finish filling container to mark. The finished product is 70 percent to 75 percent isopropyl alcohol, which is suitable for field use.

Section VII. INJECTION DOSE CALCULATIONS

1-19. INTRODUCTION

a. **Forms in Which Injections are Supplied**. Injections are found in supply either (1) in dry powder for reconstitution or (2) in a ready-made sterile solution or suspension.

b. **Labeling of Concentrations**. Drugs for injection are labeled with concentrations in various ways. Some examples might be:

(1) Morphine injection 8 mg/cc

(2) Thorazine injection 25 mg/ml

(3) Phenobarbital injection 1 grain/ml

(4) Lorfan injection 1 mg = 1 cc

(5) Kantrex injection 1 gram/3 cc

(6) Tetanus antitoxin 1500 units/cc

(7) Aramine injection one percent

NOTE: Remember that 1 cc = 1 ml

c. **Choice of Syringe**. After calculating the dose volume in milliliters, round off your answer to the nearest tenth of a milliliter. It is generally best to choose the smallest syringe capable of delivering the entire dose. For example, a 1-ml syringe would be used for doses of 1 ml or less, a 2.5-ml syringe for doses between 1.0 and 2.5 ml, a 5-ml syringe for doses between 2.6 and 5.0 ml, and a 10-ml syringe for doses between 5.0 and 10.0 ml.

1-20. SOLVING BY RATIO AND PROPORTION

a. **Like Units**. In using ratio and proportion to solve injection dose problems, we must especially remember the necessity of using like units on the same side of each ratio. For example, if our known concentration is expressed in milligrams/milliliter and we want to find the number of milliliters required to provide a 1-gram dose, it would be easiest to first express this dose as 1000 milligrams. In this manner, both the left and right sides of the equation are expressed in mg/ml.

b. **Method**. The left, or IF, side of the equation should be the concentration of the drug in stock. The right, or THEN, side of the equation should be the ratio solute dose/solution dose, or ordinarily weight dose/volume dose.

c. **Example 1**. The labeled strength of a 30 ml vial of Meperidine (Demerol) injection is 50 mg/ml. How many milliliters must be injected to provide a 75 mg dose?

$$\text{IF } \frac{50 \text{ mg}}{1 \text{ ml}} \text{ THEN } = \frac{75 \text{ mg}}{X \text{ ml}}$$

$$50 \times X = 1 \times 75$$

$$\frac{\not{50}X}{\not{50}} = \frac{75}{50}$$

$$X = 1.5 \text{ ml, answer}$$

d. **Example 2**. A preparation of Morphine is labeled with a concentration of 30 mg/cc. How many milliliters must be injected to provide a 1/8 grain dose?

First, we must convert 1/8 grain to the metric system. Using a conversion factor (1 gr = 60 mg), we calculate that 1/8 gr = 7.5 mg.

$$\text{IF } \frac{30 \text{ mg}}{1 \text{ ml}} \text{ THEN } = \frac{7.5 \text{ mg}}{X \text{ ml}}$$

$$30 \times X = 7.5 \times 1$$

$$\frac{\not{30}X}{\not{30}} = \frac{7.5}{30}$$

$X = 0.25$ (Rounding off, $X = 0.3$ ml, answer)

1-21. ANTIBIOTIC DILUTIONS

a. Antibiotic drugs such as Penicillins, Streptomycin, and the Tetracyclines often are manufactured and supplied to you in the form of a sterile powder in a vial which must be reconstituted with sterile water for injection, normal saline solution, or other suitable diluent (solvent) (Table 1-12). This presents special problems and considerations not normally seen with prepared injection solutions. Specifically, you must **STOP** and consider each of the following problems when handling antibiotics for reconstitution.

Sterile Water for Injection (SWI), 5 ml and 50 ml ampules.
Sodium Chloride Injection (Normal Saline Solution, N/S), 5 ml.
5 % Dextrose Injection (D5W).
Special diluents supplied by manufacturer.

Table 1-12. Sterile diluents for reconstitution.

(1) The volume of the vial.

(2) Stability of the dry powder.

(3) Volume of diluent (or how much water do I use?).

(4) Stability of reconstituted solution or suspension.

(5) Calculation of the volume dose.

b. It is recommended that all antibiotics that are reconstituted and are to be used later, should be labeled in the following way (see example):

(1) Hour and date reconstituted.

(2) Strength of reconstituted antibiotic.

(3) Initials of the preparer.

(1)
1400 hrs 9 Mar 01
GMcK 50,000 units/cc
(3) (2)

c. Once the antibiotic has been reconstituted, we solve for the fraction to be used as follows:

(1) What you WANT is your DOSE!

(2) What you HAVE is the LABELED STRENGTH of the antibiotic!

(3) Place the DOSE over your LABELED STRENGTH and solve as a fraction. This is the fractional part of your vial, which is your dose.

d. An example is given below:

(1) Dilute a vial of procaine penicillin G for aqueous injection labeled 300,000 units so that you can administer a dose of 75,000 units. How many milliliters must be withdrawn and injected IM to give this dose?

$$\frac{\text{WHAT (DOSE)}}{\text{HAVE (LABEL)}} = \frac{75{,}000 \text{ units}}{300{,}000 \text{ units}} = \frac{25}{100} = \frac{1}{4} \text{ of vial is your dose}$$

(2) Thus, it might be possible to dilute a vial with:

(a) Four ml and withdraw 1 ml for your dose.

(b) Eight ml and withdraw 2 ml for your dose.

(c) Two ml and withdraw 1/2 ml for your dose.

(d) One ml and withdraw 1/4 ml for your dose.

(3) All of the above are technically correct; however, you must consider the size of the vial and how easily the antibiotic is reconstituted to a solution or suspension. The manufacturer suggests and recommends that 1 ml be used to dilute this product (see Table 1-13). The vial is actually too small to accept 8 ml of diluent.

Antibiotic	Trade Name (Other Names)	Supply	Diluent I.M.	Diluent I.V. Push	Diluent I.V. Infusion	Stability Once Reconstituted Room Temp.	Stability Once Reconstituted Refrigerated
sodium ampicillin	Polycillin-N	0.5 gram	1.2 ml. SWI	5 ml. SWI	5 ml. SWI	1 hr. (I.M.) 4-8 hr. (I.V.)	Not suitable for storage
		1.0 gram	2.4 ml. SWI	10 ml. SWI	10 ml. SWI	1 hr. (I.M.) 4-8 hr. (I.V.)	Not suitable for storage
sodium cephalothin	Keflin	1.0 gram	4 ml. SWI, expands to 4.4 ml.	10 ml. SWI or N/S		6 hr. (I.M.) 6-24 hr. (I.V.)	48 hr.
		4.0 grams	For I.V. use only	N/A	20-40 ml. SWI, N/S, or D5W	6 hr. (I.M.) 6-24 hr. (I.V.)	48 hr.
erythromycin lactobionate for injection	Erythrocin	1.0 gram	Do not use I.M.	20 ml. SWI only*	20 ml. SWI only*	Not suitable for storage	Not suitable for storage
sodium methicillin for injection.[V]	Staphcillin	1.0 gram	1.2 ml. SWI, expands to 2 ml.	500 mg./ml. diluted with 25 ml. N/S per ml.	1.2 ml. SWI, then add to I.V. solution	24 hr.	4 days

*Once reconstituted with sterile water for injection, it can then be added to N/S, D5W, or other compatible solutions.

[V] Never mix another drug with solutions of methicillin.
SWI = sterile water for injection
N/S = sodium chloride injection D5W = 5% dextrose injection

Table 1-13. Reconstitution of commonly used antibiotics (continued)

Antibiotic	Trade Name (Other Names)	Supply	Diluent			Stability Once Reconstituted	
			I.M.	I.V. Push	I.V. Infusion	Room Temp.	Refrigerated
potassium penicillin G for injection	crystalline, buffered penicillin G	1,000,000 units	3.6-9.6 ml. SWI, expands 0.4 ml.	3.6-9.6 ml. N/S or D5W	3.6-9.6 ml. N/S or D5W	24 hr.	1 week
		5,000,000 units	3-23 ml. of SWI, expands 2 ml.	3-23 ml. N/S or D5W	3-23 ml. N/S or D5W	24 hr.	1 week
		20,000,000 units	Do not use I.M.	N/A	32 ml. D5W or N/S, expands to 40 ml.	24 hr.	3 days
procaine penicillin for aqueous injection	procaine penicillin G	300,000 units	1 ml. SWI	Not for I.V. use	Not for I.V. use	1 week	3 weeks
		1,500,000 units	4.5 ml. SWI, expands to 5 ml.	Not for I.V. use	Not for I.V. use	1 week	3 weeks

Table 1-13. Reconstitution of commonly used antibiotics (continued)

Antibiotic	Trade Name (Other Names)	Supply	Diluent			Stability Once Reconstituted	
			I.M.	I.V. Push	I.V. Infusion	Room Temp.	Refrigerated
streptomycin sulfate	none	1.0 gram.	2 ml. SWI or N/S	Not for I.V. use	Not for I.V. use	4 weeks	
tetracycline HCl for injection	various	0.1 gram for I.M. use	2 ml. SWI or N/S	Not for I.V. use	Not for I.V. use	24 hr.	
		0.5 gram for I.V. use	Not for I.M. use	N/A	10 ml. SWI then dilute to 100 ml.	12 hr. (initial dilution) Final dilution is adm. STAT	

SWI = sterile water for injection
N/S = sodium chloride injection
D5W = 5% dextrose injection

Table 1-13. Reconstitution of commonly used antibiotics (concluded)

Section VIII. PEDIATRIC DOSE CALCULATIONS

1-22. INTRODUCTION

a. Premature babies and other very young infants may be unusually responsive to many drugs because of the immaturity of the following.

(1) Renal function.

(2) Enzymatic mechanisms for drug inactivation.

(3) The blood-brain barrier.

(4) The brain.

NOTE: Children are often more sensitive than adults to drugs which alter the acid-base metabolism or the water-and-electrolyte balance.

b. Pediatric doses based on formal experiments or the experience of the prescriber are better than those calculated according to a general rule or formula. Unfortunately, optimal pediatric doses have not been established for most drugs. Thus, where possible, doses for younger children, and especially for infants, should be learned as such and not based merely on a formula; doses calculated with a formula (as a fraction of the adult dose based on the body weight or body surface area) are very unreliable for premature infants, but more reliable for children at least 2 years old.

1-23. DOSAGE RULES INVOLVING A FRACTION OF THE ADULT DOSE

a. **A General Rule of Dosage**.

AGE (IN YEARS)	DOSE
20 or older	the adult dose
10	1/2 the average adult dose
5	1/4 the average adult dose
2 1/2	1/8 the average adult dose
1	1/12 the average adult dose

b. **Clark's Rule**.

$$\frac{\text{weight of child (lb)}}{150} \times \text{adult dose} = \text{approximate child's dose}$$

c. **Young's Rule**.

$$\frac{\text{age of child (yr)}}{\text{age} + 12} \times \text{adult dose} = \text{approximate child's dose}$$

d. **Fried's Rule**.

$$\frac{\text{age in months}}{150} \times \text{adult dose} = \text{approximate child's dose}$$

1-24. PEDIATRIC DOSE CALCULATION BASED ON BODY WEIGHT

a. A more reliable method of pediatric dose calculation than the preceding dosage rules bases the dosage on a given amount of drug per pound or kilogram of body weight.

NOTE: Round off all body weights in kilograms to the nearest whole number.

b. Example: The parenteral dose of erythromycin injection is 10 mg/kg/24 hours. Calculate the daily dose of this drug for a 44-pound child.

(1) Step 1. Convert 44 pounds to kilograms.

$$\frac{\text{44 pounds}}{2.2} = \text{20 kilograms}$$

(2) Step 2. Multiply the client's weight by the dose.

$$\text{CHILD'S DOSE} = 20 \text{ kg} \times 10 \text{ mg/kg} = 200 \text{ mg/24 hrs (answer)}$$

1-25. PEDIATRIC DOSE CALCULATIONS BASED ON SURFACE AREA

A newer and possibly more accurate method of pediatric dose calculation is based on body surface area. Although this method is not as widely used or accepted as calculations based on body weight, most if not all drugs may have their dosage expressed per square meter of body surface area (m^2). This method of relating the surface area of individuals to dosage is simplified using a surface area nomogram in dose calculations (figure 1-1).

CHILD'S DOSE = surface area of child (m^2) $\times$ dose per m^2.

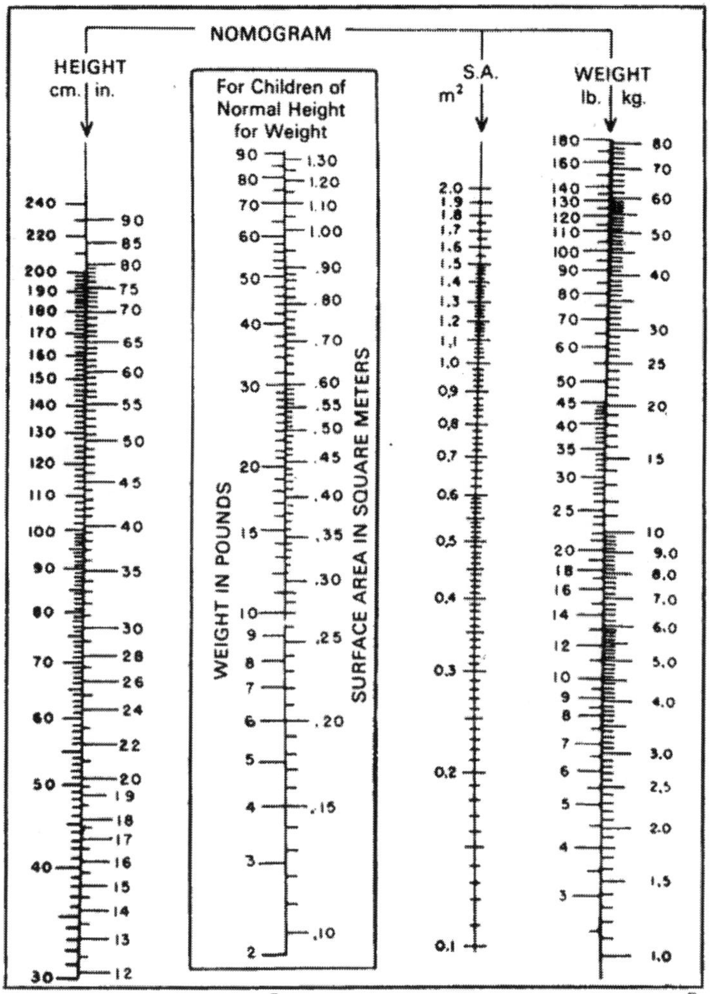

(West nomogram [for estimation of surface areas]. The surface area is indicated where a straight line connecting the height and weight intersects the surface area column, or, if the patient is roughly of average size, from the weight alone [enclosed area]. Reproduced for instructional purposes from Waldo E. Nelson, Textbook of Pediatrics, ninth edition, 1969. Written consent of the copyright owner has been obtained. Under no circumstances will this material be sold, commercially used, or copied.)

Figure 1-1. Body surface area nomogram.

a. **Example 1**. A thirty-pound child of average size is to receive Kanamycin injection with a dosage expressed as 150-450 $mg/m^2/24$ hr.

(1) Using a nomogram, calculate the client's body surface area.

SURFACE AREA = $0.6\ m^2$

(2) Multiply body surface area by the dose.

$$\text{CHILD'S DOSE} = 0.6\ m^2 \times \frac{150\text{-}450\ mg}{m^2}$$

CHILD'S DOSE = 90.0-270 mg/24 hours

b. **Example 2**. A three-month old boy who is 24.5 inches long and weighs 11 pounds, 8 ounces, is to receive Phenobarbital elixir labeled 20 mg/5 ml. The anticonvulsant dose of Phenobarbital is 125 mg/m^2 dose.

(1) Calculate the single dose of Phenobarbital in mg.

SURFACE AREA = $0.31\ m^2$

CHILD'S DOSE = 0.31×125 mg = 40 mg, approximately

(2) How many milliliters will be administered for each single dose?

$$\text{IF } \frac{20\ mg}{5\ ml} \text{ THEN } = \frac{40\ mg}{X\ ml}$$

$$20 \times X = 5 \times 40$$

$$X = \frac{200}{20} = 10\ ml\ (\text{answer})$$

NOTE: If the usual adult is assumed to have a surface area of $1.7\ m^2$, we can use the following formula for the pediatric dose if only the usual adult dose is known:

$$\text{CHILD'S DOSE} = \frac{\text{surface area } (m^2)}{1.7} \times \text{adult dose}$$

Continue with Exercises

EXERCISES, LESSON 1

INSTRUCTIONS. Answer the following exercises by marking the lettered response that best answers the question or completes the incomplete statement.

After you have completed all of these exercises, turn to "Solutions to Exercises" at the end of the lesson and check your answers. For each exercise answered incorrectly, reread the material referenced with the solution.

1. The Roman numerals LXXVII express what Arabic number?

   a. 78

   b. 77

   c. 67

   d. 64

2. The Roman numerals IVss signify what amount?

   a. 6 1/2

   b. 5 1/2

   c. 5

   d. 4 1/2

3. An order for an eye medication reads, "gtt II o.s. tid." How many times during a 24-hour period should the drug be administered?

   a. Two.

   b. Three.

   c. Four.

   d. Ten.

4. In the following equation, what is the value of X? $\frac{3}{5} = \frac{X}{10}$

a. 1.5

b. 3

c. 6

d. 17

5 In the following equation, what is the value of X? $\frac{1/2}{30} = \frac{0.6}{X}$

a. 6

b. 9

c. 18

d. 36

6. In the following equation, what is the value of X? $\frac{0.8}{2} = \frac{5}{X}$

a. 0.8

b. 1.25

c. 8

d. 12.5

7. In the following equation, what is the value of X? $\frac{0.25}{1} = \frac{1.5}{X}$

a. 6

b. 10

c. 15

d. 25

8. How many milliliters of Promethazine Hydrochloride injection labeled 25 mg/ml must be administered to provide a dose of 12.5 mg?

   a. 0.5 ml.

   b. 6.25 ml.

   c. 12.5 ml.

   d. 25 ml.

9. A 120 ml bottle of Thiabendazole oral suspension labeled 500 mg per 5 cc contains how many grams of Thiabendazole?

   a. 1.2 gm.

   b. 12 gm.

   c. 120 gm.

   d. 1200 gm.

10. Which of the following units of measure is/are expressed in the system that is official for use in the U.S. Army?

   a. Both c and d below.

   b. Both d and e below.

   c. Grain.

   d. Gram.

   e. Pound.

11. What is 0.5 gm in terms of milligrams?

a. 5 mg.

b. 50 mg.

c. 500 mg.

d. 5000 mg.

12. What is 27.3 ml in terms of liters?

a. 0.0273 liters.

b. 0.273 liters.

c. 2.73 liters.

d. 27,300 liters.

13. Approximately how many milliliters are in 8 fluid ounces?

a. 3.75 milliliters.

b. 240 milliliters.

c. 128 milliliters.

d. 120 milliliters.

14. A 10-grain dose of aspirin expressed in milligrams is approximately:

a. 10,000 mg.

b. 30 mg.

c. 60 mg.

d. 600 mg.

15. How many milliliters are there in 3 pints?

a. 1500 ml.

b. 1419 ml.

c. 195 ml.

d. 90 ml.

16. An outpatient is given a drug, which has a dosage of ten milliliters. How should the dosage be written on the label?

a. ʒx

b. 10 drams.

c. 2 teaspoonsful.

d. 2 tablespoonsful.

17. You must administer 20 grams of Mannitol from a 150 ml bottle of 15 percent (w/v) Mannitol injection. How many milliliters are required?

a. 30 ml.

b. 75 ml.

c. 133.3 ml.

d. 300 ml.

18. How many grams of dextrose are in a 250 ml bottle of five percent dextrose injection?

a. 2.0 gm.

b. 12.5 gm.

c. 50 gm.

d. 250 gm.

19. How many milliliters must be injected from a vial labeled 60 mg/cc. to give the client a dose of 1/4 grain?

a. 0.25 ml.

b. 1.5 ml.

c. 2.7 ml.

d. 15 ml.

20. Chlordiazepoxide hydrochloride (Librium) injection is supplied as a dry powder labeled 100 mg with a separate 2-ml vial of special diluent. How many should be used to administer a 30 mg dose?

a. 13.5 milliliters.

b. 2.7 milliliters.

c. 0.6 milliliters.

d. 3.3 milliliters.

21. For cyanide poisoning, a 0.3 gram dose of sodium nitrite must be administered intravenously. Your supply is a 10-ml ampule of a three percent sodium nitrite solution. What volume of the solution must you use?

a. 0.3 ml.

b. 1.0 ml.

c. 3.0 ml.

d. 10 ml.

22. You wish to infuse 50 mg of Metaraminol Bitartrate (Aramine) in 500 ml of five percent dextrose injection. How many milliliters of one percent Metaraminol Bitartrate injection must be used?

a. 5 ml.

b. 10 ml.

c. 100 ml.

d. 500 ml.

23. After reconstituting a 1 gram vial of Erythromycin Lactobionate with SWI, what fraction of the dilution must be used to provide a 350 mg dose?

a. 0.035

b. 0.05

c. 0.35

d. 0.5

24. How much sterile water for injection (SWI) should be used to reconstitute 1 gram of Erythromycin Lactobionate for injection?

a. 5 ml.

b. 10 ml.

c. 15 ml.

d. 20 ml.

25. How many milliliters of Sodium Ampicillin, reconstituted for IV administration according to table 1-13 in the subcourse, should be injected to provide a 250 mg dose?

a. 2.5 ml.

b. 25 ml.

c. 250 ml.

d. 2500 ml.

26. The pediatric antipyretic dose of Aspirin is 65 mg/kg/24 hr, divided into 4-6 doses. What should be the total daily dose of aspirin for a 55-pound child?

a. 425 mg.

b. 525 mg.

c. 715 mg.

d. 1625 mg.

27. The pediatric dose of Ampicillin for moderately severe infections in children weighing 40 kg is given as 50-100 mg/kg/24 hr, divided into 4 doses. What is the range in daily dose for a 66-pound child?

a. 2.0-4.0 gm/24 hr.

b. 3.0-4.5 gm/24 hr.

c. 4.5-6.0 gm/24 hr.

d. 6.0-7.5 gm/24 hr.

28. What is the approximate surface area of a 15-pound child whose height is normal for his weight?

a. 0.25 m^2.

b. 0.36 m^2

c. 0.42 m^2

d. 0.83 m^2

29. What is the approximate surface area of a 22-pound, 18-month-old child who is 31 inches long?

a. 0.4 m^2

b. 0.44 m^2

c. 0.48 m^2

d. 0.51 m^2

30. A 17-pound child of normal length with a resistant staphylococcal infection is to receive Sodium Oxacillin (Prostaphlin) for injection. The usual four doses and administered well-diluted, by slow IV drip. What should be the range of a single dose for this child?

a. 146-293 mg.

b. 212-424 mg.

c. 375-750 mg.

d. 431-863 mg.

SPECIAL INSTRUCTIONS FOR EXERCISES 31 THROUGH 35.

SITUATION: A 45-pound, 7-year-old girl of average height is to begin Griseofulvin therapy. The dose of this drug is 10mg/kg/24 -4 doses, orally. The average adult dose is 500 mg daily in divided doses.

Each numbered term in column A below indicates a method of solving the daily child's dose. Once you have solved the child's dose according to each method, find it in column B and enter the corresponding letter in the blank.

Column A (Method)	Column B (Daily Dose)
31. ___ Clark's Rule.	a. 184 mg
32. ___ Young's Rule.	b. 243 mg
33. ___ Calculation using mg/kg dose.	c. 205 mg
34. ___ Calculation using mg/m² dose.	d. 238 mg
35. ___ Calculation as fraction of adult dose based on surface area.	e. 150 mg

Check Your Answers on Next Page

SOLUTIONS TO EXERCISES, LESSON 1

1. b (para 1-2)

2. d (para 1-2)

3. b (para 1-2; table 1-1)

4. c (para 1-7)

$$\frac{3}{5} = \frac{X}{10}$$

$$5X = 3 \times 10$$

$$\frac{\cancel{5}X}{\cancel{5}} = \frac{30}{5}$$

$$\mathbf{X = 6}$$

5. d (para 1-7)

$$\frac{1/2}{30} = \frac{0.6}{X}$$

$$1/2\ X = 0.6 \times 30$$

$$\frac{\cancel{1/2}X}{\cancel{1/2}} = \frac{18}{1/2}$$

$$\mathbf{X =} (18/1 \div 1/2) = (18/1 \times 2/1) \mathbf{= 36}$$

6. d (para 1-7)

$$\frac{0.8}{2} = \frac{5}{X}$$

$$0.8\ X = 2 \times 5$$

$$\frac{\cancel{0.8}X}{\cancel{0.8}} = \frac{10}{0.8}$$

$$\mathbf{X = 12.5}$$

7. a (para 1-7)

$$\frac{0.25}{1} = \frac{1.5}{X}$$

$$0.25\,X = 1 \times 1.5$$

$$\frac{\not{0.25}X}{\not{0.25}} = \frac{1.5}{0.25}$$

X = 6

8. a (para 1-7)

$$\text{IF } \frac{25\text{ mg}}{1\text{ ml}} \text{ THEN } = \frac{12.5\text{ mg}}{X\text{ ml}}$$

$$25\,X = 1 \times 12.5$$

$$\frac{\not{25}\,X}{\not{25}} = \frac{12.5}{25}$$

X = 0.5 ml

9. b (paras 1-7, 1-10c, 1-11) 5 cc = 5 ml

$$\text{IF } \frac{500\text{ mg}}{5\text{ ml}} \text{ THEN } = \frac{X\text{ mg}}{120\text{ ml}}$$

$$5 \times X = 120 \times 500$$

$$\frac{\not{5}X}{\not{5}} = \frac{60{,}000}{5}$$

X = 12,000 mg = 12 gm

10. d (paras 1-9, 1-12)

11. c (para 1-11)

$$\text{IF } \frac{1000\text{ mg}}{1\text{ gm}} \text{ THEN } = \frac{X\text{ mg}}{0.5\text{ gm}}$$

$$1 \times X = 0.5 \times 1000$$

X = 500 mg

12. a (para 1-11) IF $\frac{1000 \text{ ml}}{1 \text{ liter}}$ THEN = $\frac{27.3 \text{ ml}}{X \text{ liter}}$

$1000 \times X = 1 \times 27.3$

$\frac{\cancel{1000} X}{\cancel{1000}} = \frac{27.3}{1000}$

X = 0.0273 liter

13. b (paras 1-15b, c(2)) $\frac{1 \text{ fluid ounce}}{30 \text{ milliliters}} = \frac{8 \text{ fluid ounces}}{X \text{ milliliters}}$

$1 \times X = 30 \times 8$

X = 240 milliliters

14. d (paras 1-15b, c(1)) $\frac{1 \text{ grain}}{60 \text{ milligrams}} = \frac{10 \text{ grains}}{X \text{ milligrams}}$

$1 \times X = 60 \times 10$

X = 600 milligrams

15. b (para 1-15c(2)) $\frac{1 \text{ pint}}{473 \text{ milliliters}} = \frac{3 \text{ pints}}{X \text{ milliliters}}$

$1 \times X = 473 \times 3$

X = 1419 milliliters

16. c (para 1-16; table 1-10) $\frac{1 \text{ teaspoonful}}{5 \text{ milliliters}} = \frac{X \text{ teaspoonsful}}{10 \text{ milliliters}}$

$5 \times X = 1 \times 10$

$\frac{\cancel{5}X}{\cancel{5}} = \frac{10}{5}$

X = 2 teaspoonsful

17. c (paras 1-7, 1-17)

$$\text{IF } \frac{15 \text{ gm}}{100 \text{ ml}} \text{ THEN } = \frac{20 \text{ gm}}{X \text{ ml}}$$

$$15 \times X = 20 \times 100$$

$$\frac{\cancel{15}X}{\cancel{15}} = \frac{200}{15}$$

X = 133.3 ml, approximately

18. b (paras 1-7, 1-17)

$$\text{IF } \frac{5 \text{ gm}}{100 \text{ ml}} \text{ THEN } = \frac{X \text{ gm}}{250 \text{ ml}}$$

$$100 \times X = 5 \times 250$$

$$\frac{\cancel{100}X}{\cancel{100}} = \frac{1250}{100}$$

X = 12.5 gm

19. a (paras 1-10c, 1-20; table 1-9)

60 mg/cc = 60 mg/ml.

$$\frac{60 \text{ mg}}{1 \text{ gr}} = \frac{X \text{ mg}}{1/4 \text{ gr}}$$

$$X = 15 \text{ mg}$$

IF <u>60 mg</u> THEN <u>15 mg</u>

1 ml = X ml

$$60 \times X = 1 \times 15$$

$$\frac{\cancel{60}X}{\cancel{60}} = \frac{15}{60}$$

X = 0.25 ml

20. c (paras 1-15b(2), 1-20)

$$\text{IF } \frac{100 \text{ mg}}{2 \text{ ml}} \text{ THEN } = \frac{30 \text{ mg}}{X \text{ ml}}$$

$$100 \times X = 2 \times 30$$

$$\frac{\not{100}X}{\not{100}} = \frac{60}{100}$$

$$\mathbf{X = 0.6 \text{ ml}}$$

21. d (paras 1-17, 1-20)

3 percent = 3 gm/100 ml.

$$\text{IF } \frac{3 \text{ gm}}{100 \text{ ml}} \text{ THEN } = \frac{0.3 \text{ gm}}{X \text{ ml}}$$

$$3 \times X = 0.3 \times 100$$

$$\frac{\not{3}X}{\not{3}} = \frac{30}{3}$$

$$\mathbf{X = 10 \text{ ml}}$$

22. a (paras 1-17, 1-20)

$$1 = 1 \text{ g/100 ml} = \frac{1000 \text{ mg}}{100 \text{ ml}} = 10 \text{ mg/ml}$$

$$\text{IF } \frac{10 \text{ mg}}{1 \text{ ml}} \text{ THEN } = \frac{50 \text{ mg}}{X \text{ ml}}$$

$$10 \times X = 1 \times 50$$

$$\frac{\not{10}X}{\not{10}} = \frac{50}{10}$$

$$\mathbf{X = 5 \text{ ml}}$$

23. c (paras 1-10b, 1-21)

1 gram = 1000 mg

$$\frac{\text{WANT}}{\text{HAVE}} = \frac{350 \text{ mg}}{1000 \text{ mg}} = 0.35$$

24. d (table 1-13)

25. a (paras 1-11, 1-21; table 1-13) 0.5 g = 500 mg.

$$\frac{\text{WANT}}{\text{HAVE}} = \frac{250\text{ mg}}{500\text{ mg}} = \frac{1}{2}$$

Volume of diluent = 5 ml

1/2 × 5 ml = **2.5 ml** (answer)

26. d (para 1-24) $\frac{55\text{-lb}}{2.2\text{-lb/kg}}$ = 25 kg.

25 kg × 65 mg/kg = **1625 mg** (answer)

27. a (paras 1-11, 1-24) 40 kg × 50 mg/kg = 2000 mg

40 kg × 100 mg/kg = 4000 mg

Range: 2000 - 4000 mg/24 hr

= 2.0 - 4.0 gm/24 hr (answer)

28. b (fig 1-1) Note on the enclosed column of the nomogram that the number 15 on the left scale is adjacent to the notch for 0.36 on the right scale.

29. c (fig 1-1) A straight edge, connecting the 22-pound mark on the weight column and the 31-inch mark on the height column, intersects

30. a (paras 1-11, 1-25; fig 1-1) The surface area corresponding to 17 pounds on the enclosed column of the nomogram is about 0.39 m^2.

$0.39\ m^2 \times 1.5\ gm/m^2 = 0.585\ gm = 585\ mg$

$0.39\ m^2 \times 3.0\ gm/m^2 = 1.17\ gm = 1170\ mg$

$\frac{585\text{ mg}}{4}$ = **146 mg**

$\frac{1170\text{ mg}}{4}$ = 292.5 mg = **293 mg,** approximately

31. e (para 1-23b) $\text{CHILD'S DOSE} = \frac{\text{weight of child (lb)}}{150} \times \text{adult dose}$

$$= \frac{45}{150} \times 500 \text{ mg} = \frac{22{,}500 \text{ mg}}{150} = \mathbf{150\ mg}$$

32. a (para 1-23c) $\text{CHILD'S DOSE} = \frac{\text{age of child (yrs)}}{\text{age} + 12} \times \text{adult dose}$

$$= \frac{7 \times 500 \text{ mg}}{7 + 12} = \frac{3500 \text{ mg}}{19}$$

= 184 mg, approximately

33. c (para 1-24) $\frac{45\text{-lb}}{2.2\text{-lb/kg}} = 20.5 \text{ kg}$

CHILD'S DOSE = 20.5 kg × 10 mg/kg = **205 mg**

34. b (para 1-25; fig 1-1) Note on the enclosed column of the nomogram that a point for 45 on the left scale would correspond to a point for 0.81 on the right. Thus, a 45-lb child of normal height has a surface area of about 0.81 m^2.

CHILD'S DOSE = 0.81 m^2 × 300 mg/m^2 = **243 mg**

35. d (para 1-25; fig 1-1) Note on the enclosed column of the nomogram that a point for 45 on the left scale would correspond to a point for 0.81 on the right scale. Thus, a 45-lb child of normal height has a surface area of about 0.81 m^2.

$$\text{CHILD'S DOSE} = \frac{\text{surface area } (m^2)}{1.7} \times \text{adult dose}$$

$$= \frac{0.81 \times 500 \text{ mg}}{1.7} = \frac{405 \text{ mg}}{1.7} = \mathbf{238\ mg}$$

End of Lesson 1

LESSON ASSIGNMENT

LESSON 2	Basic Pharmacology; Antiseptics and Disinfectants; Other Topical Drugs; Gastrointestinal Agents; Respiratory Drugs; Local Anesthetics.
LESSON ASSIGNMENT	Paragraphs 2-1 through 2-45.
LESSON OBJECTIVES	Upon completion of this lesson, you should be able to define terms commonly used in pharmacology; describe common dosage forms; name and describe important factors affecting drug action; and discuss the actions, uses, untoward effects, administration, cautions, and contraindications for common antiseptics, disinfectants, antacids, cathartics, antidiarrheals, antitussives, expectorants, and local anesthetics.
SUGGESTION	After studying the assignment, complete the exercises at the end of this lesson. These exercises will help you to achieve the lesson objectives.

LESSON 2

BASIC PHARMACOLOGY; ANTISEPTICS AND DISINFECTANTS; OTHER TOPICAL DRUGS; GASTROINTESTINAL AGENTS; RESPIRATORY DRUGS; LOCAL ANESTHETICS

Section I. INTRODUCTION TO PHARMACOLOGY

2-1. DEFINITIONS

a. **Drug**. A drug may be broadly defined as any substance or group of substances that affects living protoplasm. However, the term is used most often to refer to any substance used to prevent, diagnose, or treat disease or to prevent conception. A drug of choice is the most effective or most commonly used drug for achieving a desired therapeutic effect.

b. **Pharmacology**. Pharmacology is the study of drugs in all their respects.

c. **Therapeutics**. Therapeutics is the science and art of healing.

d. **Poison**. A poison is a substance which when absorbed or ingested into the body may alter physiology to a mild or a critical extent by damaging body tissues or cells.

e. **Toxicology**. This is the study of poisons, their actions, the treatment of poisoning, and the use of antidotes.

f. **Pharmacy**. This is the art and science of preparing and dispensing drugs for medical purposes. Pharmaceutical is a adjective which means pertaining to pharmacy.

g. **The United States Pharmacopeia and The National Formulary (U.S.P/ N.F.)**. This one reference contains standards and tests for quality, purity, strength, packaging, and labeling of drugs in the United States. The U.S.P./N.F. has information which is useful to persons whose jobs require them to work with various medications. Annual supplements to the reference ensure that it contains the latest information on drugs.

h. **Official Drug or Preparation**. An official drug or preparation is one that is listed in the U.S.P./N.F.

2-2. DOSAGE FORMS

a. **Discussion**. Drugs are compounded into various types of preparations depending upon the physical characteristics of the drugs, the purpose for which intended, and the method by which they are to be administered. Some drugs are prepared in more than one form and may therefore be administered in several ways.

b. **Solid Preparations**.

(1) Powder. A drug that is ground up and used in powder form.

(2) Capsule. A drug placed in a gelatin container (figures 2-1C and D).

(3) Tablet. A molded or compressed solid mass of one or more medicinal substances, often diluted and bound together by other ingredients. The shape, usually discoid, may vary considerably from one tablet to another (figure 2-1A).

(4) Suppository. A drug that is molded into shape for insertion in a body opening and which melts or dissolves at body temperature (figure 2-1B).

(5) Ointment. A drug suspended in lard, Vaseline, lanolin, or other solid or semisolid base, intended for external application.

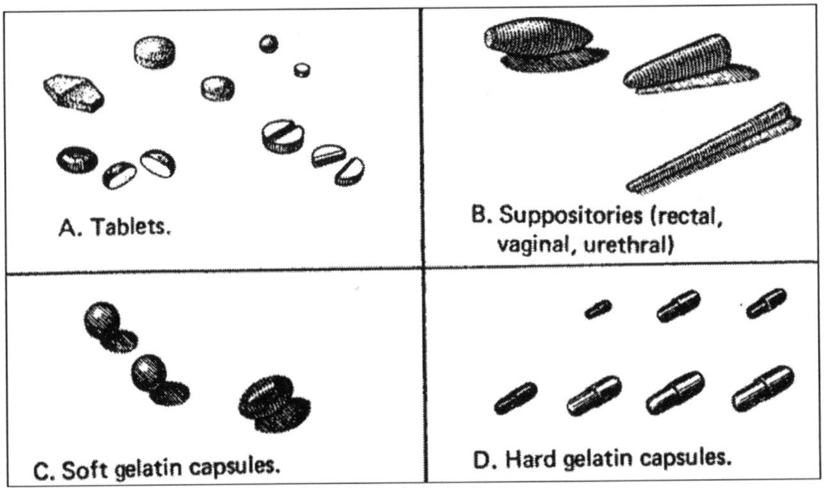

Figure 2-1. Solid dosage forms.

c. **Fluid Preparations**. Fluid drugs for oral and external use are packaged in bottles; those for injection are packaged sterile in vials or ampules.

(1) Fluidextracts. Alcoholic or hydroalcoholic solutions of the active constituents of vegetable drugs. They are usually prepared so that each milliliter of the finished preparation contains the extractive from 1 gm of the crude drug. These drugs should be kept in dark bottles because many of them precipitate in light. They are not to be used if precipitate has formed.

(2) Spirit. An alcoholic solution of volatile substances.

(3) Elixir. A solution containing alcohol, sugar, and flavoring substance in which one or more drugs may be dissolved.

(4) Tincture. Alcoholic or hydroalcoholic solution or ostrichtion of a drug. Tinctures of potent drugs are 10 percent in strength; of most other drugs, 20 percent in strength.

(5) Emulsion. A mixture of two liquids, usually oil and water, one of which is dispersed as droplets in the other. Any emulsion should have a "SHAKE WELL" label on the container.

(6) Suspension. A liquid preparation containing undissolved material. A "SHAKE WELL" label is applied to the container.

(7) Syrup. A highly concentrated sugar solution containing a flavoring agent into which a drug may be incorporated.

(8) Liniment. A solution of drugs in a soapy, oily, or alcoholic base, intended for external application with friction.

(9) Lotion. An aqueous preparation, usually containing suspended insoluble matter, to be applied externally. A "SHAKE WELL" label should be on the container.

d. **Cautions Concerning Certain Fluid Drugs**. Fluidextracts, spirits, elixirs, and tinctures (paragraph 2-2c(1)-(4) above) are preparations that are generally potent and, hence, the dosage is likely to be small. The usual dose range is from a few drops up to 2 to 4 ml. In addition, these drugs are never to be injected. Fluid drugs containing alcohol should not be applied to open lesions.

2-3. POSOLOGY

Posology is the science of dosage. It deals with the amount of drug necessary to produce a desired physiological, therapeutic, or prophylactic effect.

a. The average dose, also called the usual dose, is the amount of drug that ordinarily produces the effect for which the drug is intended. In addition to the usual dose, the usual dose range is often indicated for many drugs in standard pharmacy references. This provides a guide to dispensing personnel in deciding whether the prescriber should be consulted about the correctness of a prescribed dose. The usual dose range is the range of doses that consistently produce the effect for which the drug is intended.

b. The minimum dose is the smallest dose that produces a therapeutic effect.

c. The maximum dose is the largest dose that can be safely administered.

d. The toxic dose is the dose that produces harmful effects.

e. The lethal dose is the dose that will result in death. The minimum lethal dose (MLD) is the smallest amount that will cause death.

f. The single dose is the amount of a drug taken at one time. The daily dose is the total amount of a drug taken in 24 hours. A continuous dose consists of small doses taken at short intervals. A maintenance dose is that amount of drug taken to replace previous doses that have been inactivated, detoxified, or excreted. The purpose of a maintenance dose is to maintain the required concentration of the drug in the body.

2-4. FACTORS AFFECTING DRUG ACTION

In drug administration, many factors affect the action of the medication. These factors also affect the dose to be administered. The usual adult dose of medication as listed in standard references, is based on the assumption that the adult weighs 150 pounds, but since the following variables influence the action of the medication, they also may alter the quantity of the drug necessary to produce the desired results.

a. **Weight**. Heavy, burly clients require larger doses than weak, emaciated ones. The doses of many drugs are calculated on a weight basis; a specified number of grams or milligrams are administered per pound or kilogram of body weight.

b. **Age**. As a rule, the very young and the very old require less than the normal adult dose. As you recall from lesson 1, several formulas are available for estimating a child's dose when the average adult dose is known.

c. **Sex**. Females usually require smaller doses than males. Iron preparations and other hematinics are exceptions to this rule because of the blood lost by women during menstruation.

d. **Race**. Race can be a factor affecting drug action, since enzyme systems, body chemistry, and stature may vary.

e. **Temperament**. The high-strung, nervous, always-busy type of individual requires smaller amounts of stimulants but larger amounts of sedatives than the phlegmatic (dull, apathetic) individual.

f. **Climate**. Cathartics seem to be effective in smaller doses in warm climates than in cold.

g. **Occupation**. Men who work outdoors and who engage in strenuous, physical activity usually require larger doses than those who are engaged in sedentary or indoor work.

h. **Disease**. Some pathological conditions require changes in dosage. People in extreme pain need more analgesic and sedative drugs than those suffering only mild pain. The extremely weak or debilitated client may require smaller doses of some medications.

i. **Tolerance**. The therapeutic effects of some medications are lessened in individuals after prolonged use. Thus, a person who has used such a drug for a long time needs larger doses than he did when he first began to take it in order to realize the same therapeutic effects from it. This is called tolerance. Users of opium, morphine, cocaine, amphetamines, and barbiturates fall into this category. Cross-tolerance develops when the use of one drug causes a tolerance to another. Alcoholics, barbiturate habitues, and narcotic addicts develop a cross-tolerance to sedatives and anesthetics. These individuals require very large amounts of anesthetics before surgical anesthesia can be attained.

j. **Mode of Administration**. Generally, drugs given parenterally are used in smaller quantities and those given rectally are used in greater quantities than the usual oral dose.

k. **Frequency of Administration**. Drugs given at frequent intervals are administered in smaller doses than those given at wide intervals.

l. **Time of Administration**. Some drugs given by the oral route are absorbed more rapidly before a meal (on an empty stomach) than they would be if they were administered immediately after a meal.

m. **The Drug**. Many factors of the drug itself can influence its action. They may alter its potency, making some preparations weaker and others stronger. The form of a drug, that is, solution, powder, or suspension, may alter the amount of the drug necessary and the effects derived from it.

n. **Additive Effect**. If two drugs exhibit the same overt effect and their combined effects are equal to the sum of their individual effects, they are additive.

o. **Synergism**. Synergism is the joint action of two or more drugs such that their combined effects are greater than the sum of their individual effects. A reduced dosage may be necessary.

p. **Antagonism**. If only one of two drugs exhibits an effect, but that effect is decreased when the two drugs are given in combination, they are antagonistic. An increased dosage of the active component may be necessary.

q. **Accumulation**. When the body is unable to detoxify and excrete a drug as rapidly as it is being absorbed, or when a drug is stored in the tissues for an appreciable length of time, pronounced drug effects and poisoning can follow. Usually this is noticed when a number of doses are administered over a period of time. This may require progressively smaller doses (or "rest" days between doses) to allow the accumulated drug to be expended.

r. **Side Effects**. Most drugs are not singular in action. They may produce several different physiological responses at the same time. Antihistamines used for their anti-allergic effect tend to produce drowsiness, which is a side effect of the drug. Amphetamines are sometimes used to appease appetite in weight control, but at the same time they cause nervousness and insomnia, which are side effects to the diet client. Thus, to minimize undesirable side effects, a lower dose may be given, or another drug may be given concomitantly to antagonize the side effect.

s. **Drug Allergy (Hypersensitivity)**. A few individuals may be allergic, or hypersensitive, to a drug because of prior contact with a particular substance called an allergen (perhaps the same drug). This phenomenon of acquiring an allergy is called sensitization. The symptoms of an allergic reaction are not related to the ordinary effects of the drug. Thus, the allergic individual should not be confused with the individual who is highly responsive to a drug and thus requires only a small dose to achieve the desired therapeutic effect. Allergic reactions to a drug may range in severity from a mildly irritating skin rash to a fatal state of shock (anaphylaxis). One drug to which many clients are allergic is penicillin.

Section II. ANTISEPTICS AND DISINFECTANTS

2-5. DEFINITIONS

The antiseptic and disinfectant drugs are used extensively by both medical personnel and the general public. These drugs act locally to produce their effects.

a. **Antiparasitic**. A preparation used to eliminate body parasites.

b. **Antiseptic**. A preparation that checks or prevents the growth or development of pathogenic (disease-producing) bacteria. Antiseptics are primarily intended for use upon animate (living) objects. Antiseptics usually act as bacteriostats.

c. **Bactericide**. A drug that kills bacteria.

d. **Bacteriostat**. A drug that inhibits the growth of bacteria.

e. **Disinfectant**. A preparation that kills infectious organisms, but does not necessarily destroy their spores. Disinfectants are primarily intended for use upon inanimate (nonliving) objects. For the most part, disinfectants act as bactericides.

f. **Fungicide**. A drug used to kill fungus that infects the body surface.

g. **Fungistat**. An agent that inhibits the growth of fungous organisms without necessarily killing them.

h. **Pediculicide**. A preparation used to kill lice.

i. **Scabicide**. A preparation used to kill itch mites (scabies).

j. **Sterile**. An object is sterile if it is free from all living organisms. The appropriate use of antiseptics and disinfectants will greatly reduce the number of pathogenic (disease-producing) organisms present, but these agents will seldom sterilize objects.

2-6. ALCOHOLS

a. **Discussion**. Both ethyl alcohol and isopropyl alcohol have an antiseptic action when applied to the skin. Alcohol is commonly applied to the skin prior to giving an injection to cleanse the infection site. In addition, alcohol may be used for the disinfection of some medical equipment, such as thermometers. Isopropyl alcohol is a more effective antiseptic agent than ethyl alcohol.

b. **Strength**. For both ethyl alcohol and isopropyl alcohol, the optimum concentration for antiseptic purposes is 70 percent. If this concentration is varied, either higher or lower, these products become less effective. Stronger concentrations of ethyl alcohol may result in the formation of spores.

c. **Other Uses**.

(1) Both ethyl alcohol and isopropyl alcohol may be applied to the skin as a cooling rub in concentrations of 35 percent-70 percent.

(2) Alcohol may be ordered to be taken internally. Only alcohol, USP (ethanol, ethyl alcohol), is to be taken internally. Receipts and expenditures of ethyl alcohol must be accounted for in the narcotic and controlled drug register.

d. **Precautions**.

(1) When the alcohols are used to disinfect metal instruments, an antirust agent (such as sodium nitrite) should be put into the solution. Ethyl alcohol produces more rusting than does isopropyl alcohol.

(2) Both alcohols are flammable in concentrations over 50 percent; therefore, these solutions should not be used in the presence of open flames, nor when there is danger of electrostatic sparks.

(3) Isopropyl alcohol is not to be given internally.

(4) Both alcohols should be kept covered when not being used, because the alcohols will evaporate rapidly if left in an open container.

e. **Supply**. Both ethyl and isopropyl alcohol are ordinarily supplied in quarts.

2-7. BENZALKONIUM CHLORIDE

a. **Action and Uses**.

(1) Benzalkonium chloride (Zephiran) has either a bacteriostatic or a bactericidal action, depending upon the concentration of the solution. Both the aqueous solution and the tincture act as a bactericide when used in a concentration of 1:1000.

(2) Benzalkonium chloride is used to prepare the skin for surgery, and to prepare an injection site. It is also used to disinfect surgical instruments and polyethylene tubing.

b. **Precautions**.

(1) An antirust agent should be used when benzalkonium chloride is being used for the disinfection of instruments.

(2) Care must be taken to carefully rinse articles that have been washed before soaking them in benzalkonium chloride, since soap and other anionic detergents will inactivate it.

(3) Benzalkonium chloride is not to be taken internally.

c. **Supply**.

(1) Benzalkonium chloride solution is supplied in a 10 percent concentration that must be diluted to the proper concentration before it is used. To make a 1:1000 solution, 10 ml of the drug is combined with enough water to make 1 liter of solution.

(2) Benzalkonium chloride tincture is supplied tinted, so that it is readily identified as containing alcohol. It is available in both 10-ml and 2-ml bottles with applicator tip, in a 1:1000 concentration.

2-8. HYDROGEN PEROXIDE

a. **Action and Uses**. Hydrogen peroxide is an antiseptic agent that is used as a mouthwash, as a germicide, and as a mechanical cleansing agent for wounds. The antiseptic action of hydrogen peroxide is produced by the release of oxygen when the drug is applied to a wound. The drug is an effective antiseptic only as long as oxygen is being released. The bubbling, effervescent action of oxygen affords a mechanical means for the removal of debris from a wound. Particles of dirt and dead skin are brought to the surface of the wound and allowed to be washed away. Such mechanical cleansing is thought to be more valuable than the antiseptic action. Medicinal hydrogen peroxide contains 3 percent hydrogen peroxide in water.

b. **Precautions**.

(1) It is dangerous to use hydrogen peroxide in wounds or in body cavities from which the released oxygen cannot freely escape.

(2) Care must be taken to use only medicinal (3 percent) peroxide. Bleaching peroxide, used for the hair, is a 20 percent solution and will cause irritation if used for medicinal purposes. (Bleaching peroxide is not a standard item, but it may be available at some installations.)

(3) Hydrogen peroxide should be stored in tight, light-resistant containers to prevent deterioration.

c. **Supply**. Hydrogen peroxide solution is available in a 3 percent concentration. It is packaged in one-pound (pint) bottles.

2-9. HEXACHLOROPHENE (SURGICAL DETERGENT AND SURGICAL SOAP)

a. **Action and Uses**. Hexachlorophene is the active ingredient of surgical soap and surgical detergent (pHisoHex). Surgical detergent cleanses the skin, and hexachlorophene is effective against staphylococci and other gram-positive bacteria. Cumulative antibacterial effect develops with continued use. Surgical detergent is indicated for use as a surgical scrub and a bacteriostatic skin cleanser. It is often used for preoperative cleansing of clients. It may be used to control an outbreak of gram positive infection in the nursery when ordinary procedures have failed, but only as long as necessary to control the infection.

b. **Precautions**.

(1) The residue of hexachlorophene should not be rinsed from the skin by the subsequent use of alcohol, soaps, or others cleansers which contain no hexachlorophene.

(2) Hexachlorophene products should not be used on burned or denuded skin.

(3) They should not be used as a wet pack, occulsive dressing, or lotion.

(4) They should not be routinely used for prophylactic total body bathing.

(5) They should not be used on any mucous membranes (such as a vaginal pack or tampon).

(6) Persons who evidence sensitivity to the drug (such as the appearance of a skin rash) should discontinue its use. Sensitivity occurs infrequently.

(7) Products containing hexachlorophene are for external use. If a large amount is swallowed, the drug can be harmful.

c. **Supply**.

(1) Surgical detergent contains 3 percent hexachlorophene and is supplied in 5-ounce and 1-gallon containers.

(2) Surgical soap, containing 2 percent hexachlorophene, is available in 1.75-ounce and 4-ounce bars. A liquid surgical soap containing 1 percent hexachlorophene is available in 1-pint and 1-gallon containers.

2-10. THIMEROSAL

Thimerosal (Merthiolate) is a general purpose antiseptic or disinfectant depending upon the concentration. It also has mild fungistatic properties. The drug can be used safely as a skin antiseptic on abraded skin in concentrations of 1:1000. Aqueous solutions of the drug in the appropriate concentrations can be used on mucous membranes such as the urethra, the nasal mucosa, and the eye. The tincture is for use on the skin only. Thimerosal tincture should not be used in the presence of open flames, as tinctures are flammable. An occasional person may be sensitive to the mercury contained in the drug, but such a sensitivity is rare. Thimerosal is supplied as an aqueous solution in pint bottles, a tincture in pint bottles, and as a solid in 1/4-ounce quantities.

2-11. DISINFECTANT--GERMICIDAL AND FUNGICIDAL CONCENTRATE (WESCODYNE)

Wescodyne (trade name) is a general purpose germicide, suitable for hand cleansing as well as for disinfecting thermometers and instruments, washing furniture, floors, and equipment. The concentrate must be diluted to make a 75 parts-per-million (ppm) solution. This 75-ppm solution is made by adding 18 ml. of concentrate to 4 liters (1 gallon) of water. The clear, dark amber color of this solution is an indication of its germicidal effectiveness; when the color fades, a fresh solution must be prepared.

2-12. POVIDONE-IODINE

Povidone-iodine (Betadine, Isodine) slowly releases its iodine after it has been applied to a surface. However, a 10 percent solution is equivalent to only 1 percent of available iodine. The attenuated effect is claimed to compensate for the decreased concentration of free iodine. It is effective as an antiseptic. Povidone-iodine may be used to disinfect inanimate objects, but it is not very effective against spores or fungi.

2-13. FORMALDEHYDE SOLUTION (FORMALIN)

Formaldehyde solution (37 percent by weight) is used as a disinfectant and deodorant. It is not only effective against vegetative bacteria and fungi, but also against spores and viruses. A solution of 20 percent formaldehyde and 50 percent ethanol is even more effective.

Section III. OTHER TOPICAL DRUGS

2-14. ALUMINUM ACETATE SOLUTION (BUROW'S SOLUTION)

Aluminum acetate solution is diluted with 10 to 40 parts of water for use as an antiseptic dressing and astringent.

2-15. ZINC OXIDE OINTMENT

Zinc oxide has a mild astringent and antiseptic action and is used in treatment of disorders of the skin, such as impetigo, eczema, ringworm, pruritis, varicose ulcers, and psoriasis. The drug is applied directly to the area affected. Zinc oxide ointment is supplied in 1-ounce and 1-pound containers.

2-16. CALAMINE LOTION, PHENOLATED AND MENTHOLATED

This lotion acts as a mild astringent and antiseptic agent, as described for zinc oxide ointment. In addition, it has a soothing effect upon irritated or itchy skin. The lotion should be shaken thoroughly before being applied, and it should be patted on the skin area to be treated. Calamine lotion is available in 53-ml (1.8-fl. oz.) and 118-ml (4-fl. oz.) sizes.

2-17. COMPOUND BENZOIN TINCTURE

Compound benzoin tincture is used as a protective agent (demulcent) to alleviate irritation of the skin or mucous membranes. When mixed with glycerin and water, it is used for bedsores, cutaneous ulcers, fissures of the lips or anus, and cracked nipples. On sugar, it may be used for throat and bronchial infection. When it is mixed with boiling water, the vapor may be inhaled as a soothing expectorant for croup and acute laryngitis. Compound benzoin tincture is supplied in 1-pt containers.

2-18. HYDROCORTISONE CREAM

Hydrocortisone cream is used topically to suppress the inflammatory response in numerous skin diseases. The antibiotic neomycin is included in some preparations to protect against bacterial infections that might be favored by this suppression and to clear up infections secondary to the inflammation.

2-19. SODIUM FLUORESCEIN APPLICATORS

Sodium fluorescein is an ophthalmic diagnostic aid with which damaged parts of the cornea appear green and foreign bodies are surrounded by a green ring. A yellow hue indicates loss of substance on the conjunctiva. Merely dipping the paper strips into the lacrimal fluid releases an adequate amount of this highly soluble drug.

Section IV. ANTACIDS

2-20. INTRODUCTION

Antacids are agents used to neutralize excess hydrochloric acid in the stomach, especially to treat ulcers. Antacids are often abused; many people unwisely take antacids at the first sign of gastrointestinal (GI) discomfort.

a. **Systemic Antacids**. Systemic antacids are those which are readily absorbed from the GI tract and thus produce changes throughout the body. Prolonged use or overdose of systemic antacids, such as sodium bicarbonate, may injure the health. Forexample, a predisposition to kidney stones may result. Systemic antacids can cause systemic alkalosis, a potentially dangerous change in the acid-base balance of the body in which the base predominates.

b. **Nonsystemic Antacids**. Fortunately, not all antacids are systemic. A nonsystemic antacid contains a cation, for example, aluminum, calcium, or magnesium, which is not easily absorbed by the lining of the stomach. The accompanying anion, for example, a hydroxide or carbonate ion, helps neutralize the extra acid concentration in the stomach. The cations from the antacid react with anions in a portion of the small intestine called the jejunum, where the pH is basic, and the compound thus formed may produce additional antacid effects in the small intestine.

2-21. SODIUM BICARBONATE

a. **Action and Uses**. Sodium bicarbonate, a systemic antacid, may be used to combat systemic acidosis or render the urine alkaline. As a gastric antacid, it has several disadvantages: its duration of action is short; its reaction with hydrochloric acid produces carbon dioxide, which may cause stomach pains or exacerbate an ulcer, and it will produce systemic alkalosis.

b. **Usual Dose**. The usual dose is 300 mg to 2 grams, 1 to 4 times daily.

c. **Supply**. Sodium bicarbonate is supplied as 600-mg tablets and as a powder. It is also available as a tablet combined with charcoal and peppermint.

2-22. ALUMINUM HYDROXIDE GEL

a. **Action and Uses**. Aluminum hydroxide (Amphojel) is not an adsorbent, but it does act chemically to neutralize gastric acidity. It is a nonsystemic antacid.

b. **Administration**. The drug is usually given orally 1 hour after meals or when needed. The average single dose of tablets is 0.6 gm (2 tablets). The tablets are chewed thoroughly before being swallowed. The usual dose of the liquid is 5 to 15 ml. The bottle is shaken thoroughly before the drug is poured.

c. **Untoward Effects**. Constipation occurs in some people who take aluminum compounds. However, there are no systemic effects, since the drug is not absorbed from the gastrointestinal tract.

d. **Cautions and Contraindications**. The liquid preparation should be kept from freezing.

e. **Supply**. The drug is supplied as a liquid suspension (320mg/5ml) in one-pint bottles and as 300 mg and 600 mg flavored tablets.

2-23. ALUMINUM HYDROXIDE GEL AND MAGNESIUM HYDROXIDE

a. **Action and Uses**. Magnesium hydroxide is an antacid that acts both by chemically reacting with stomach acid and by adsorbing it. This preparation is used to treat hyperacidity and ulcers of the stomach. The drug is not adsorbed from the intestinal tract. A preparation of magnesium hydroxide combined with aluminum hydroxide gel (Gelusil) is available. The untoward effect of constipation that may occur with the administration of aluminum compounds is generally offset by the laxative action of the magnesium. Such a combined preparation is standard for the Army.

b. **Administration**. The drug is given orally in a usual dosage of 2 tablets or 5 to 15 ml. of the liquid preparation four times a day. Greater dosages are sometimes prescribed. The tablets should be chewed thoroughly and the liquid suspension shaken as was described for aluminum hydroxide gel.

c. **Untoward Effects**. Slight diarrhea may result due to local irritation of the bowel by the magnesium salt. Since the drug is not absorbed, no systemic side effects are seen.

d. **Cautions and Contraindications**. The liquid preparation should not be allowed to freeze, and the tablets are subject to deterioration as noted on the manufacturer's label.

e. **Supply**. This drug is supplied in both liquid and tablet form.

2-24. MILK OF MAGNESIA

Preparations containing magnesium hydroxide, such as milk of magnesia, are fairly effective in reducing gastric acidity, but they may also cause diarrhea. For this reason, magnesium hydroxide is often used also as a cathartic by increasing the dosage.

2-25. ALUMINUM HYDROXIDE AND MAGNESIUM HYDROXIDE

Aluminum hydroxide and magnesium hydroxide are both nonsystemic antacids. They are included together in many familiar over-the-counter preparations (Maalox, Mylanta, Aludrox, Bidrox, Wingel, Creamalin, and so forth). The constipating effect of the aluminum hydroxide is counteracted by the laxative effect of the magnesium hydroxide.

2-26. CHOICE OF AN ANTACID

Since antacids are available without a prescription, many individuals develop their own preference for a particular antacid. This choice is logically based on flavor, texture, dosage form, and laxative or constipating effects. It is important to choose an antacid that does not adversely affect the consistency or frequency of bowel movements or to train the client to use more than one antacid as needed. The precaution against systemic antacids, such as sodium bicarbonate, is also important.

Section V. CATHARTICS

2-27. INTRODUCTION

a. Cathartics, agents that promote evacuation of the bowels, are frequently self-prescribed and misused. The occasions when cathartics are therapeutically useful are infrequent. However, they are overused due to the misconception that a periodic cleansing of the bowels is necessary for good health, that a regular frequency of bowel movements must be maintained, or to a neurotic preoccupation with bowel movements.

b. Catharsis is naturally followed by a period in which there are no bowel movements. The individual may construe this as an indication that a cathartic is needed once again. This may lead to the formation of the "cathartic habit," in which the individual depends upon a cathartic again and again to induce a bowel movement.

c. Constipation occurs more frequently among older people, due in part to inactivity, dietary factors, and inadequate water intake. However, their attitudes, formed when "regular bowel habits" were viewed as a key to good health, also play an important part.

2-28. INDICATIONS AND CONTRAINDICATIONS FOR CATHARTICS

a. Cathartics may be used for specific situations of brief duration. The following are a few examples of situations in which cathartics may be used:

(1) To relieve constipation caused by the use of opiate drugs.

(2) To soften the stool, thereby reducing irritation of hemorrhoids or following hemorrhoidectomy.

(3) To avoid straining in clients confined to bed for an acute illness such as myocardial infarction.

(4) To prepare an individual for proctoscopy.

b. Milk cathartics such as the hydrophilic colloids may be useful for bedridden clients who become constipated because of lack of activity. However, people who are habitually constipated should generally not be given cathartics. Cathartics are useful for softening the stool of clients with hemorrhoids, diverticulitis, hernias, or cardiac disease. Castor oil is useful in treating some clients for poisoning and in preparing others for special examinations.

c. Cathartics should **NOT** be used when the client has an undiagnosed intestinal pain such as cramps, nausea, or vomiting; a cathartic may cause an inflamed appendix to rupture. Nor should cathartics be used when the GI tract is mechanically obstructed; the intestine may rupture. Pregnant clients should ordinarily not be given cathartics.

2-29. STIMULANT (IRRITANT) CATHARTICS

Stimulant cathartics function either by irritating the mucous membranes of the intestines or directly stimulating the nerves and muscles concerned with bowel movement. Since individual reactions to stimulant cathartics vary, the usual dose may in some clients cause excessively severe effects, including diarrhea and intestinal cramps, and in other clients have no effectiveness.

a. Aromatic cascara fluidextract is a mild, effective stimulant laxative that takes about 8 hours to take effect, since it acts on the colon rather than the small intestines. Another stimulant laxative containing cascara sagrada is cascara tablets. After about 8 hours, these preparations produce a single evacuation of the bowels.

b. Bisacodyl (Dulcolax) is another stimulant cathartic that acts primarily on the colon. Bisacodyl cleanses the bowel thoroughly enough to obviate the need for an enema.

c. The one stimulant cathartic that stimulates the small intestine is castor oil. Castor oil is not used routinely but only when prompt, thorough evacuation of the bowels is desired, such as for a special examination.

2-30. SALINE CATHARTICS

Saline cathartics, salts which draw water into the GI tract and thereby increase the bulk of the intestinal contents, usually take about 3 to 6 hours to produce a bowel evacuation, which is watery or fluid-like. Saline cathartics, unless administered with sufficient amounts of water, tend to dehydrate the body and are sometimes used for this purpose alone. In order to avoid magnesium poisoning, cathartics containing magnesium compounds must never be given to clients with impaired kidney function. Cathartics containing sodium compounds should not be administered to clients with congestive heart disease.

a. A mild saline cathartic is milk of magnesia, which contains magnesium hydroxide and which is also used as an antacid. The cathartic dose is 15-30 ml.

b. Magnesium sulfate (epsom salt) is a widely used saline cathartic. Its main disadvantage is its bitter taste, which can be masked to some extent by mixing with ice water or orange juice. The usual dose is 15 grams.

2-31. FECAL SOFTENERS

During prolonged bed rest and dietary change, it may be necessary to prevent dessication, hardening, or impaction of feces within the colon and facilitate defecation by maintaining a soft stool. Fecal softeners include agents that mix with the intestinal contents and others which serve as emulsifying agents.

a. Mineral oil (heavy liquid petrolatum), also known as an emollient cathartic, softens the fecal material by becoming emulsified with it. It is probably harmless when taken on an occasional basis. However, if it is taken chronically, it may impair the appetite and interfere with the absorption of fat-soluble vitamins. The usual dose is 15 ml.

b. Dioctyl calcium sulfosuccinate (Surfak) is an emulsifying ("surface-acting" or "wetting") agent that probably causes the fats and water in the intestine to mix and form a soft stool. It should not be used with mineral oil since it might facilitate absorption of mineral oil into the body. It is widely used in persons who should not strain at stool, such as those with hemorrhoids, and in older persons to avoid constipation. The usual dose is 240 mg.

c. Dioctyl sodium sulfosuccinate (Colace) lowers surface tension and is thought to soften the contents of the intestines by causing the contents to absorb water. It should not be used with mineral oil since it might facilitate absorption of mineral oil into the body.

d. Psyllium dycrophilic mucilloid (Metamucil) is a light-colored, slightly granular powder with only a slight acid taste. It consists of the mucilaginous portion of blond psyllium seeds. It acts as a fecal softener, is demulcent, nonirritating, and may be used over long periods. Not only does it increase intestinal activity, but it has psychological value for some clients in that it increases the bulk of the stool. The usual dose is 4-7 grams (1 rounded teaspoonful), 1-3 times daily, in a glass of liquid followed by another glass of liquid.

Section VI. ANTIDIARRHEALS

2-32. KAOLIN MIXTURE WITH PECTIN

Kaolin is an adsorbent; pectin is considered a protective. Pectin is capable of creating a viscous colloidal solution in water. Kaolin mixture with pectin may provide relief from mild diarrhea, especially among children. However, it is of little use in severe diarrhea such as that associated with ulcerative colitis. The usual adult dose is 4 to 8 tablespoons after each loose bowel movement.

2-33. DIPHENOXYLATE HYDROCHLORIDE AND ATROPINE SULFATE TABLETS

The trade name for diphenoxylate hydrochloride and atropine sulfate is Lomotil. Diphenoxylate is a synthetic drug similar to the narcotic meperidine (Demerol), but diphenoxylate is more highly constipating. Since diphenoxylate cannot be taken by the parenteral route, and since it is mixed with atropine, it is not as likely to be abused as other narcotics. There is no evidence of addiction liability in therapeutic doses. Lomotil is used in the management of diarrhea due to gastroenteritis, functional hypermotility, ulcerative colitis, drugs, and food poisoning. Each Lomotil tablet contains 2.5 mg of diphenoxylate hydrochloride and 0.025 mg of atropine sulfate. The usual dose for initial control is two tablets, 4 times daily. This may be decreased after control has been established.

2-34. PAREGORIC

Paregoric (camphorated opium tincture) contains 0.4 percent to 1 percent opium. In the Army it is subject to the same controls as ethyl alcohol and "hard" narcotics (this is indicated in the Federal Supply Catalog by a note R or Q). Opium induces spasm of the colon, increases tone, and prevents propulsive movement. Therefore, paregoric is used as an antidiarrheal agent and also as a weak agent for coughing, abdominal pains, and nausea. The usual dose is 5-10 ml, one to four times daily.

Section VII. RESPIRATORY DRUGS

2-35. ANTITUSSIVES

An antitussive is a drug used to suppress coughing. We are all familiar with the traditional antitussive remedies, such as hard candies, cough drops, and lozenges. By stimulating the flow of saliva, these agents help reduce the irritation which causes a cough. In this paragraph, however, we will discuss only those antitussives that produce a significant part of their effect after being absorbed into the body tissues (for example, from the GI tract). Many of these act directly on the nerve connections in the medulla which are responsible for the cough reflex.

a. **Narcotics**. The narcotic antitussives are very effective and have been in use for some time. The fact that they are narcotics is not normally a decisive contraindication for their use. However, they should not be used in the treatment of a chronic (prolonged) cough or the cough of a client who tends to become psychologically dependent on drugs. Among the cough remedies, it is possible to become addicted to codeine (or its salts, such as codeine sulfate or codeine phosphate). This frequently used antitussive will be discussed in a later section.

b. **Other Antitussives**. Other antitussives include the following:

(1) Dextromethorphan hydrobromide. This antitussive is a morphine derivative, but it has few of the observable properties of a narcotic. No cases of addiction or severe central nervous system depression have been reported with it.

(2) Benzonatate (Tessalon). This drug has an effect on the mucous membranes of the respiratory system similar to that of a local anesthetic. In addition, like the other antitussives discussed, it has an effect on the nerve connections in the medulla concerned with the cough reflex. It does not appear to be as effective clinically as codeine.

2-36. EXPECTORANTS

Expectorants are drugs that increase the volume of secretions from the mucous membranes of the respiratory tract below the epiglottis. They also help liquefy the mucous secretions, which are subsequently spat out by the client. Expectorants are useful in treating coughs. Since some of the difficulty of asthma arises from obstruction of breathing by mucus, expectorants are sometimes useful in treating asthma.

a. **Potassium Iodide**. Potassium iodide is one of the most effective expectorants. Mild side effects, including weeping of the eyes and nose, sometimes occur, but serious side effects are rare. Potassium iodide is also used to treat iodine deficiencies.

b. **Ipecac Syrup**. This preparation may be used as an expectorant, but the dose is lower than when it is used as an emetic. It is useful when the client has unpleasant reactions to potassium iodide.

c. **Ammonium Chloride**. As is part of the effect of potassium iodide, the expectorant effect of ammonium chloride is due to its irritation of the stomach lining. Large doses may cause nausea.

d. **Guaiafenesin**. In large doses, this is an effective expectorant. It is an ingredient in many cough syrups.

e. **Terpin Hydrate**. This drug can be used as an expectorant but terpin hydrate elixir, NF, does not contain enough terpin hydrate to make the elixir a useful expectorant.

Section VIII. LOCAL ANESTHETICS

2-37. INTRODUCTION

Pain can be abolished by inducing unconsciousness with the general anesthetics or by preventing painful impulses from reaching the cortex by blocking the sensory nerve impulses from a localized area. This loss of feeling and sensation to a localized portion of the body is known as local anesthesia. It is accomplished by using local anesthetic drugs. Local anesthetics can be broken down into two main categories; those that lower skin temperature and those that have a specific effect on sensory nerves.

a. **Skin Refrigerants**. The local anesthetics that create anesthesia through the production of cold are liquids of low boiling point. Since ethyl chloride evaporates from the skin rapidly, it quickly reduces skin temperature and thereby produces its anesthetic action. Dichlorotetrafluoroethane also belongs to this group.

b. **Specifics**. The specific local anesthetics are those drugs that have a specific effect on the sensory nerve or on nerve endings. This category can be further subdivided into drugs of the water-soluble group that are intended for injection, such as procaine hydrochloride, and those that are only slightly water-soluble which are intended for topical use, such as benzocaine. Local anesthetics are detoxified by the liver. In the later discussion of specific local anesthetics, notice that almost all the names end in "caine." When you see a drug name with this suffix, you should immediately recognize it as a probable local anesthetic.

2-38. METHODS OF ADMINISTRATION

The ways in which local anesthetic agents may be applied so that they will produce their anesthetizing action are as follows:

a. Topical application to the skin or mucous membrane may be used.

b. The drug may be infiltrated (injected) into the tissue, thus anesthetizing adjacent nerves.

c. The drug may be injected into or around a nerve trunk, producing regional anesthesia (the region of the body supplied by the nerve trunk is anesthetized).

d. The drug may be introduced into the spinal canal (spinal block anesthesia), or at certain sites around the spinal canal (such as peridural or caudal anesthesia). Use of this method results in a more extensive area of anesthesia than is possible with the other methods above.

2-39. OVERDOSAGE TOXICITY

All local anesthetic agents are toxic to some degree. Therefore, the smallest amount of anesthetic solution compatible with successful anesthesia should be used. The toxicity of local anesthetic agents depends not only upon the strength of the solution and the total dose given, but also upon the rate of absorption (rapid absorption of an agent increases its toxicity). As all local anesthetic agents are potentially toxic, it is imperative that anyone using them be familiar with, and have the facilities for the treatment of overdosage toxicity and true allergic reactions. However, true allergic reactions occur infrequently.

a. **Symptoms of Overdosage Toxicity**. The symptoms may begin with brief or persistent central nervous system (CNS) stimulation, followed by CNS and cardiovascular depression, or there may be depression without apparent prior CNS stimulation.

(1) Early CNS stimulation. This stage is characterized by anxiety, nausea, slightly lowered pulse rate, slightly elevated blood pressure, increased respiratory rate and depth, and pale, moist skin.

(2) Profound CNS stimulation. With greater CNS stimulation, there may be muscular twitching leading to convulsions. Blood pressure and pulse rate rise. Breathing may be rapid, shallow, and less effective even between convulsions.

(3) Depression and shock. The client may go into depression and shock due to depression of the medulla, vasodilation, and postconvulsive depression. This state may involve are flexia (absence of reflexes), coma, extreme hypotension, and respiratory failure.

b. **Treatment**. Oxygen and assisted respiration help the client to tolerate the convulsive period. Shock is treated as any other form of shock, but the need for assisted respiration is much greater.

2-40. PROCAINE HYDROCHLORIDE

a. **Action and Uses.** Procaine hydrochloride (Novocaine Hydrochloride) is an effective, local anesthetic when given by injection. It is not useful as a topical anesthetic because of its poor penetrating power but is used for infiltration, nerve block, peridural, and spinal anesthesia. Generally, procaine is combined with epinephrine hydrochloride, which delays absorption, prolongs anesthesia, reduces toxic effects, and promotes hemostasis. In addition to its use as a local anesthetic, procaine can also be used intravenously, in special cases (with great caution), as an analgesic in cases of burn, fracture, or trauma.

b. **Administration**. Procaine solutions of 0.25 percent to 0.5 percent, often combined with epinephrine 1:50,000, are used for infiltration anesthesia. For nerve block, a 1 percent to 2 percent solution is used. To produce spinal anesthesia, a dosage up to 150 mg may be used; the actual dosage varies with the technique used. The onset of surgical anesthesia requires 5 to 15 minutes and the duration is 45 to 90 minutes.

c. **Untoward Effects**. Procaine is one of the least toxic of the injectable local anesthetics. However, untoward reactions to the drug occur occasionally and may be manifested as discussed previously. Treatment of reactions has also been discussed in paragraph 2-39b.

d. **Cautions and Contraindications**. Care must be taken to have available facilities for combating overdosage. If symptoms of overdosage appear while the drug is being given, its administration should be stopped immediately. Procaine should not be administered to people allergic to it. An intradermal skin test should be administered to any person suspected of being allergic to the drug. (NOTE: An intradermal skin test will yield information concerning allergy only. It will not indicate a person's susceptibility to toxic effects.) The use of procaine is contraindicated during therapy with sulfonamide drugs because these have an antagonistic effect.

e. **Supply**. Procaine hydrochloride is supplied in 100 mg and 1 gram quantities of sterile crystals in ampules and as a parenteral 1percent solution in 2 ml ampules.

2-41. LIDOCAINE HYDROCHLORIDE

a. **Actions**. Lidocaine hydrochloride (Xylocaine) is a potent local anesthetic agent which produces a prompt (5 to 15 minutes for the onset of operating analgesia), intense, and extensive anesthesia. Unlike procaine, lidocaine is effective when applied topically. Its anesthetic potency and area of anesthesia are greater than those of procaine hydrochloride. At a concentration of 0.5 percent, lidocaine has approximately the same toxicity as does procaine, but as the concentration of lidocaine is increased, its toxicity exceeds that of procaine. Moreover, lidocaine diffuses rapidly, a property that may increase the incidence of systemic reactions. Lidocaine is dissimilar to procaine in its chemical structure and, hence, may be used for persons sensitive to procaine. In addition, it produces effective anesthesia without the use of epinephrine, and so it may be used for persons allergic to epinephrine.

b. **Uses of Lidocaine Hydrochloride**. This agent is useful for topical, infiltration, and nerve block anesthesia. Lidocaine is also used for peridural block anesthesia. Its effect lasts from 1 1/2 to 3 hours with low dosage. This agent is often used in individuals sensitive to procaine. The drug is administered according to the type of local anesthesia to be induced. The onset of mucosal anesthesia may require 5 to 15 minutes, and depending on the procedure and the amount used, the anesthesia may persist for 30 minutes. The jelly form of the drug may be applied by means of cotton pledgets or applicators to the mucous membrane of the oral cavity and the urethra. An ointment containing lidocaine is used topically in treatment of burns and abrasions, as well as for minor dermatological, anorectal, and otological conditions.

c. **Administration**. Lidocaine solutions of 0.5 percent, often combined with epinephrine, are usually administered for infiltration anesthesia. Solutions of 1percent to 2 percent are used to produce nerve block. For topical anesthesia, 2 percent to 5 percent preparations are used. A 1 percent solution is generally used for peridural anesthesia.

d. **Untoward Effects**. Central nervous system stimulation followed by depression may occur as with the use of procaine. In addition, a drowsy, sleepy state may occur as an aftereffect of the use of lidocaine.

e. **Cautions and Contraindications**. Care should be taken not to administer the drug intravenously. The commercially prepared lidocaine-epinephrine solution should not be withdrawn ahead of time. This preparation should be injected immediately upon its withdrawal into a syringe. Lidocaine preparations deteriorate at or before 36 months from the date on the package, and they are damaged by freezing.

f. **Supply**. Lidocaine hydrochloride is supplied in 0.5 percent to 2 percent solutions, with and without epinephrine, and as a 2 percent jelly. Lidocaine is also available as a 5 percent ointment.

2-42. DIBUCAINE OINTMENT

a. **Action and Uses**. Dibucaine (Nupercaine) is the most potent, most toxic, and the longest acting of the local anesthetic agents available as standard items. It is about 15 times as potent and as toxic as procaine; its anesthetic action lasts about 3 times as long as that of procaine. The drug is employed topically for the relief of pain associated with conditions such as sunburn and hemorrhoids.

b. **Administration**. For topical application a 1 percent ointment is used, and it is applied to the painful surface.

c. **Cautions and Contraindications**. Caution should be exercised in the use of this drug because of its potential toxicity.

d. **Supply**. Dibucaine is supplied as a 1 percent ointment with rectal applicator.

2-43. TETRACAINE

Tetracaine hydrochloride (Pontocaine Hydrochloride) is an all-purpose anesthetic with a longer duration of action than procaine. Found in field sets are tetracaine hydrochloride ophthalmic solution (0.5 percent) and tetracaine ointment (0.5 percent).

2-44. EUGENOL

a. **Action and Uses**. Eugenol (oil of cloves) is a pale yellow liquid obtained from clove oil. It is used as a surface anesthetic and an antiseptic. Its chief use is in the temporary relief of toothache and in the disinfection of root canals.

b. **Supply**. The drug is supplied in 1-ounce bottles.

2-45. DICHLOROTETRAFLUOROETHANE ANESTHETIC

This agent is a skin refrigerant. It is included in the field dispensary medical instrument and supply set. The loss of sensation that results when this agent is sprayed onto the skin enables minor surgical procedures to be done with relative freedom from pain. Its duration of action is less than 1 minute. The drug is supplied in an 8-ounce aerosol dispenser.

Continue with Exercises

EXERCISES, LESSON 2

INSTRUCTIONS. Answer the following exercises by marking the lettered response that best answers the question or completes the incomplete statement.

After you have completed all of these exercises, turn to "Solutions to Exercises" at the end of the lesson, and check your answers. For each exercise answered incorrectly, reread the material referenced with the solution.

1. A drug that is compressed into a small disk is a:

   a. Pill.

   b. Capsule.

   c. Tablet.

   d. Suppository.

2. When a standard pharmacy reference lists the usual adult dose of a particular drug, the dose is specifically appropriate for a normal adult whose weight is:

   a. 120-lbs.

   b. 150-lbs.

   c. 180-lbs.

   d. 210-lbs.

3. A client who has been taking a drug discovers one evening that the customary dose is no longer effective. He now requires a larger dose. This reaction, due to the chronic use of the drug, is called:

   a. Addiction.

   b. Dependence.

   c. Habituation.

   d. Tolerance.

4. Some drugs remain within the body for extended periods. In order to prevent the accumulation of excessive amounts of such a drug in the body, it is often necessary for the physician to prescribe:

   a. Any drug which is excreted faster.

   b. Great volumes of water to free the body of the accumulated drug.

   c. Smaller doses later in therapy.

   d. Special drugs to counteract the effects of the accumulated drug.

5. What is the function of a bacteriostat?

   a. The destruction of bacteria.

   b. The inhibition of bacteria.

   c. The isolation of bacteria.

   d. Microscopic examination of bacteria.

6. A preparation that kills pathogenic bacteria but does not necessarily kill their spores is called:

   a. An antiseptic.

   b. A disinfectant.

   c. A pediculicide.

   d. A scabicide.

7. Pediculicides are agents used to destroy:

   a. Amoebas.

   b. Fungi.

   c. Lice.

   d. Protozoa.

8. Ethyl alcohol should not be used in a stronger concentration than that needed for use as an antiseptic agent because stronger concentrations:

   a. Produce burns.

   b. Result in spore formation.

   c. Freeze tissue.

   d. Bleach clothing.

9. An alcohol that should NOT be given internally is:

   a. Alcohol, USP.

   b. Ethyl alcohol.

   c. Ethanol.

   d. Isopropyl alcohol.

10. When an alcohol solution or a Benzalkonium Chloride Solution is used for the disinfection of metal instruments, an agent should be put into the solution to protect the instruments from:

   a. Rust.

   b. Pathogenic bacteria.

   c. Discoloration.

   d. Spores.

11. The effectiveness of Benzalkonium chloride is radically reduced by the presence of even a very small amount of:

   a. Acetone.

   b. Alcohol.

   c. Soap.

   d. Water.

12. In the concentration in which it is supplied, how much Benzalkonium Chloride Solution is required to make 4000 ml of a 1:1000 solution?

a. 10 ml

b. 20 ml

c. 40 ml

d. 100 ml

13. The antiseptic action of Hydrogen Peroxide is due to the release of:

a. Iodine.

b. Oxygen.

c. Histamine.

d. Carbon dioxide.

14. What concentration of hydrogen peroxide is for medicinal use?

a. 3 percent

b. 10 percent

c. 20 percent

d. 50 percent

15. The active ingredient in surgical detergent is:

a. Benzalkonium chloride.

b. Hydrogen peroxide.

c. Hexachlorophene.

d. Thimerosal.

16. Residue of Hexachlorophene should not be rinsed from the skin because the residue:

   a. Continues to act against bacteria.

   b. Forms a mechanical barrier against bacteria.

   c. Protects the skin from discoloration.

   d. Makes further washing unnecessary.

17. A drug that is contraindicated for persons with ulcers is:

   a. Aluminum hydroxide gel.

   b. Magnesium trisilicate.

   c. Sodium bicarbonate.

   d. Belladonna.

18. A normal bowel frequency may be once or twice a day for one individual, once or twice a <u>week</u> for another individual. However, many people take drugs to produce bowel movements, often inadvisably. These drugs are called:

   a. Adsorbents.

   b. Cathartics.

   c. Demulcents.

   d. Digestants.

19. Magnesium Sulfate should NOT be given to clients with which of the following conditions?

   a. Edema.

   b. Impaired kidney function.

   c. Congestive heart disease.

   d. Impaired function of the lungs.

20. A cathartic that may interfere with the absorption of certain vitamins is:

a. Magnesium sulfate.

b. Cascara sagrada.

c. Mineral oil.

d. Dioctyl calcium sulfosuccinate.

21. Which of the following is the most desirable cathartic to give a person with bleeding hemorrhoids?

a. Bisacodyl.

b. Castor oil.

c. Magnesium sulfate.

d. Dioctyl calcium sulfosuccinate.

22. Which of the following drugs is effective in the control of diarrhea?

a. Diphenoxylate.

b. Dextromethorphan.

c. Sodium bicarbonate.

d. Magnesium hydroxide.

23. Which of the following is an expectorant which is also used to relieve deficiencies of iodine?

a. Iodine.

b. Ipecac.

c. Guaiafenesin.

d. Potassium Iodide.

24. Which of the following local anesthetic agents is not effective if applied topically?

    a. Lidocaine.

    b. Procaine.

    c. Dibucaine.

    d. Eugenol.

25. A drug used for the relief of pain associated with hemorrhoids is:

    a. Procaine.

    b. Eugenol.

    c. Dibucaine.

    d. Dichlorotetrafluoroethane.

Check Your Answers on Next Page

SOLUTIONS TO EXERCISES, LESSON 2

1. c (para 2-2b(3))

2. b (para 2-4)

3. d (para 2-4i)

4. c (para 2-4q)

5. b (para 2-5d)

6. b (para 2-5e)

7. c (para 2-5h)

8. b (para 2-6b)

9. d (para 2-6c(2), d(3))

10. a (paras 2-6d(1); 2-7b(1))

11. c (para 2-7b(2))

12. c (para 2-7c(1)) 10 ml of a 10 percent concentration makes 1000 ml of a 1:1000 solution.

$$\text{IF } \frac{10 \text{ ml}}{1000 \text{ ml}} \text{ THEN } = \frac{X \text{ ml}}{4000 \text{ ml}}$$

$$\frac{\not{1000}X}{\not{1000}} = \frac{40,000}{1,000}$$

X = 40 ml

13. b (para 2-8a)

14. a (para 2-8a)

15. c (para 2-9a)

16. a (para 2-9a, b(1))

17. c (para 2-21a)

18. b (para 2-27a)

19. b (para 2-30)

20. c (para 2-31a)

21. d (para 2-31b)

22. a (para 2-33)

23. d (para 2-36a)

24. b (para 2-40a)

25. c (para 2-42a)

End of Lesson 2

LESSON ASSIGNMENT

LESSON 3	Central Nervous System Drugs
LESSON ASSIGNMENT	Paragraphs 3-1 through 3-32
LESSON OBJECTIVES	Upon completion of this lesson, you should be able to discuss the actions, uses, untoward effects, administration, cautions, and contraindications for common sedative- hypnotics, antipsychotic tranquilizers, narcotic analgesics, nonaddictive analgesics, amphetamines, and naloxone.
SUGGESTION	After studying the assignment, complete the exercises at the end of this lesson. These exercises will help you to achieve the lesson objectives.

LESSON 3

CENTRAL NERVOUS SYSTEM DRUGS

Section I. THE CENTRAL NERVOUS SYSTEM

3-1. PARTS OF THE CENTRAL NERVOUS SYSTEM

The central nervous system (CNS) includes the brain and spinal cord. It is divided into the following levels based on anatomical position and function.

a. **Cerebrum**. The cerebrum consists of two hemispheres and contains the cerebral cortex, which is the site of consciousness, memory, sensation, some conditioned reflexes, and inhibition of certain reflexes. Nerve fibers extend to the lower portion of the brain and spinal cord. Transverse fibers connect the two hemispheres.

b. **Midbrain (Mesencephalon)**. The midbrain carries pathways that connect the cerebrum and lower parts of the brain and the spinal cord. It also contains the thalamus and hypothalamus portion of the brain. Visual and audio reflexes are received here. Movement of the head and eyes in response to retinal stimuli originates here.

c. **Pons**. The pons is that part of the brain stem that is behind the midbrain and above the medulla oblongata. It carries various nerve pathways. The pons is connected with all portions of the brain.

d. **Medulla Oblongata**. The medulla is an oblongated portion at the base of the brain, which can be considered an upward continuation of the spinal cord. It contains the "vital centers"--the cardiac, vasomotor, and respiratory control centers--as well as controls for swallowing, vomiting, and coughing.

e. **Cerebellum**. The cerebellum, situated behind the brain stem (midbrain, pons, and medulla), is concerned with voluntary movements, although it plays no part in initiating them. Removal of the cerebellum would cause lack of muscular control, with shaky, jerky movements, and loss of equilibrium.

f. **Spinal Cord**. The spinal cord contains a central mass of gray matter surrounded by columns of white matter, which are bundles of nerve fibers. The cord serves as a reflex center and provides a series of ascending and descending pathways to and from the brain.

(1) <u>Ascending</u>. The ascending pathways carry stimuli of conscious muscle sense, pain, heat, and cold.

(2) Descending. The descending pathways carry stimuli for voluntary and involuntary functions.

3-2. PHARMACOLOGIC CONSIDERATIONS OF THE CNS

The CNS is more sensitive to the action of drugs than any other system in the body. Drugs act on it either by stimulation or by depression. Stimulation may range from mild alertness to convulsions; depression may range from mild sedation to loss of consciousness. The parts of the CNS respond to the presence of drugs with specific action. When given in ordinary doses, drugs may affect only one specific portion of the CNS, but when they are given in larger doses, they may affect the entire system. The following are examples of this:

a. Caffeine given in small doses stimulates the psychic center; given in larger doses, it stimulates the respiratory center; and given in very large doses, it may induce convulsions.

b. Alcohol depresses the inhibitory centers in the cerebral cortex; large doses depress the medulla, causing a slowing of respiration, sometimes even to the point of death.

c. Anesthetics depress sensory and motor areas of the cortex and the reflex centers in the spinal cord. Given in large doses, they depress the respiratory center in the medulla.

d. Phenobarbital depresses sensory and motor areas of the cortex; large doses depress the respiratory center in the medulla.

e. Morphine gives relief from pain by acting primarily on sensory areas in the cerebral cortex. Given in large doses, it causes respiratory depression.

Section II. SEDATIVE-HYPNOTICS

3-3. EFFECTS OF SEDATIVE-HYPNOTICS

A hypnotic, also called a soporific or somnifacient, is an agent that induces sleep. A sedative is an agent that produces relaxation, lessens excitement, and slows motor activity. However, a drug that falls into one of these categories generally falls into the other also and is thus called a sedative-hypnotic. The effect of a sedative-hypnotic depends on the dose. A small dose produces sedation; a large dose produces sleep. However, because of differences in duration of action, some of these drugs are preferable for use as hypnotics and others as sedatives. The effects that sedative-hypnotics produce depend to some extent on the traits of the particular client, but we can still give a description of the effects generally to be expected. Sedative-hypnotics are not useful as analgesics (pain-killers). The effect of a small dose is to produce sedation, a state of calmness in which the client tends to be less active and less responsive and possibly even sleepy. With a slightly greater dose, he tends to lose feelings of anxiety and inhibition, and lose some muscular coordination. His eyes may begin to move irregularly. If the dose is large enough, he will go to sleep. With a very large dose, he may enter a state similar to surgical anesthesia or die of respiratory depression. If large, but nonlethal doses are regularly given to a client for an extended period of time and then administration of the drug is discontinued, the client is likely to experience a withdrawal state in which he is hyperexcited and may even go into convulsions. Thus, sedative-hypnotics can cause physical dependence. There is a possibility of habituation (psychological dependence) with either small or large doses.

3-4. USES OF SEDATIVE-HYPNOTICS

a. **Situational Anxiety**. Anxiety is sometimes a normal response to a particular situation. If the situation is one in which a high level of physical or mental performance is necessary, a sedative--hypnotic may produce in the client a generalized feeling that he is performing well although his proficiency is, in fact, impaired. Nevertheless, there are situations in which sedative-hypnotics are valuable for reducing anxiety. One frequently recurring example is the use of a sedative-hypnotic to prepare a client for an unpleasant or painful medical or dental procedure.

b. **Neurotic Anxiety**. Neurotic anxiety is anxiety in which there is not an external situation sufficient to account for the dread and fear felt by the client. This anxiety is manifested in some clients as obsessive behavior, phobias (abnormal fears), depression, or excessive fatigability. Though sedative-hypnotics are useful in treating the symptoms of neurotic anxiety, they should never be used as a substitute for psychotherapy, where the client will not associate the administration of the drug too closely with relief of his anxiety, it is a good idea to use a longer-acting drug, such as phenobarbital, which does not have to be administered as frequently as some sedative-hypnotics. This helps reduce the likelihood of habituation, or psychological dependence.

c. **Induction of Sleep**. The pattern of a client's insomnia is important to the physician in determining how it should be treated. If the client has trouble only in going to sleep, a rapidly acting hypnotic which lasts only for a short time is desirable. A client who has trouble only in staying asleep or who has trouble in both going to sleep and staying asleep may be given an intermediate-acting hypnotic, or he may be given a short-acting hypnotic with instructions to take a second dose upon awakening. The intermediate-acting hypnotic carries with it the possibility of a hangover the next morning. (Sedative--hypnotics cannot be expected to induce sleep in clients experiencing severe pain.)

d. **Other Uses**. Some drugs, such as epinephrine, and some maladies, such as hyperthyroidism, cause excitement or hyperactivity that can be reduced by the use of sedative-hypnotics. Sedative-hypnotics are sometimes desirable to reduce the activity of a client; for example, a sedative-hypnotic may be used to make bed rest less frustrating. Sedative-hypnotics are sometimes used as muscle relaxants, anticonvulsants, and even general anesthetics.

3-5. SIDE EFFECTS

All of the sedative-hypnotics are capable of causing drowsiness, impaired judgment, and loss of coordination. These effects correspond to those of alcohol administered in amounts of comparable strength. In fact, alcohol and sedative-hypnotics have an additive effect in the body. The use of sedative-hypnotics, especially the long-acting ones, may be followed by a hangover, that is, a feeling of fatigue or grogginess. As previously mentioned, a withdrawal state may occur when a client is removed from a regimen of high doses given over an extended period. This withdrawal state corresponds to delirium tremens in alcoholics. It includes such symptoms as weakness, tremors, high blood pressure, fast breathing, fast pulse, and possibly convulsions, confusion, and hallucinations. Thus, it is possible to become physically dependent on sedative-hypnotics, as well as psychologically habituated to them. Tolerance to a nightly hypnotic dose does not usually develop to the point where increased doses are required. However, when these drugs are used continually as sedatives, tolerance may develop rapidly.

3-6. OVERDOSES OF SEDATIVE-HYPNOTICS

An intentional overdose of "sleeping pills" is frequently chosen as a means to commit suicide. When an individual ingests as little as eight times the hypnotic dose of a sedative-hypnotic, he may die of circulatory collapse or respiratory depression (slowing or cessation of breathing). However, if a client who has received even a very large overdose is given proper treatment soon after the overdose, he will probably not die. The lethal doses of the less potent sedative- hypnotics are so large that successful suicides are rare. The risk of death is greater if the person is under the influence of additional CNS depressants, such as alcohol.

3-7. SUMMARY OF INDIVIDUAL AGENTS

The use of barbiturates, a group of chemically related organic compounds, as sedative-hypnotics, began in 1903 with the introduction of barbital (Veronal). This was followed in 1912 by the introduction of phenobarbital (Luminal), still one of the most widely used CNS depressants. Today, out of about 50 barbiturates sold for clinical use, only about a dozen are widely used and a selected group of 5 or 6 is sufficient to meet the requirements of most prescribers. In addition, there are a number of nonbarbiturate sedative-hypnotics. These include the time-proven chloral hydrate and several newer drugs. (The nonbarbiturates discussed below are distinguishable from the barbiturates because the names of the barbiturates end with "-al.")

a. **Long-Acting Sedatives**. The long-acting sedatives have a duration of action of 6 to 8 hours. When used as hypnotics, they should induce a sleep of at least 4 to 6 hours, followed by a hangover.

(1) Phenobarbital (Luminal). This drug is widely used as a sedative. In addition, it is used to induce sleep and to treat the symptoms of epilepsy, particularly grand mal epilepsy. Most other barbiturates are not effective in the treatment of epilepsy. This drug is less expensive than the other long-acting sedatives discussed here, but in comparable doses its therapeutic effectiveness is at least equivalent.

(2) Chlordiazepoxide hydrochloride (Librium). A distinctive trait of chlordiazepoxide is the slowness with which it is excreted from the body; this gives it a longer duration of action than phenobarbital. Otherwise, its effects are similar to those of phenobarbital in comparable doses.

(3) Oxazepam (Serax). This drug is very similar to chlordiazepoxide above.

(4) Flurazepam (Dalmane). This drug is very similar to chlordiazepoxide.

b. **Intermediate-Acting Sedative-Hypnotics**. These drugs produce sedation for 4 to 6 hours. Like short-acting sedatives, these drugs have a greater potential for abuse than do the long-acting sedatives.

(1) Sodium amobarbital (Amytal Sodium). This drug is typical of the intermediate-acting sedative-hypnotics. Doses may be varied to produce anything from mild sedation to preanesthetic hypnosis.

(2) Meprobamate (Equanil; Miltown). This drug is nearly equivalent in its effects to amobarbital.

(3) Glutethimide (Doriden). A few clients experience convulsions while using this drug. When used as a hypnotic, glutethimide may cause a hangover.

(4) Diazepam (Valium). Though this drug is very similar chemically to chlordiazepoxide (Librium), its effect begins more quickly and its action is of shorter duration.

(5) Lorazepam (Ativan). This drug is chemically similar to both diazepam and chlordiazepoxide. It has a short duration of action and onset of action.

c. **Short-Acting Hypnotics**. The short-acting sedative-hypnotics are used almost exclusively as hypnotics. Since the duration of action is only 2 to 4 hours, a client using one of these drugs as a sedative might become psychologically dependent on it because of the frequency with which his anxiety or discomfort is rapidly relieved by taking it. An advantage of these short-acting drugs as hypnotics is that after a full night's sleep the client is likely to experience no hangover; the action of these drugs is completely exhausted after about 4 hours.

(1) Chloral hydrate. Sometimes, this old and very effective hypnotic is used as a sedative. However, it occasionally causes irritation of the stomach, and it should not be given to clients with serious heart, kidney, or liver disease.

(2) Paraldehyde. Paraldehyde is a very effective hypnotic, but it has an unpleasant taste and some of it is exhaled from the lungs of the client. This causes an odor more offensive to those dealing with the client than to the client himself. Since paraldehyde is infrequently used, care must be taken to avoid the use of deteriorated stock, which may be very acidic. Once opened, paraldehyde must be refrigerated.

(3) Sodium pentobarbital (Nembutal). Pentobarbital is the standard of the short-acting hypnotics.

(4) Sodium secobarbital (Seconal Sodium). Both sodium pentobarbital (above) and sodium secobarbital are effective short-acting hypnotics.

(5) Triazolam (Halcion). This drug is similar to chlordiazepoxide but has a short onset of action and short duration. Clients are less likely to experience hangover effects.

3-8. PHENOBARBITAL

a. **Action and Uses**. Phenobarbital is a long-acting barbiturate, requiring 30 to 60 minutes to become effective and acting over a period of 6 hours or more. The drug has many uses. It can be used as a sedative in times of mental stress or anxiety. It is often used in conditions such as hyperthyroidism, hypertension, peptic ulcer, and menopause. It is used as a hypnotic drug for insomnia and as an anticonvulsant in certain kinds of epilepsy.

b. **Administration**. The drug can be given orally, intramuscularly, or intravenously as indicated by the clinical situation. Unless there is specific indication for giving the drug parenterally, the oral route is preferred. The usual dose as a sedative is 16 to 32 mg. As a hypnotic, it is given in a dose of 100 mg. Dosage as an anticonvulsant varies with the needs of the client, but usually ranges from 16 mg to 64 mg.

c. **Untoward Effects**. Clients can become addicted to phenobarbital as they can to any potent sedative-hypnotic. This drug may exert a toxic effect upon the kidney, resulting in depressed kidney function. Overdosage may result in the typical symptoms of shock, respiratory complications (including respiratory failure), and kidney failure.

d. **Cautions and Contraindications**. Care must be taken not to give an overdose of the drug. The drug should not be used in clients with kidney disease.

e. **Supply**. Phenobarbital is supplied as 16-mg and 32-mg tablets; as a 1-ounce powder; as sodium phenobarbital injection in 2-ml ampules containing 162 mg per ml; and as a sterile powder in 125-mg ampules.

3-9. SODIUM SECOBARBITAL (SECONAL SODIUM)

a. **Action and Uses**. This drug is a short-acting barbiturate that becomes effective in 15 to 30 minutes and produces sleep lasting 2 to 4 hours. It is used in people who have difficulty in falling asleep, and as a preanesthetic agent.

b. **Administration**. The usual adult dose for treatment of insomnia is 100 mg given orally at bedtime. As a preanesthetic agent, 200 to 300 mg is given one to two hours before surgery.

c. **Cautions and Contraindications**. The drug should not be given to people who state they are allergic to it. Use of this drug may result in liver damage, since it is detoxified mainly by the liver. It should not be used on people with disorders of the liver.

d. **Supply**. The drug is supplied as 100-mg capsules.

3-10. SODIUM PENTOBARBITAL (NEMBUTAL)

a. **Action and Uses**. Since sodium pentobarbital and sodium secobarbital are both short-acting barbiturates, sodium pentobarbital has essentially the same actions and uses as sodium secobarbital, discussed above.

b. **Administration**. The usual hypnotic dose, oral or intravenous, is 100 mg.

c. **Cautions and Contraindications**. The cautions and contraindications are the same as with sodium secobarbital.

d. **Supply**. Sodium pentobarbital is supplied in 100-mg tablets and capsules. Sodium pentobarbital injection is supplied in 2-ml and 5-ml ampules containing 50 mg per ml.

3-11. DIAZEPAM (VALIUM)

a. **Action and Uses**. Diazepam is widely used as a daytime sedative. In addition, it has muscle relaxant properties and may be used to relieve muscle spasm (reflex spasm to muscle or joint inflammation or trauma), muscle spasticity (such as in cerebral palsy or paraplegia), athetosis, tetanus, and stiff-man syndrome. It can be used adjunctively in the treatment of convulsive disorders.

b. **Administration**. The usual oral dose is 2 to 10 mg, 2 to 4 times daily. The usual intramuscular or intravenous dose is 2 to 10 mg, repeated in 3-4 hours if necessary, but no more than 30 mg in an 8-hour period.

c. **Untoward Effects**. The untoward effects of diazepam are similar to those of other sedative-hypnotics. Skin rashes have also been reported.

d. **Supply**. Diazepam is supplied in 2 mg, 5 mg, and 10 mg tablets. Diazepam injection is supplied in 2 ml and 10 ml containers that contain 5 mg/ml.

Section III. ANTIPSYCHOTIC TRANQUILIZERS AND RELATED ANTIDEPRESSANTS

3-12. INTRODUCTION

The tranquilizers discussed in this section apparently stimulate the higher areas of the CNS to depress the lower areas and thus produce a tranquilizing effect. Sedatives, which are often called "tranquilizers" and which we discussed in the previous section, directly depress the CNS. To distinguish the type of tranquilizer discussed here from sedatives, we use the term antipsychotic tranquilizer or phenothiazine-type tranquilizer. These tranquilizers are used primarily in the treatment of psychoses, severe mental disorders. The sedative-hypnotics discussed previously are used to combat anxiety, but they are of little use in psychoses.

3-13. EFFECTS OF ANTIPSYCHOTIC TRANQUILIZERS

a. Unlike the sedative-hypnotics, some of the antipsychotic tranquilizers can cause convulsions when given in large doses. This is characteristic of CNS stimulants. However, in normal doses, these drugs produce a type of sedation in which the client is apathetic and unemotional but never as sedated as in anesthesia. Thus, an actively disturbed client would require less restraint after having received an antipsychotic tranquilizer. It is true, however, that a highly excited client might become a different type of problem upon receiving one of these drugs--that is, an immobile, inactive person. Nevertheless, these drugs are very useful. In addition to their use with actively disturbed clients, they can affect the thinking of unexcited schizophrenics as well.

b. Side effects of the synthetic antipsychotic tranquilizers (except reserpine) include dryness of the mouth, dilated eyes, lessening of near vision, constipation, and a fast pulse rate. The main group of antipsychotic tranquilizers, the phenothiazines, tend to cause a fall in body temperature except in the extremities; they dilate the blood vessels, which may produce hypotension or postural hypotension (low blood pressure which occurs when the client sits up or stands up). Some endocrine effects, such as a change in the menstrual cycle or lactation, may result.

c. The antipsychotic tranquilizers are neither habituating nor do they cause physical dependence. However, the sedative effects for a given dose decrease with prolonged use. That is, tolerance to the sedative effects (but not to the antipsychotic effects) develops rapidly. All in all, the experience of taking an antipsychotic tranquilizer is usually unpleasant to the client, since it makes him feel listless and easily fatigued.

3-14. TOXICITY CAUSED BY LARGE DOSES

In addition to the unpleasant side effects already discussed, there are other side effects that may result from the large doses of phenothiazine-type drugs ordinarily used. These include parkinsonism in which the muscles become rigid and there may be fine tremors. The degree of muscle rigidity may vary from impairment of facial expression to complete immobility of the body. Other effects may include dystonia (in which muscle tonicity is disordered) and akathisia (a feeling of restlessness). These effects -- parkinsonism, dystonia, and akathisia--are collectively called extrapyramidal effects. Other possible adverse effects of these drugs are dizziness, slate-colored pigmentation of the body and impaired vision (rarely). Allergic reactions to particular drugs may occur; for example, jaundice may result from the use of chlorpromazine.

3-15. THERAPEUTIC USES

The phenothiazine-type drugs are useful in controlling excited activity and hostile behavior in psychotic clients. In addition to sedation, these drugs produce other beneficial changes in the behavior of psychotics, including non-excited schizophrenics. Clinical records seem to indicate that schizophrenic clients tend to have a shorter stay in mental hospitals when they are given phenothiazine-type tranquilizers. These drugs are also useful in treating severe depression.

3-16. CHLORPROMAZINE HYDROCHLORIDE

a. **Action and Uses**. Chlorpromazine hydrochloride (Thorazine) acts to depress the central nervous system and to relieve the symptoms of nausea and vomiting. It is used to relieve anxiety, tension, and hyperactivity in psychotic and psychoneurotic clients. It is used to treat nausea and vomiting associated with recovery from an anesthetic, the action of certain drugs, radiation therapy, nitrogen mustard therapy, acute infections, cancer, and uremia. Also, it is used to relieve hiccups.

b. **Administration**. The drug may be given orally, intramuscularly, or intravenously. The usual oral dose is 25 to 100 mg. The usual parenteral dose for mild nausea and vomiting is 25 mg daily, given intramuscularly. For the severely disturbed manic client, dosage is much higher, up to 400 mg daily. Because this drug is irritating to tissue, it should be injected slowly, deep into the muscle. It is not to be given subcutaneously. The site should be massaged to help reduce local irritation.

c. **Untoward Effects**. Sedation and drowsiness are untoward effects in some instances, but in others they are the effects desired. Other side effects are dryness of the mouth, skin rash, sensitivity to light, nausea and vomiting, and nasal stuffiness. Low blood pressure may result, especially when the drug is given intravenously. Therefore, the client should remain in bed for an hour or two following parenteral administration. As a rule, these effects do not require that administration of the drug be stopped. Untoward effects that do require immediate stopping of the drug are the development of extrapyramidal effects (tremulousness, drooling, muscular rigidity, blank facial expression, and peculiar, stiff-legged gait), as well as jaundice, fever, sore throat, leukopenia (too few white blood cells), and anemia.

d. **Cautions and Contraindications**. The drug is not to be given to a comatose client. It should be used with caution when given with drugs that it potentiates (such as ethyl alcohol, morphine, and phenobarbital). Caution in its use should also be observed for clients in whom a sudden drop in blood pressure is considered dangerous. The drug should not be used on people who have liver disease.

e. **Supply**. Chlorpromazine hydrochloride is supplied in 25-mg, 50-mg, and 100-mg tablets; in 150-mg capsules; in 4-fl oz (118-ml) bottles of concentrated, flavored solution containing 30 mg per ml; and as a solution for injection containing 25 mg per ml in 2-ml ampules.

3-17. SUMMARY OF RELATED AGENTS

a. The following are phenothiazines with effects very similar to chlorpromazine:

(1) Promazine hydrochloride (Sparine Hydrochloride). The therapeutic effects of promazine hydrochloride seem to be identical to those of chlorpromazine hydrochloride, but the toxic effects are apparently less. However, the same degree of caution should be used.

(2) Thioridazine hydrochloride (Mellaril). This drug produces the same effects as chlorpromazine hydrochloride, except it does not have an antiemetic effect and it does not produce extrapyramidal effects (parkinsonism, dystonia, and akathisia) in ordinary doses.

b. The drugs listed here tend to have more pronounced extrapyramidal and antiemetic effects than other antipsychotic tranquilizers.

(1) Trifluoperazine hydrochloride (Stelazine Hydrochloride).

(2) Perphenazine (Trilafon).

(3) Haloperidol (Haldol).

c. Promethazine hydrochloride (Phenergan), discussed elsewhere with the antihistamines, has antihistaminic and highly sedative properties, which are sometimes employed to enhance the action of analgesics given concurrently. It may be used for sedation both before and after an operation.

d. The following two mildly sedative drugs are used mainly on senile clients. They are used to relieve headaches and muscle spasms and in conjunction with other drugs to treat arthritis and angina pectoris.

(1) Hydroxyzine hydrochloride (Atarax).

(2) Hydroxyzine pamoate (Vistaril).

e. In addition to their use as antipsychotic tranquilizers, the following drugs are also used as antiemetics to control mild or severe nausea and vomiting:

(1) Prochlorperazine maleate (Compazine). The antiemetic effects of this drug are equal to those of a dose of chlorpromazine five times as large. The side effects are generally mild; extrapyramidal symptoms may occur, but they can usually be relieved by reduction of the dose, concurrent administration of an antiparkinsonism drug, or temporary withdrawal of the drug. Prochlorperazine edisylate (Compazine Ethanedisulfonate) can be injected IM, as well as given orally. Prochlorperazine (Compazine) suppositories are given rectally.

(2) Thiethylperazine maleate (Torecan). This weakly tranquilizing agent is used to treat nausea and vomiting.

f. Trimeprazine tartrate (Temaril) has both antipruritic and tranquilizing properties. An antipruritic is a drug that relieves or prevents itching.

3-18. RELATED ANTIDEPRESSANTS

The drugs listed below are pharmacologically similar to the group of antipsychotic tranquilizers called phenothiazines, but they are used in less potent doses to improve the state of mind of severely depressed clients. The side effects, also similar, may include dry mouth, constipation, weakened bladder, blurred vision, and increased pressure within the eye. Allergies may be revealed by symptoms such as skin rash and itching. Orthostatic hypotension (postural hypotension), low blood pressure when the client sits up or stands up, may occur. The client may feel weak and drowsy. Doses of these drugs, at first smaller than ordinary, are gradually built up until therapeutic effects are observed or the maximum dose is reached. Usually, it takes 1-3 weeks to observe any improvement in a severely depressed client. Therapy may continue as long as 3 months, after which the drug should be gradually withdrawn. These drugs probably do not cause physical dependence.

a. Amitriptyline Hydrochloride (Elavil Hydrochloride). This drug can be given at bedtime since it has a significant sedative effect.

b. Imipramine Hydrochloride (Tofranil).

c. Desipramine Hydrochloride (Norpramin; Pertofrane).

d. Nortriptyline Hydrochloride (Aventyl).

Section IV. NARCOTIC ANALGESICS

3-19. EFFECTS OF NARCOTIC ANALGESICS

Morphine is the standard of comparison for all addictive, or narcotic, analgesics (painkillers). Morphine is an ingredient of opium, which in its crude state is a sticky brown gum from a particular type of poppy. Though addiction to morphine and its derivatives, particularly to illegal heroin, is a serious social problem, morphine and its derivatives are essential to the practice of medicine. Heroin, however, is not used for therapeutic applications.

a. **Analgesia**. The first reactions to morphine are muscle relaxation and perhaps euphoria, a general feeling of well being. The pain-killing effects of morphine are of three different types. The first of these is an indifference to perceived pain. Though the client is aware of a pain, he does not react with fright, anxiety, or action. This effect has been compared to a temporary prefrontal lobotomy. The second source of relief is an actual reduction of perceived pain. Morphine does this by raising the "threshold" to pain stimuli so that a stimulus must be of greater intensity to be perceived. Thus, morphine is more effective against continuous pains than against intermittently sharp pains (which are occasionally great enough to get past the threshold raised by the morphine). Third, if the morphine is in a large enough dose, the client will become lethargic and perhaps go to sleep.

b. **Respiratory Depression**. Morphine slows the rate of breathing. In the case of an overdose, breathing may cease altogether, with death soon following.

c. **Nausea**. Soon after the drug is administered, the client may experience nausea. Morphine stimulates the vomiting center during its onset of action and thereafter depresses it. If the client vomits, he usually does so without great emotion or discomfort.

d. **Antitussive Action**. Morphine depresses the cough reflex.

e. **Postural Hypotension**. When the client sits up or stands up, he may experience the effects of low blood pressure. That is, he may become dizzy and even faint. This is called postural hypotension or orthostatic hypotension.

f. **Constipation**. Since morphine has a constipating effect, paregoric, which contains opium, is used to treat diarrhea.

g. **Miosis**. Morphine causes the pupils to contract.

3-20. TOLERANCE, ADDICTION, AND HABITUATION

a. Tolerance is the condition which develops after the continued use of a drug and which requires the use of progressively larger doses of the drug to achieve the same effect. Tolerance does not occur with all drugs, but it does occur with narcotic analgesics. Tolerance is not the same as addiction.

b. Addiction (physical dependence) occurs when a drug must be present in the body to maintain physiological balance. If administration of the drug stops, the individual experiences a withdrawal state. A withdrawal state is characterized by excitement, anxiety, nasal discharge, sweating, and goose-flesh, and -- in the case of severe withdrawal state -- pain in the muscles, joints, abdomen, fever, and even convulsions. Normally, this severe degree of withdrawal is seen only in addicts who have been unable to make a "connection" or who have been put in prison. In a controlled situation, when the client has been receiving narcotics for valid medical reasons, withdrawal is usually mild, and the client usually does not even realize the source of his discomfort. (Once an addict has endured the withdrawal state, however, he is still not free from his compulsion to use narcotics. In fact, the typical addict lives a life in which he repeatedly withdraws and returns to the use of narcotics.)

c. Habituation is a psychological dependence on drugs. We have seen how individuals may become habituated to the use of sedatives because they mentally associate relief from anxiety with the administration of the sedative. When the addict injects heroin, he experiences a pleasurable "rush." The addict, even after withdrawal, may be convinced that the use of heroin is essential to a feeling of well being, that without it he is unable to cope with his life and environment. (The addict typically has serious anxieties related to pain, sexuality, and feelings of aggression.) These factors may cause the addict to remain psychologically dependent on, that is, habituated to, narcotics even when he is no longer physically dependent on them.

3-21. CAUTIONS FOR THE USE OF NARCOTIC ANALGESICS

a. One of the main contraindications for the use of narcotic analgesics is a client's lack of sufficient respiratory reserve to withstand the respiratory depressions caused by narcotic analgesics. This is especially true of clients with emphysema, kyphoscoliosis (in which the spine is curved backwards or to the side), corpulmonale (heart disease secondary to lung disease), and sometimes extreme obesity.

b. Extreme caution should be used when treating clients who have asthma, impaired liver function, or a low volume of blood.

c. It is generally unwise to treat migraine or arthritis with narcotic analgesics since these maladies are chronic and thus increase the possibility of addiction. However, narcotic analgesics are useful in relieving the pains of terminal cancer, but they should be used in doses as small as practicable with as long a delay as possible between doses. This extends the period over which the drug is effective.

3-22. MORPHINE

a. **Action and Uses**. Morphine, which is the most potent of the drugs derived from opium, is a powerful central nervous system depressant, having a selective action on respiration and pain sensation. These functions are greatly reduced by amounts of morphine that have only moderate effect upon general consciousness. The drug exerts a narcotic action manifested by analgesia, drowsiness, changes in mood, and mental clouding. The relief of pain following administration of morphine is often accompanied by euphoria. The combined properties of pain relief and euphoria make morphine a useful drug for relieving severe heart pain. Morphine also exerts an antidiarrheal action, but it is not used in the treatment of diarrhea. The opiate used for this purpose is paregoric.

b. **Indications for Morphine**. Only when simple measures fail and severe pain continues, or when a severely injured person must be moved quickly (as from a wrecked vehicle or aircraft) or in the event of a heart attack, is it wise to give morphine at once. However, if the use of morphine is indicated, it should be given without hesitation. Its ability to stop pain may be lifesaving. Severe pain can increase the severity of shock, and shock is deadly.

c. **Administration**. The drug is most often given parenterally. The usual dose for adults is 10 mg, 4 to 6 times a day as necessary. The dose given, route of administration, and the time should be entered on the client's record immediately after the drug is given.

d. **Untoward Effects**. Whenever morphine is administered, a number of toxic effects may occur, the most severe and dangerous of which is depression of respiration. This reaction is especially likely in people with asthma and other chronic bronchial conditions. Naloxone hydrochloride (Narcan), discussed later in this section, may be given as directed for the treatment of depressed respiration. Other reactions include vomiting (which results from the stimulation of the vomiting center in the brain), dryness of the mouth, constipation, urinary retention, and possibly physical dependence upon the drug.

e. **Morphine Poisoning**. Acute morphine poisoning results from an over dosage of the drug. A delayed type of morphine poisoning may occur from the intramuscular injection of the drug into chilled skin areas, burned clients, or into clients with low blood pressure and shock. In such clients, the drug is incompletely absorbed or its absorption is delayed; therefore, the client may continue to complain of pain, and an additional dose may be given. When the circulation is improved, an excessive amount of morphine may suddenly be absorbed.

(1) Symptoms. When coma, depressed respiration, and pinpoint pupils appear concurrently in a client who has been given morphine, it is likely that he has morphine poisoning. The client is usually asleep or stuporous; he may be in a profound coma if the overdose is large. The respiratory rate is very low, sometimes only 2 to 4 per minute, and the client may be cyanotic. The blood pressure is normal at first, then falls progressively. The pupils are pinpoint in size, unless oxygen depletion is severe; in that case, they will be dilated. Urine formation is depressed; body temperature falls; and the skin becomes cold and clammy. The skeletal muscles are lax and soft, the jaw is relaxed, and the tongue may fall back and block the airway.

(2) Treatment. The prompt restoration of normal respiration is of first importance, since death in morphine poisoning is nearly always because respiratory failure. The client's airway must be kept open, and artificial respiration is too slow to provide adequate oxygenation. Naloxone may be given as directed to treat the respiratory depression. Cold towels may be used to keep the client awake. If the client has taken the morphine orally, he may be treated with emetics and gastric lavage. A careful record of the client's intake and output should be made, because overdosage of morphine may damage the kidneys and cause suppression of urine. After the danger has passed, a laxative may be indicated to relieve constipation.

f. **Cautions and Contraindications**. There are a number of contraindications to the use of morphine, as follows:

(1) Abdominal pain. A person's life may depend upon the correct diagnosis of abdominal disease, and pain is an important symptom. Relief of pain causes the true picture of the symptoms to become blurred. A diagnosis made on this basis may not be accurate. Therefore, morphine should not be given for any undiagnosed abdominal condition.

(2) Injuries of the head. Morphine is contraindicated because it distorts the symptom picture and interferes with diagnosis. Morphine also causes an increase in intracranial pressure.

(3) Chest injuries or depressed respiration. Morphine should not be given to anyone with a chest injury, or whose respiratory rate is under 12 per minute. In such a case, the drug would cause further respiratory depression, and this might be fatal.

(4) Unconsciousness. Morphine is contraindicated when the person is unconscious.

(5) A prior dose of morphine. A dose of morphine never should be repeated within 2 hours. It should not be repeated at all, unless necessary to control pain. It should not be repeated if there is any reason to believe that the first dose has not been absorbed. Sometimes when a client is in shock, his circulation is so poor that injected drugs are not absorbed. If a dose of morphine is repeated in such a case, both injections will be absorbed at once when circulation is restored, and morphine poisoning will result.

(6) Pending surgery. If there is a possibility that the client may soon be operated on, morphine should not be given, unless ordered by a medical officer. Morphine and surgical anesthesia both act to depress the respiration.

(7) Sedative. Morphine should not be used as a sedative in the treatment of anxiety, fear, or hysteria.

(8) Walking wounded. Morphine should not be given in the field to walking wounded. The drug will cause some to become confused and nauseated, and will increase disability in other ways.

(9) Shock. Morphine should not be used in shock, unless severe pain is present and is retarding the effect of shock treatment. If morphine is ordered for a client in shock, it should be given intravenously (by a medical officer) rather than intramuscularly.

(10) Liver disease. Morphine should not be given to persons with hepatic (liver) disease or infection.

g. **Supply**. Morphine injection is supplied in sterile cartridge- needle units containing 8, 10, and 15 mg of the drug. This form of issue should be protected from freezing, and in addition, the date on the package should be checked, since this drug is subject to deterioration in 24 months or less. Available for field use is a collapsible tube with needle attached (syrette), containing 16 mg of the drug (figure 3-1).

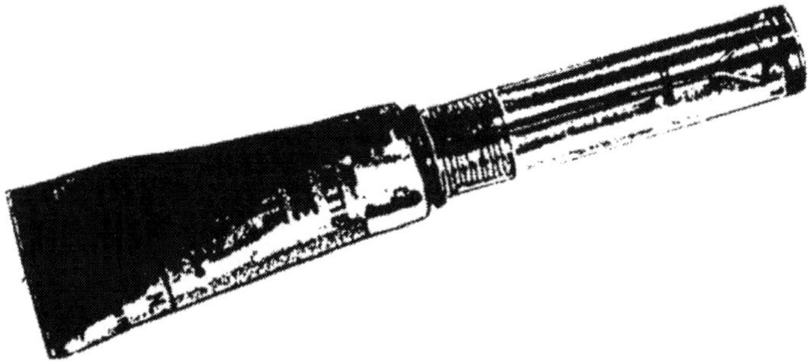

Figure 3-1. Morphine syrette.

3-23. CODEINE

a. **Action and Uses**. Codeine, also derived from opium, exerts a narcotic action similar to that of morphine, though far less potent. When codeine is given concurrently with aspirin, its analgesic effect is greatly enhanced. Besides its analgesic activity, codeine has a selective action on the cough center and is often used as an antitussive, especially for the relief of nonproductive coughs.

b. **Administration**. For analgesia, codeine is given in a dose of 30 to 60 mg orally every 4 to 6 hours. As an antitussive, it is used in a dose of 15 to 30 mg orally every 4 to 6 hours.

c. **Untoward Effects**. Toxic reactions that occur with the use of codeine and with over dosage of codeine are the same as those that occur with morphine, but they are less severe. The treatment of such reactions is as described for the treatment of morphine poisoning.

d. **Cautions and Contraindications**. Codeine is an addicting drug, though it is less addicting than morphine. The same cautions and contraindications should be observed as those observed with the use of morphine.

e. **Supply**. Both codeine phosphate and codeine sulfate are supplied in injection and solution forms. Further, codeine is marketed in combination with aspirin as Empirin with Codeine #2, #3, and #4. Codeine is also combined with Tylenol in the products Tylenol with Codeine #1, #2, #3, and #4.

3-24. MEPERIDINE HYDROCHLORIDE

a. **Action and Uses**. Meperidine (Demerol) is a synthetic narcotic analgesic drug. Its analgesic properties are excellent, but it is not useful for the treatment of cough. It has a shorter duration of action than morphine, and this feature makes it preferable to morphine in certain clinical situations. These include certain diagnostic procedures, such as cystoscopy, retrograde pyelography, and gastroscopy. In addition, meperidine may be used as a preanesthetic medication, and in obstetrical analgesia. It is generally not used as an antidiarrheal or antitussive.

b. **Administration**. The usual dose of meperidine is 50 to 100 mg, given orally or by intramuscular injection, 4 to 6 times daily.

c. **Untoward Effects**. Some untoward effects that may occur after therapeutic doses of meperidine include dizziness, sweating, flushing of the skin, dryness of the mouth, constipation, and nausea and vomiting. Over dosage with this drug may result in severe respiratory depression and coma, or it may produce tremors and convulsions; the treatment is that described for treatment of over dosage with morphine.

d. **Cautions and Contraindications**. This drug is addicting and should be used with the same caution that is necessary with the opiates. The contraindications to the use of the drug are the same as those for morphine.

e. **Supply**. Meperidine hydrochloride is supplied as 50-mg tablets, in 30-ml vials containing 50 mg per ml, and in cartridge- needle units in a size of 1 or 2 ml, both sizes containing only 1 ml of solution. The strength of the solutions in either size may be 50 mg, 75 mg, or 100 mg per ml. The use of the cartridge-needle units requires the precautions cited previously. The period of potency of the drug in these units is 24 months.

3-25. PROPOXYPHENE HYDROCHLORIDE

a. **Action and Uses**. Propoxyphene (Darvon) is chemically and pharmacologically related to a narcotic called methadone. It possesses analgesic properties, but not anti-inflammatory or antipyretic effects. It is indicated for mild to moderate pain, but its superiority to aspirin for relief of pain is questionable.

b. **Usual Dosage**. The usual dosage is 65 mg, 3 to 4 times daily as needed for pain.

c. **Cautions and Warnings**.

(1) This preparation may impair the mental and/or physical abilities required to drive a car or operate machinery, especially during the first few days of therapy.

(2) This drug should be used cautiously in pregnant women and children due to the fact that adequate data on safety with these clients is lacking.

(3) Clients who receive this product for long periods of time may develop physical dependence, psychological dependence, and tolerance.

(4) Clients who have received other narcotic drugs for long periods of time may have developed physical dependence, and the sudden substitution of propoxyphene may cause acute withdrawal symptoms, because of the fact that propoxyphene will not support dependence upon other narcotics.

d. **Adverse Reactions**.

(1) Nausea, vomiting, sedation, dizziness, constipation, and skin rash are the more common adverse reactions.

(2) Development of morphine-type drug dependence has been reported.

(3) Excessive doses may cause confusion, muscle fasciculations, respiratory depression, coma, or convulsions.

(4) Euphoria may occur.

e. **Treatment of Overdosage**. Naloxone hydrochloride (Narcan), discussed later, is the specific antidote for propoxyphene.

f. **Supply**. This drug is supplied in 32 and 65 mg (Darvon) capsules and in propoxyphene hydrochloride, aspirin, and caffeine (Darvon Compound) capsules, which contain 389 mg of aspirin, 32 mg of propoxyphene hydrochloride, and 32.4 mg of caffeine.

3-26. NALOXONE HYDROCHLORIDE INJECTION--NARCOTIC ANTAGONIST

a. **Action and Uses**. Naloxone (Narcan) is a nonagonist or complete antagonist which will reverse most of the effects of narcotics, including respiratory depression, without the risk of producing agonistic or morphine effects of its own. It is indicated for the complete or partial reversal of narcotic depression, including respiratory depression, induced by:

(1) Natural and synthetic narcotics.

(2) The narcotic-antagonist analgesic, pentazocine (Talwin).

(3) Propoxyphene (Darvon).

NOTE: Naloxone may also be used for the diagnosis of suspected acute opiate overdosage.

b. **Administration**. In an emergency, Naloxone should be administered intravenously at a dosage of 0.01 mg/kg of body weight (about 0.8 mg) for an adult. The onset of action of naloxone IV is within 2 to 3 minutes. This dose may be repeated once or twice at 5-minute intervals. This drug may also be administered IM or SC. Failure to obtain significant improvement after 2 or 3 doses suggests that the condition may be due partly or completely to other disease processes or non-narcotic drugs. (In the newborn, naloxone in 10 to 15 mcg/kg doses may be injected directly into the umbilical vein, if the newborn shows evidence of narcotic-induced respiratory depression.)

c. **Cautions and Warnings**.

(1) In addition to naloxone, other resuscitative measures such as maintenance of a free airway, artificial ventilation, cardiac massage, and vasopressor agents should be employed when necessary to counteract acute narcotic poisoning.

(2) Naloxone may precipitate acute withdrawal symptoms in clients physically dependent on narcotics.

(3) Repeated doses of naloxone may be necessary since the duration of action of some narcotics (that is, methadone) may exceed that of naloxone.

(4) Naloxone is not effective against respiratory depressions that is, to nonnarcotic drugs.

(5) Naloxone will not produce tolerance nor cause physical or psychological dependence.

d. **Supply**. Naloxone is available in 1-ml ampules containing 0.4 mg of naloxone hydrochloride.

Section V. NONADDICTIVE ANALGESICS AND ANTIPYRETICS

3-27. INTRODUCTION

a. **Analgesics**. An analgesic is a drug that relieves pain without causing a loss of consciousness; nonaddictive analgesics raise the threshold to pain stimuli. The threshold is the degree of intensity a stimulus must have in order to be perceived. (A local anesthetic is not considered an analgesic; it works by preventing the conduction of nerve impulses, which would be perceived as pain by the CNS. A general anesthetic is not an analgesic; it works by stopping consciousness.) Some analgesics relieve only specific types of pain, for example, integumental pain, characterized by its sharp, piercing quality, or visceral pain, which is dull, burning, and aching, and tends to depress the person.

b. **Antipyretics**. An antipyretic is an agent that is capable of lowering abnormally high body temperatures. That is, antipyretics are useful in relieving fever. They do not greatly affect the body temperature when it is already normal. Most of the nonaddictive analgesics have antipyretic effects.

c. **Anti-inflammatory Agents**. Many of the nonaddictive analgesics also have anti-inflammatory effects. That is, they reduce inflammation occurring in such maladies as rheumatoid arthritis and rheumatic fever.

3-28. ASPIRIN

A common name for aspirin is ASA (acetylsalicylic acid).

a. **Action and Uses**. Aspirin is the drug of choice when a mild analgesic is needed. It is useful in treating headache, neuralgia (paroxysmal pain, extending along the course of a nerve or nerves), myalgia (muscle pain), arthralgia (joint pain), and other pains arising from integumental structures. It is also useful in relieving the discomfort of dysmenorrhea (painful menstruation), sore throat, toothache, and influenza. It is an effective anti-inflammatory agent for acute rheumatic fever, rheumatoid arthritis, and degenerative joint disease. It is an effective antipyretic agent. Uricosuric effects (excretion of uric acid) may be achieved with daily doses of 5-6 grams.

b. **Usual Dosage**. The usual adult oral dose is 0.3-1.0 gm, 4-6 times a day, as necessary.

c. **Adverse Effects**. Irritation of the gastric mucosa is common. Peptic ulceration, blood loss sufficient to cause iron-deficiency anemia, and massive gastrointestinal hemorrhage occur rarely. Dyspepsia, nausea, vomiting, and occult bleeding are the most common adverse effects with ordinary doses. During therapy with large doses of salicylates for prolonged periods, salicylism may occur; it is characterized by nausea, vomiting, tinnitus, decrease in auditory acuity, dizziness, sweating, thirst, and confusion. A small number of clients are hypersensitive to aspirin, and ordinary doses may cause skin eruptions, urticaria, or asthmatic-type anaphylactoid reactions.

d. **Overdosage**. Serious intoxication usually follows the ingestion of at least 1 grain per pound of body weight (about 150-175 mg/kg). Toxicity is characterized by hyperthermia, CNS stimulation followed by depression and coma, acid-base disturbances, hypoprothrombinemia, and gastroenteritis. Respiratory alkalosis appears first, followed by metabolic acidosis. The minimum lethal dose (M.L.D.) is 5-10 grams.

e. **Treatment of Overdosage**.

(1) Obtain a blood pH to determine acid-base balance.

(2) Treat dehydration and alkalosis with normal saline and potassium as indicated.

(3) Metabolic acidosis can be corrected with fluids and adequate sodium bicarbonate as determined by blood pH.

(4) Perform gastric lavage if client is received within 4 hours after ingestion.

(5) Vitamin K, 50 mg IV, should be administered for hypothrobinemia.

(6) Treat fever with tepid water sponge baths.

(7) Short-acting barbiturates should be given cautiously, if convulsions occur.

(8) Support respiration.

(9) In presence of cardiovascular collapse, maintain blood pressure with fluids.

f. **Cautions and Warnings**.

(1) Aspirin is contraindicated or should be used with caution in clients with hemorrhagic tendencies, diabetes, gastric ulcer, gastrointestinal irritation, and hepatic disease.

(2) Aspirin should not be given concurrently with coumarin, since it will prolong the prothrombin time.

(3) In sensitive clients or when prolonged high doses of aspirin are required, gastric irritation can be reduced by using enteric-coated tablets such as Ecotrin, designed to dissolve in the intestine.

(4) Gastrointestinal effects may be reduced or eliminated by taking aspirin with food, milk, or a full glass of water.

(5) Children and teenagers should not use aspirin (salicylates) for chickenpox or flu-like symptoms before a doctor is consulted about Reyes Syndrome, a rare but serious illness.

g. **Supply**. Aspirin is available in 80 mg tablets for pediatric use and in 325 mg tablets. It is also available in 325 mg enteric-coated (Ecotrin) tablets, 325 mg suppositories, and in various combinations such as aspirin with codeine (Ascodeen) and aspirin with magnesium oxide and aluminum hydroxide (CAMA).

3-29. ACETAMINOPHEN

a. **Action and Uses**. Acetaminophen (Tempra; Tylenol; APAP) is a mild analgesic used for temporary relief of minor muscular aches and pains, headache myalgia, arthralgia, dysmenorrhea, and discomfort and fever associated with common cold and viral infections. It is the mild analgesic of choice in clients allergic or sensitive to aspirin, ulcer clients, and clients receiving an anticoagulant or a uricosuric agent, such as probenecid. Acetaminophen does not possess anti-inflammatory or uricosuric action.

b. **Usual Dosage**. The usual dosage is 325 to 650 mg, every 4-6 hours as needed, not to exceed 2.6 grams per 24-hour period. The pediatric dose is as follows (see Table 3-1).

0-3 months	40 mg
4-11 months	80 mg
1-2 years	120 mg
2-3 years	160 mg
4-5 years	240 mg
6-8 years	320 mg
9-10 years	400 mg
11 years	480 mg

Table 3-1. Pediatric dose of Acetaminophen.

c. **Adverse Effects**. Gastrointestinal irritation is negligible. Prolonged administration may cause methemoglobinemia and other abnormal pigmentation, hemolytic anemia, and with large doses, hepatic toxicity.

d. **Cautions and Warnings**.

(1) Do not exceed the recommended dosage. Consult a physician for use in children under three years or for oral use longer than 10 days.

(2) Chronic daily ingestions have resulted in liver damage.

e. **Supply**. Acetaminophen is supplied as an elixir, containing 160 mg per 5 ml; as a 10 percent solution in a bottle for pediatric use, supplied with a dropper calibrated at 0.6 ml; as 325 mg and 500 mg tablets, and as 120 mg, 325 mg, and 650 mg suppositories.

Section VI. CNS STIMULANTS

3-30. INTRODUCTION

In this lesson, we have discussed many drugs that are depressant to the CNS. There are many more that we did not mention. Drugs that are used to stimulate the CNS, on the other hand, are few in number. They stimulate various portions of the CNS and differ in site and mechanism of action. They are not employed exclusively as CNS stimulants because they have many other actions. The CNS can be stimulated only for a brief period, because the excitation is soon followed by depression.

3-31. AMPHETAMINES

The amphetamines are discussed in this subcourse primarily because of their drug abuse potential.

a. **Action and Uses**. The amphetamines are sympathomimetic amines with potent CNS stimulant properties. The amphetamines have a significant potential for abuse. They should be used with extreme caution and only for limited periods of time in weight reduction programs. The amphetamines are indicated only in the following situations:

(1) Attention deficit-hyperactivity disorder (AD-HD), formerly called minimal brain dysfunction in children.

(2) Narcolepsy.

(3) In exogenous obesity, as a short-term (a few weeks) adjunct in a regimen of weight reduction based on caloric restriction.

b. **Usual Dosage of Dextroamphetamine Sulfate**.

(1) Narcolepsy: 5-60 mg in divided doses.

(2) Attention deficit-hyperactivity disorder: Not recommended in children under 3 years of age. For children 3-5 years of age: 2.5 mg daily, increased in increments of 2.5 mg weekly, until optimum response is obtained. For children 6 years of age and older: Ten mg once or twice daily, increased in increments of 10 mg weekly until optimum response is obtained.

(3) Obesity: 5-30 mg per day in divided doses.

c. **Adverse Effects**.

(1) Cardiovascular: Palpitation, tachycardia, elevation of blood pressure.

(2) CNS: Overstimulation, restlessness, dizziness, insomnia, euphoria, dysphoria, tremor, headache; rarely, psychotic reactions at therapeutic doses.

(3) Other: Dryness of mouth, unpleasant taste, diarrhea, urticaria, impotence, changes in libido.

d. **Overdosage**. Restlessness, confusion, assaultiveness00, hallucinations, and panic states are manifestations of acute poisoning. Fatigue and depression usually follow the central stimulation. Cardiovascular effects such as arrhythmias, hypertension or hypotension, and circulatory collapse may be seen. Fatal poisoning usually terminates in convulsions and coma.

e. **Treatment of Overdosage**.

(1) Lavage, if drug has been orally ingested, and sedate with a barbiturate or diazepam (Valium).

(2) Maintain a high volume of acid urine.

(3) Use saline cathartic if the drug has been orally ingested.

(4) Give artificial respiration if cyanosis is present.

(5) Maintain blood pressure with fluids in the presence of cardiovascular collapse.

(6) Administer as an alternative chlorpromazine (Thorazine), 1 mg/kg IM for sedation.

f. **Cautions and Warnings**.

(1) Amphetamines are contraindicated in advanced arteriosclerosis, symptomatic cardiovascular disease, moderate to severe hypertension, hyperthyroidism, and known hypersensitivity or idiosyncracy to the sympathomimetic amines.

(2) Do not administer to clients with a history of drug abuse.

(3) Do not use during or within 14 days following the administration of MAO inhibitors.

(4) Tolerance to anorectic (appetite-reducing) effect usually develops within a few weeks.

(5) Amphetamines may impair the ability of the client to engage in potentially hazardous activities.

(6) Tolerance and extreme psychological dependence have occurred.

(7) Abrupt cessation following prolonged high dosage results in extreme fatigue and mental depression.

(8) Manifestations of chronic intoxication include severe skin diseases, marked insomnia, irritability, hyperactivity, and personality changes, including psychosis often clinically indistinguishable from schizophrenia.

(9) Amphetamines are not recommended for pregnant women. Annual studies have suggested that the amphetamines are potentially embryotoxic and teratogenic (tending to produce physical defects in the developing embryo).

(10) Amphetamines may decrease the hypotensive effect of guanethidine.

3-32. SPECIFIC AMPHETAMINES AND RELATED PREPARATIONS

a. Amphetamine Sulfate (Benzedrine).

b. Dextroamphetamine Sulfate (Dexedrine).

c. Methamphetamine Hydrochloride (Desoxyn, Methedrine).

d. Methylphenidate Hydrochloride (Ritalin).

e. Diethylpropion Hydrochloride (Tenuate; Tepanil).

f. Phenmetrazine Hydrochloride (Preludin).

g. Chlorphentermine (Pre-Sate).

Continue with Exercises

EXERCISES, LESSON 3

Answer the following exercises by marking the lettered response that best answers the question or completes the incomplete statement.

After you have completed all of these exercises, turn to "Solutions to Exercises" at the end of the lesson and check your answers. For each exercise answered incorrectly, reread the material referenced with the solution.

1. What factor determines whether a sedative-hypnotic is more useful as a sedative or more useful as a hynotic?

   a. Its length of action.

   b. Its potency per milligram.

   c. The rapidity with which it takes effect.

   d. Its specific effect on the electric currents in the brain.

2. What effect should a moderate dose of a sedative-hypnotic have on the performance of a student taking a difficult examination?

   a. Immediate sleep.

   b. Improved performance due to enhanced powers of concentration.

   c. Unjustified feeling of performing well.

   d. No effect.

3. When a client is being treated for neurotic anxiety with a sedative, why is a long--acting sedative usually preferred?

   a. To avoid psychological dependence on the drug.

   b. To avoid the troublesome labor of frequently administering a drug.

   c. To restore the client's confidence in himself.

   d. To utilize the greater potency of long-acting sedatives.

4. A dose of a long-acting sedative sufficient to induce sleep is given to a client. In the morning, he is likely to experience:

   a. A hangover.

   b. Delirium tremens.

   c. A withdrawal state.

   d. Fears of persecution.

5. Comparable doses of the drugs below produce similar sedative effects. Which of these long-acting sedatives is the least expensive?

   a. Chlordiazepoxide.

   b. Oxazepam.

   c. Phenobarbital.

   d. Dichlorobenzamine.

6. Which of the following is a contraindication for phenobarbital?

   a. Psychosis.

   b. Epilepsy.

   c. Pregnancy.

   d. Kidney disease.

7. Two effective short-acting hypnotics are:

   a. Diazepam and chlordiazepoxide.

   b. Amobarbital and meprobamate.

   c. Secobarbital and pentobarbital.

   d. Phenobarbital and oxazepam.

8. To the client, the overall effects of a phenothiazine are:

   a. Intolerable.

   b. Unpleasant.

   c. Imperceptible.

   d. Pleasurable.

9. Which of the following is a drug used specifically, but not solely, in the therapy of psychotic clients?

   a. Chlorpromazine.

   b. Diazepam.

   c. Pentobarbital.

   d. Phenobarbital.

10. Which of the following drugs is NOT used clinically?

    a. Codeine.

    b. Heroin.

    c. Morphine.

    d. Opium.

11. Which of the following is NOT a significant pain-alleviating effect attributable to morphine?

    a. Hypnotic effect.

    b. Less objection to perceived pain.

    c. Reduction of perceived pain.

    d. Reduction of pain-generating toxins.

12. What effect does morphine have on respiration?

    a. Depression.

    b. Stimulation.

    c. Increase in muscular tone.

    d. Occurrence of rhythmic irregularities.

13. Which of the following drugs tends to constipate?

    a. Aspirin.

    b. Diazepam.

    c. Paregoric.

    d. Phenobarbital.

14. A client in a hospital has been receiving moderate doses of a narcotic analgesic regularly for therapeutic purposes. When the pain for which it has been administered has ceased and the drug is discontinued, the probable result will be:

    a. Postural hypotension.

    b. Convulsions.

    c. Angry demands for more narcotics.

    d. Discomfort, with the cause unknown to the client.

15. Which of the following does NOT contribute to the tendency of heroin to produce psychological dependence?

    a. Anxieties about sex, aggression, and pain.

    b. Feelings of inability to survive emotionally without narcotics.

    c. The need for increasingly large doses to maintain physiological balance.

    d. A pleasurable surge immediately after injection.

16. A client in shock who is given intramuscular injections of morphine may suffer which of the following, as a result of the injection.

    a. Morphine poisoning.

    b. Heart attack.

    c. Anemia.

    d. Damaged peripheral circulation.

17. A client who has been given morphine is presumed to have morphine poisoning whenever there is concurrent appearance of coma, depressed respiration, and:

    a. Flushed face.

    b. Pinpoint pupils.

    c. Cyanosis.

    d. Vomiting.

18. Morphine should NOT be used in the treatment of emergency clients whose symptoms include:

    a. c, d, e, or f below.

    b. d, e, or f below.

    c. Pain in abdomen.

    d. Head injury.

    e. Chest injury.

    f. Unconsciousness.

19. When codeine is used as an antitussive, the single dose falls within a range of:

a. 2--4 mg.

b. 15--30 mg.

c. 32--64 mg.

d. 0.25--0.5 gm.

20. The oral analgesic dose of codeine is:

a. 2--4 mg.

b. 15--30 mg.

c. 30--60 mg.

d. 0.25--0.5 gm.

21. The contraindications to the use of morphine are also contraindications to the use of:

a. Aspirin.

b. Meperidine.

c. Secobarbital.

d. Chlorpromazine.

22. Which of the following will reverse most of the effects of narcotics?

a. Caffeine.

b. Naloxone.

c. Epinephrine.

d. Dextroamphetamine.

23. When aspirin is given to a client whose body temperature is normal, his temperature will:

    a. Stay the same.

    b. Increase.

    c. Decrease.

24. Which of the following drugs acts as both an analgesic and antipyretic?

    a. Mephobarbital.

    b. Meprobamate.

    c. Morphine.

    d. Aspirin.

Check Your Answers on Next Page

SOLUTIONS TO EXERCISES, LESSON 3

1. a (para 3-3)

2. c (para 3-4a)

3. a (para 3-4b)

4. a (para 3-5)

5. c (para 3-7a(1))

6. d (para 3-8d)

7. c (paras 3-7c(4), 3-9a, 3-10a)

8. b (para 3-13c)

9. a (paras 3-15, 3-16)

10. b (para 3-19)

11. d (para 3-19a

12. a (para 3-19b)

13. c (para 3-19f)

14. d (para 3-20b)

15. c (para 3-20c)

16. a (para 3-22e)

17. b (para 3-22e(1))

18. a (para 3-22f(1)-(4))

19 b (para 3-23b)

20. c (para 3-23b)

21. b (para 3-24d)

22. b (para 3-26a)

23. a (paras 3-27b, 3-28a)

24. d (para 3-28a)

End of Lesson 3

LESSON ASSIGNMENT

LESSON 4	Autonomic and Cardiovascular Drugs
LESSON ASSIGNMENT	Paragraphs 4-1 through 4-35
LESSON OBJECTIVE	Upon completion of this lesson, you should be able to discuss the basic types of autonomic drugs and discuss the actions, uses, untoward effects, administration, cautions, and contraindications for common anticholinergics, adrenergics, vasodilators, antihistamines, drugs used in fluid and electrolyte therapy, hydrocortisone, and mannitol.
SUGGESTION	After studying the assignment, complete the exercises at the end of this lesson. These exercises will help you to achieve the lesson objectives.

LESSON 4

AUTONOMIC AND CARDIOVASCULAR DRUGS

Section I. THE AUTONOMIC NERVOUS SYSTEM

4-1. INTRODUCTION

The autonomic nervous system is the part of the nervous system that controls the automatic or involuntary functions of the body. Its nerves lead to the heart, blood vessels, glands, stomach, intestines, and other organs that have muscular actions independent of conscious will. The autonomic nervous system is divided into two parts, the sympathetic nervous system and the parasympathetic nervous system. These have nerves leading to the same organs, but the effects of the nerves belonging to each system are different. The basic differences in functions of the two systems are depicted in Table 4-1. Note that the sympathetic nervous system induces a state characteristic of fear or anger and prepares the body for coping with danger by "fight or flight," and the parasympathetic system induces a state characteristic of calmness and security. These states are produced by chemical substances released by the nerve endings of the two systems. The nerve endings of the sympathetic nervous system release norepinephrine, chemically similar to epinephrine (Adrenalin). The nerve endings of the parasympathetic system release acetylcholine (ACh). When these substances are released, the characteristic effects of their respective nervous systems are produced. Norepinephrine produces adrenergic effects, characteristic of fear and stress. ACh produces cholinergic effects, also called muscarinic effects, characteristic of calm, unstrenuous life. In the body, ACh is rapidly hydrolyzed (broken down in a reaction with water) by the action of an enzyme called acetylcholinesterase.

4-2. TYPES OF AUTONOMIC DRUGS

A sympathomimetic (adrenergic) is a drug that mimics the action of norepinephrine, the substance produced by the nerve endings of the sympathetic nervous system. A sympatholytic (antiadrenergic) is a drug that blocks the response of the effector organs to adrenergic stimulation. A parasympathomimetic (cholinergic) is a drug that mimics the action of acetylcholine (ACh), the substance produced by the nerve endings of the parasympathetic nervous system. A parasympatholytic (anticholinergic) is a drug that blocks the parasympathomimetic (muscarinic) effects of ACh.

Sympathetic (Adrenergic)	Parasympathetic (Cholinergic)
1. Dilates pupils.	1. Contracts pupils.
2. Lessens tonus of ciliary muscles, so that the eyes are accommodated to see distant objects.	2. Contracts ciliary muscles, so that the eyes are accommodated to see objects near at hand.
3. Dilates bronchial tubes.	3. Contracts bronchial tubes.
4. Quickens and strengthens the action of the heart.	4. Slows the action of the heart.
5. Contracts blood vessels of the skin and viscera so that more blood goes to the muscles Where it is needed for "fight or flight."	5. Dilates blood vessels.
6. Inhabits peristalsis. Food "sits like a lump" in the stomach.	6. Increases peristalsis. (Thus, digestion is promoted.)
7. Decreases secretions of glands (except the sweat glands and the adrenal glands, which secrete more).	7. Increases secretions of glands (except the sweat glands and the adrenal glands). Glands Involved in digestion are stimulated.
8. Causes contraction of sphincters to prevent emptying of bowels or bladder.	8. Relaxes sphincters so that waste matter can be removed.

Table 4-1. Functions of the sympathetic and parasympathetic nervous systems.

Section II. ANTICHOLINERGIC (PARASYMPATHOLYTIC) DRUGS

4-3. ATROPINE AS THE STANDARD ANTICHOLINERGIC DRUG

Atropine is the best known of the anticholinergic or parasympatholytic drugs, which inhibit the parasympathetic nervous system. Atropine is an extremely poisonous drug derived from a plant called belladonna. A tincture, an extract, and a leaf fluid extract are still official drugs. Their therapeutic value lies chiefly in their atropine content.

a. **Effects**. Small doses of atropine cause bradycardia (slow heartbeat), and larger doses cause tachycardia (fast heartbeat). Atropine relaxes all smooth muscles (for example, the muscles lining the intestines) except those of the blood vessels. It decreases the rate of secretion of glands of the respiratory tract, gastric glands, salivary glands, and some sweat glands.

b. **Adverse Effects**. The side effects of atropine and other parasympatholytics may include dry mouth, blurred vision, fatigue, light- headedness, and dizziness. Older men may suffer urinary retention. These effects may limit the amount of these drugs, which can be given chronically. However, extremely dangerous reactions from normal doses of these drugs are rare with adults, but more frequent with children. Very large doses tend to cause sedation, a disturbed mental state, and even respiratory depression and convulsions. Some clients may acquire a dry, flushed skin, and a high body temperature, which is very dangerous in children.

c. **Uses**. Atropine and other parasympatholytics have been frequently used in the treatment of peptic ulcer, which they ameliorate by reducing acid secretions in the stomach when it is empty and by decreasing the strength of smooth muscle contractions. They are also used to treat some other GI disturbances, which are not associated with organic disease--diarrhea, belching, spasm of the pylorus (opening through which the stomach empties into the intestine), and "stomach ache" because of overactivity of the GI smooth muscles. These drugs also relieve cystitis (bladder inflammation) by relaxing smooth muscles of the bladder. These drugs are used in the eye to dilate it and to paralyze accommodation (that is, temporarily prevent the eye from focusing). Atropine is sometimes used to counteract some of the effects of cholinergic drugs during or after their use in therapy. One significant use of atropine in the military is to counteract the effects of nerve gas. Atropine is used preoperatively to decrease the amount of saliva and respiratory secretions, especially when an inhalation anesthetic is to be used.

d. **Contraindications**. A client with glaucoma should never be given a parasympatholytic, except for small doses such as those given just before anesthesia. These drugs should not be given to clients over 35 with a shallow anterior chamber (between the cornea and the lens of the eye). These drugs are not necessary for eye dilation in routine eye examinations. Sympathomimetics are better for this purpose.

e. **Administration**. Atropine sulfate is a very poisonous drug. Therefore, when it is administered to a client, extreme care should be used to ensure that an overdose is not given.

(1) Belladonna is given orally, often in combination with other drugs as an antispasmodic. The usual dose of the tincture is 0.6-ml, while the usual dose of the tablet is one or two tablets three times a day at mealtime and one or two tablets at bedtime.

(2) Atropine is given orally, parenterally, or topically (in the eye). The usual adult dose preoperatively is 0.5-mg (1/120-gr) given intramuscularly together with the preoperative analgesic. The usual dose given to treat persons exposed to nerve gas is 2 mg given at 10-minute intervals for three doses. In addition, one percent atropine sulfate ophthalmic ointment is applied in the victim's eyes after first irrigating them with water for 30 seconds.

f. **Storage**. Belladonna tincture should be stored in tightly closed, light-resistant containers away from extreme heat or cold. Atropine for injection should not be allowed to freeze, and atropine sulfate ophthalmic solution is subject to deterioration as indicated on the manufacturer's label.

g. **How Supplied**.

(1) Belladonna is supplied as a tincture and in tablets with phenobarbital combined.

(2) Atropine is supplied for injection in automatic plastic injectors and in collapsible tubes with needles attached, each containing 2-mg of atropine. Atropine sulfate injection is supplied in 25-ml vials (2-mg per ml) and in 20-ml vials (0.4-mg per ml). There are 1-mg tablets for the treatment of nerve gas casualties only. Atropine is also supplied as a one-percent ophthalmic ointment and as a one-percent ophthalmic solution.

4-4. PROPANTHELINE

a. **Action and Uses**. Propantheline bromide (trade name: Pro-Banthine) is an antispasmodic similar in action to atropine, but having a longer duration of action, and a greater ability to decrease gastric secretion. It is used for the symptomatic treatment of peptic ulcer; it does not cure ulcers.

b. **Administration**. The drug is given orally or by injection. The usual dose is 15 mg with meals, and 15 to 30 mg at bedtime. The effects of a therapeutic dose of this drug last for about 6 hours.

c. **Untoward Effects**. The untoward effects of this drug are the same as those with belladonna and atropine, but not as severe.

d. **Cautions and Contraindications**. This drug is contraindicated for persons with glaucoma.

e. **How Supplied**. The drug is supplied as 15-mg tablets and as sterile propantheline bromide in 30-mg vials, which must be diluted for intramuscular or intravenous injection, according to the manufacturer's instructions.

4-5. HOMATROPINE HYDROCHLORIDE OPHTHALMIC OINTMENT

Homatropine hydrochloride ophthalmic ointment paralyzes visual accommodation for ophthalmological procedures. Recovery from this effect is complete in one day. It must be used with care in persons disposed to glaucoma.

Section III. ADRENERGIC (SYMPATHOMIMETIC) DRUGS

4-6. INTRODUCTION

The sympathomimetic drugs stimulate the structures innervated by the sympathetic (adrenergic) nerves and produce effects similar to those caused by stimulation of these nerves. The basic compound to which sympathomimetic, or "sympathetic-mimicking," drugs are generally compared is epinephrine. Other drugs in this class have actions similar to epinephrine. For this reason, epinephrine will be discussed first and the other drugs compared to it. (The amphetamines, which also are sympathomimetics, are used primarily as CNS stimulants and are, therefore, discussed in the section on CNS stimulants.)

4-7. EPINEPHRINE

The most important actions of epinephrine (Adrenalin) are on the heart and blood vessels.

a. **Actions**. Epinephrine is not effective orally, as it is destroyed in the stomach before it can be absorbed. When injected or inhaled, the actions of epinephrine include:

(1) Acceleration of the heart and increase in cardiac output. The cardiac rhythm is altered.

(2) Constriction of blood vessels in some areas and dilation in others. The vessels in the skin and in the mucosa are constricted after local application of the drug, while those of the skeletal muscles are dilated by injection.

(3) Relaxation of the bronchial musculature and the muscles of the GI tract and urinary bladder.

(4) When applied locally to the eyes, occasionally a mydriatic effect (dilation of the pupils) will occur.

b. **Therapeutic Uses**. Epinephrine is used to control hemorrhage from minor cuts, but it is not effective when a vein or artery is involved. It relieves nasal congestion by vasoconstriction for a short duration. It is used in conjunction with local anesthetics to prolong their action and to lessen the possibility of hemorrhage. Epinephrine is valuable in treating bronchial asthma, as an injection or by inhalation. It is also used frequently to relieve such allergic disorders as urticaria, serum reactions, and anaphylactic shock, for which epinephrine is the most often used drug. Certain heart failures can be corrected by injecting epinephrine directly into the heart. However, epinephrine is not of much value in the treatment of hemorrhagic, cardiogenic, or traumatic shock or circulatory collapse, and it may be harmful.

c. **Administration**. For the treatment of anaphylactic shock, epinephrine may be given IM as 1.0 ml of the 1:1000 solution. In general, the solutions for injection may be given SC, IM, or IV. However, the suspension in oil is preferably administered IM, though it may be given subcutaneously.

d. **Untoward Effects**. Some undesirable effects of this drug include insomnia, nervousness, anxiety, tremors, headache, and rapid heartbeat.

e. **Cautions and Contraindications**. Extreme care should be used to ensure that a dosage of epinephrine prepared for a client is in the appropriate concentration and amount. Because of its powerful vasopressor action, overdosage is especially dangerous in a client with an open wound, since fresh hemorrhage may result when the blood pressure is markedly elevated. Epinephrine is contraindicated for persons with heart disorders. An epinephrine preparation should be clear and colorless. If the solution is colored or has a sediment, it should not be used. All epinephrine preparations should be kept from freezing, and the package should be checked for the expiration date.

f. **How Supplied**. Epinephrine is available in strengths of 1:1000 for injection (in 1 ml cartridge-needle units and 1 ml ampules), 1:2600 for injection (in 1 ml ampules), and a 1:500 suspension in oil for intramuscular injection (in 1 ml ampules). It is also available in 1 percent and 2 percent ophthalmic solutions.

4-8. EPHEDRINE

a. **Action and Uses**. Ephedrine occurs naturally in various plants. This drug is very similar to epinephrine in its action. The administration of ephedrine results in vasoconstriction and stimulation of the heart that produces an elevation of blood pressure. Although this effect upon the blood pressure is not as great as that produced by the administration of epinephrine, it lasts seven to 10 times as long. The use of ephedrine produces relaxation of bronchial muscles that is less prominent than that obtained with epinephrine, but is sustained for a much longer time. This action of sustained bronchial relaxation is responsible for the greatest use of ephedrine--to facilitate breathing in chronic asthmatic conditions, and in treatment of hay fever and colds. Ephedrine (or compounds very similar to it in action) is commonly used in many preparations for the treatment of colds. Also, this drug may be given by intramuscular or intravenous injection prior to the administration of spinal anesthesia, because this use of the drug will enable blood pressure to be maintained during the operation. Ephedrine has a stimulating effect upon the central nervous system that is greater than that obtained with epinephrine. Ephedrine also acts to relieve nasal congestion.

b. **Administration**. The usual dose to be given either orally or parenterally is 25 to 50 mg. Two or three drops of a one- percent solution are usually given as nose drops.

c. **Differences Between Epinephrine and Ephedrine**. Although ephedrine and epinephrine are quite similar in action, there are a number of differences that are important clinically.

(1) Ephedrine is effective when given orally, whereas epinephrine must be given by injection (except when used as a spray or inhalation for asthmatic attacks.)

(2) Ephedrine has a longer duration of action than epinephrine does, but ephedrine also has a slower onset of action. These properties make ephedrine better suited for the treatment of chronic asthma and of colds.

(3) Epinephrine has a greater vasoconstricting effect than ephedrine.

(4) A tolerance to ephedrine may be acquired but not to epinephrine.

(5) Ephedrine has a greater stimulating effect upon the central nervous system than does epinephrine.

(6) Ephedrine has a much lower potency than epinephrine.

d. **Untoward Effects**. The main toxic effect of ephedrine is anxiety. A tolerance to the drug may be acquired.

e. **Cautions and Contraindications**. Clients may acquire a tolerance to the drug. If ephedrine is to be used in nose drops, the drug should be dissolved in water and not in oil. Continuous use of an oily preparation in the nose can cause lipid pneumonia (pneumonia due to the aspiration of oil). Liquid preparations of ephedrine should be protected from freezing. Like epinephrine, ephedrine should be used with caution, if at all, in clients with heart disease, high blood pressure, hyperthyroidism, and diabetes mellitus.

f. **How Supplied**. Ephedrine sulfate is supplied as a powder, as a 25-mg capsule, and as an injection which contains 25 or 50-mg of the drug per ml.

4-9. METARAMINOL BITARTRATE INJECTION

a. **Action and Uses**. Metaraminol (Aramine) is a vasopressor drug used to raise the blood pressure of clients in some types of hypotensive states. Metaraminol has a longer duration of action than epinephrine: The vasopressor effect of an intramuscular dose of 5 mg of metaraminol lasts for about 1 1/2 hours.

b. **Administration**. This drug can be given by either intramuscular or intravenous injection. It should not be given subcutaneously, as tissue sloughing may result when it is so administered. The usual dose is 1 ml of a one percent preparation, which is 10 mg of the drug. The drug may be included in solution for intravenous infusion, the rate of flow being regulated according to the client's response to the drug.

c. **Untoward Effects**. Toxic reactions to a therapeutic dose of the drug are rare, but hypertension may result, if too much is given. Hypertension is especially dangerous in a client with an open wound, since the elevated blood pressure may lead to fresh hemorrhage.

d. **Cautions and Contraindications**. This drug should not be given by subcutaneous injection, since tissue sloughing may result from such administration. Metaraminol deteriorates after 60 months; therefore, the date on the package should be checked before the drug is given. When this drug is given in a solution by the intravenous route, the client's blood pressure should be monitored frequently (5 to 10 minute intervals) and the rate of flow adjusted to the client's response.

e. **How Supplied**. Metaraminol bitartrate injection is supplied in 10-ml vials, each milliliter containing 10-mg of metaraminol.

4-10. PHENYLEPHRINE HYDROCHLORIDE

Phenylephrine (Neo-Synephrine) is similar in structure and action to epinephrine and has a vasopressor action when injected or taken orally. When applied locally to mucous membrane, it acts as a vasoconstrictor, reducing swelling and congestion, and is the most widely used nose drop preparation for decongestion. It is often combined with local anesthetics in a similar manner to epinephrine. Phenylephrine is also used in eye solutions as a conjunctival decongestant, vasoconstrictor, and mydriatic. Its action is superior to that of ephedrine in maintaining blood pressure during spinal anesthesia.

4-11. MISCELLANEOUS SYMPATHOMIMETICS

a. **Levarterenol Bitartrate Injection** (norepinephrine; Levophed). Levarterenol is provided in the Field Shock Treatment Surgical Instrument and Supply Set as a 0.2 injection in 4-ml ampules. It produces general vasoconstriction without stimulating the heart. (In the treatment of shock, one ampule may be added to 1000 ml of a dextrose solution and given by intravenous infusion. Rate of flow must be carefully regulated to obtain and maintain the desired effect. Blood pressure readings must be taken at 5 to 15 minute intervals to avoid overdosage. Someone must stay with the client continuously to see that the drug does not leak into the subcutaneous tissue, because dangerous necrosis of tissue can result from such leakage.) However, the first definitive treatment of shock, after obvious bleeding has been controlled, is the restoration of adequate blood volume. When levarterenol is used to treat shock, despite adequate restoration of blood pressure, failures occur in approximately 50 percent of cases. The rationale of its use is questionable.

b. **Isoproterenol Hydrochloride** (Isuprel Hydrochloride). Isoproterenol is very closely related chemically to epinephrine, but it is a pure vasodilator. It is used in the symptomatic relief of asthma. Unreliable when administered orally, it is usually given by inhalation.

c. **Oxymetazoline Hydrochloride** (Afrin Hydrochloride). Oxymetazoline hydrochloride is included as a 0.05 percent solution in the Battalion Aid Station Medical Equipment Set. It is used as a decongestant for allergic rhinitis (inflammation of the mucous membranes of the nose).

d. **Phenylpropanolamine Hydrochloride** (Propradrine). This drug has actions similar to ephedrine, but with slightly longer action and less CNS stimulation. It is used in nasal congestion and bronchial asthma.

e. **Propylhexedrine** (Benzedrex). This is a decongestant used by inhalation.

f. **Xylometazoline Hydrochloride** (Otrivin Hydrochloride). This is a nasal decongestant.

Section IV. VASODILATOR DRUGS

4-12. INTRODUCTION

The nitrites and organic nitrates are a group of drugs whose basic action is to relax smooth muscles. They produce vasodilation, which results in a lowering of blood pressure, venous dilatation and pooling, and a decreased cardiac workload. Their chief use is in the relief of attacks of angina pectoris (spasmodic suffocative chest pain), and they may be used to relieve acute attacks of hypertension and asthma. These drugs have a relatively short duration of action, however, and are not suited for the treatment of chronic hypertension. Because better drugs are available, they are not routinely used in the treatment of asthma. Untoward effects of these drugs include flushing of the skin, headache, nausea, vomiting, dizziness, fainting, and a faster heartbeat. A tolerance to these drugs is easily acquired; therefore, a client may need to increase the dosage progressively to obtain the desired response from the drug.

4-13. AMYLNITRITE

a. **Action and Uses**. Amyl nitrite has the action discussed above. In addition to its therapeutic use in the treatment of angina pectoris, it may be used to combat the effects of cyanide gas poisoning.

b. **Administration**. This drug is administered by inhalation. The pearl (ampule covered with a cloth mesh) is crushed in a handkerchief or in paper tissue and placed over the client's nose. The client inhales the fumes two or three times. When he has inhaled about 0.3 ml of the drug (average dose), there is onset of action within 20 seconds, which lasts for 7 to 10 minutes. When administered to a victim of cyanide gas poisoning, two pearls should be crushed and placed inside his gas mask. The original dose of two pearls is repeated three times (eight ampules).

c. **Caution**. Amyl nitrite should not be used in the presence of flame, because it is a very flammable agent.

d. **How Supplied**. The drug is supplied in 0.33-ml pearls, which should be kept refrigerated but protected from freezing. The drug is subject to deterioration after 24 months.

4-14. NITROGLYCERIN TABLETS

a. **Action and Uses**. Nitroglycerin tablets (glyceryl trinitrate tablets) are used chiefly to give relief from the pain associated with angina pectoris attacks. This drug may also be used as an aid in the diagnosis of migraine.

b. **Administration**. The tablets are administered sublingually (placed under the tongue and allowed to dissolve) in a dose of 0.3 to 0.6 mg. The onset of action of the drug commonly takes about 30 seconds, and its effects last for 20 to 30 minutes.

c. **How Supplied**. Nitroglycerin is available as soluble tablets, 0.3 mg, 0.4 mg, and 0.6-mg in strength.

Section V. FLUID AND ELECTROLYTE THERAPY

4-15. FLUID VOLUME REPLACEMENT

a. **Discussion**. The essential need in hypovolemic (oligemic) shock is restoration of the depleted fluid volume. When fluid volume is restored, the improvement in the circulation permits the most effective use of the blood that the client has not lost.

b. **Choice of Replacement Fluid**. The choice of replacement fluid is based on the type of fluid lost (whether whole blood, plasma, or water and electrolytes), the availability of specific fluids, and laboratory facilities. Whole blood is often the most effective, but other fluids should be given until completion of the necessary laboratory work and acquisition of the correct type of blood. A frequent course in hypovolemic shock is to immediately administer 500-2000 ml of sodium chloride injection (physiologic saline), Ringer's injection, lactated Ringer's injection, or five percent dextrose in saline rapidly intravenously, while making preparations of plasma protein fraction, serum albumin, or whole blood.

c. **General Precautions for Intravenous Solutions**.

(1) Do not overload the client with fluids.

(2) Check expiration date of solution.

(3) Do not administer a solution which is discolored or contains sediment.

(4) Do not administer if leakage from the bag is detected.

(5) Check urine output per hour.

4-16. NORMAL HUMAN SERUM ALBUMIN

a. **Action and Uses**. The albumin content in normal human serum albumin is a large-molecule protein extracted from human blood. It is an effective but potentially harmful blood volume substitute in emergencies; it is useful when the client has lung injury, because it acts by drawing fluid into the blood vessels from the surrounding tissues. This preparation is used also in other clinical situations where protein replacement therapy is indicated--such as nephrosis, certain skin diseases, and others. One vial of 25 percent albumin (100 ml) is equivalent to 500 ml of plasma.

b. **Administration**. Albumin is administered by intravenous infusion. The usual dose is 100 ml of 25 percent solution or 500 ml of a five-percent solution.

c. **Untoward Effects**. There are no untoward reactions to the administration of albumin in therapeutic amounts. However, unless this drug is given concurrently with infusions of saline or dextrose solutions, it will worsen the condition of a dehydrated client by drawing additional fluid from his tissues.

d. **Cautions and Contraindications**. This preparation should be refrigerated, however, it is damaged by freezing. The 25 percent solution has a potency period of 120 months when the drug is refrigerated, but its life is only half this long if it is not refrigerated. It should not be used if no vacuum is detected when the intravenous hookup is inserted into the bottle. As noted above, the preparation should be administered simultaneously with solutions of saline and dextrose when used in the treatment of dehydrated clients.

e. **How Supplied**. The 25 percent solution is supplied in vacuum-sealed cans containing 100 ml of the drug in an infusion bottle, with the equipment for sterile intravenous infusion. The 5 percent solution is provided in 500-ml bottles, also with an intravenous injection set.

4-17. PLASMA PROTEIN FRACTION

a. **Action and Uses**. Plasma protein fraction, derived from human donor plasma, is a 5 percent solution of plasma proteins, mainly albumin, but excluding certain unstable globulins. Its use and effects are very similar to normal human serum albumin, discussed above. It is used for a plasma substitute in treating shock and as a source of protein for intravenous feeding. Of course, it contains no clotting factors.

b. **Administration**. The usual minimum dose is 250-500 ml by IV infusion, not exceeding 8 ml per minute. Continued administration is dependent on the client's response to therapy.

c. **Cautions**. The period of potency is 60 months when stored at a temperature not exceeding 30°C (86°F).

d. **How Supplied**. Plasma protein fraction is supplied as a 5 percent solution in 250-ml and 500-ml bottles, with an intravenous injection set.

4-18. DEXTROSE SOLUTIONS

a. **Actions and Uses**. Dextrose (glucose), often 5 percent in water, is given to correct nutritional and water deficiency when the oral route cannot be used. Five-percent solutions of dextrose have nearly the same osmotic pressure as the body fluids. In addition to their use in the treatment of dehydration, five-percent dextrose solutions in saline (dextrose and sodium chloride injection, dextrose in lactated Ringer's injection, or dextrose in Ringer's injection) may be used in the emergency treatment of hypovolemic shock until preferred fluids are available. A 50-percent dextrose injection acts as a diuretic and is used in the relief of edema.

b. **Administration**. Dextrose solutions are most commonly given by intravenous infusion. Rarely, they may be given orally or rectally. One to three liters of a 10-percent solution (about 400 calories) are usually given for nutritional deficiency. One to two liters of a 5 percent solution in saline is usually used as a plasma expander. Fifty to 100-ml of a 50 percent solution are usually given to produce a diuretic effect.

c. **Untoward Effects**. Too much dextrose solution with sodium chloride can cause edema. Too much dextrose solution without sodium chloride can cause a clumping of the red blood cells.

d. **Cautions and Contraindications**. Dextrose solutions should be kept from freezing. They should not be used if there is sediment in the bottle. Use cautiously in diabetics. A client receiving dextrose solutions by intravenous infusion should be observed for signs of edema. Puffing of the hands and feet indicates that the client is becoming edematous. In addition, the infusion site should be observed for infiltration of the solution into the tissues, as indicated by swelling of the tissues around the needle. Should infiltration occur, the infusion should be discontinued and restarted at a new site.

e. **How Supplied**.

(1) Dextrose and sodium chloride (NaC1) injection. Various preparations are available: 0.5 percent dextrose in 0.45 percent NaC1; five-percent dextrose in 0.2-percent, 0.33 percent, 0.45-percent, or 0.9-percent NaC1; and 10-percent dextrose in 0.9-percent NaC1. Most of the preparations are available in transparent, flexible plastic, single-dose containers. The most frequently used preparations contain five-percent dextrose in 0.9-percent NaC1, available in 250-ml, 500-ml, and 100-ml bags. A solution of 2.5-percent dextrose in 0.45 percent NaC1 is supplied in 250-ml bags for pediatric use.

(2) Dextrose and sodium chloride injection, modified. This solution contains five-percent dextrose in 0.9-percent NaC1. It is supplied in a 1000-ml transparent, flexible plastic, single-dose container with graduation intervals at each 100-ml. An infusion set and swab-type antiseptic ampule are included in the carton, which converts to an arm board.

(3) Dextrose in lactated Ringer's injection. This five-percent dextrose solution is supplied in 500-ml and 1000-ml flexible plastic containers.

(4) Dextrose in Ringer's injection. This five-percent dextrose solution is supplied in 500-ml and 1000-ml flexible plastic containers.

(5) Dextrose injection, modified. This five-percent dextrose solution is supplied in 1000-ml flexible plastic containers similar to that for dextrose and sodium chloride injection, modified (see (2) above).

(6) Dextrose injection. Dextrose injection is available in five percent, 10 percent, and 50 percent strengths in various types and sizes of containers.

4-19. SODIUM CHLORIDE INJECTION

a. **Action and Uses**. Sodium chloride injection (normal saline solution; physiological salt solution) is a 0.9-percent solution of sodium chloride, which gives it the same osmotic pressure (makes it isotonic with) as the body fluids. This preparation is of great value in the treatment of dehydration, which is frequently associated with shock. Also, it will replenish body salt (electrolyte) loss. Since it passes out of the circulatory system very quickly, it is only briefly effective as a volume replacement fluid in hypovolemic shock. Normal saline solution is also used to irrigate wounds, because it is not irritating to tissue.

b. **Administration**. Sodium chloride injection is given parenterally. About 2000 ml, or more, of sodium chloride per day by intravenous infusion is required to keep the client's urine output at a desired amount of 1200 to 1500 ml of urine for each 24-hour period.

c. **Untoward Effects**. The intravenous infusion of sodium chloride can lead to edema, acidosis, and loss of potassium--especially when therapy is continued over a prolonged period.

d. **Cautions and Contraindications**. This preparation should be kept from freezing. It should not be used for intravenous infusion if it is discolored, or it contains sediment, or if no vacuum is detected when the intravenous assembly is attached.

e. **How Supplied**. Sodium chloride injection is supplied in 5-ml-ampules, in an infusion bag containing 250-ml for pediatric parenteral use, and in infusion bags containing 1000 ml for parenteral use. It is also supplied in 150-ml, 250-ml, 500-ml, and 1000-ml. transparent, flexible plastic, single-dose containers. Sodium chloride injection, modified, is supplied in 1000-ml flexible plastic containers with graduation intervals at each 100-ml, including an infusion set, swab-type antiseptic ampule, and a carton that converts into an armboard.

4-20. RINGER'S INJECTION

a. **Action and Uses**. Ringer's injection is an isotonic solution which supplies the three important cations: sodium, potassium, and calcium. It has a slightly greater therapeutic value as a fluid and electrolyte replenisher than sodium chloride injection. However, large volumes of Ringer's injection, like sodium chloride injection, alter the acid-base balance.

b. **Administration**. The usual dose by intravenous infusion is 1000-ml.

c. **How Supplied**. Ringer's injection is supplied in 500-ml and 1000-ml transparent, flexible plastic, single-dose containers.

4-21. LACTATED RINGER'S INJECTION

a. **Action and Uses**. Lactated Ringer's injection is used as a fluid and electrolyte replenisher. Designed to avoid the tendency of sodium chloride injection to cause acidosis, it also supplies the important cations: sodium, potassium, and calcium. Sodium lactate is included because lactate eventually metabolizes to bicarbonate and thus alkalinizes the body fluids. However, bicarbonate itself is not included because it tends to hasten the calcium ions as calcium carbonate in heated solutions.

b. **Administration**. The usual dose by intravenous infusion is 1000-ml.

c. **How Supplied**. Lactated Ringer's injection is supplied in 1000-ml transparent, flexible plastic, single-dose containers.

4-22. POTASSIUM CHLORIDE INJECTION

a. **Action and Uses**. Potassium chloride injection is used to treat hypokalemia, a deficiency of potassium in the blood. Hypokalemia may result from prolonged vomiting or diarrhea, treatment with adrenal steroids or diuretics (especially the thiazides), and kidney tubule malfunction.

b. **Administration**. It is important to confirm adequate renal function when administering potassium, since the kidney is the principle route of excretion. Except in an emergency in which serum K is extremely low and cardiac and respiratory muscle activity is seriously impaired, the rate of administration should be 10-20-mEq per hour, or less. A total dose of 1-3 mEq/kg/24 hours may be given in glucose or saline solutions.

c. **Effects of Overdose**. The symptoms of overdose include paresthesias (abnormal sensations), general weakness or paralysis, mental confusion, hypotension, cardiac arrhythmias, and heart block.

d. **How Supplied**. Potassium chloride injection is supplied in 10-ml ampules. Each milliliter contains two milliequivalents of potassium ion.

4-23. SODIUM BICARBONATE INJECTION

a. **Action and Uses**. Sodium bicarbonate is specific in the treatment of systemic acidosis, since the salt is composed of the two ions essential to correct this condition. Large quantities of sodium bicarbonate are needed only in unusual and threatening conditions.

b. **Administration**. It is difficult to set a general dosage schedule for sodium bicarbonate in the treatment of metabolic acidosis. In chronic, stable conditions, it is possible to begin with very small doses and find the correct dose empirically. The drug is usually administered in 5 percent dextrose in water in concentrations from 44 to 176-mEq/L.

c. **Precautions**. An overdose may result in systemic alkalosis. Clients with renal failure may demonstrate circulatory failure or tetany during alkali therapy.

d. **How Supplied**. Sodium bicarbonate injection is supplied in 50-ml ampules. Each ampule contains 44.6-milliequivalents of sodium.

Section VI. ANTIHISTAMINES

4-24. INTRODUCTION

In order to understand the role of the histamine-antagonizing agents (antihistamines), you must be familiar with histamine and its effects on the body. Histamine, a basic amine, may be found wherever protein is broken down into its component amino acids in the presence of putrefactive organisms; thus, it is found in the intestines, and in the putrefaction of meats. It occurs as well in all body tissues and is present in the highest concentration in the lungs. Histamine is not normally found in the bloodstream. It is released at the time of their injury.

4-25. HISTAMINE POISONING

When injected into the body, histamine causes swelling and itching. The affected area may be very sensitive to pressure. Headache and congestion of the head occur. Breathing becomes difficult. The body systems are affected as follows:

a. **Circulatory**. After histamine is injected, there is a short initial rise in blood pressure due to direct action on the smooth muscle, followed by a marked fall in pressure because of dilation of the capillaries. The walls of the capillaries lose tone and become distended with blood. The client "bleeds" into his own capillaries, and shock and collapse follow.

b. **Respiratory**. Histamine causes constriction of smooth muscle (with the exception of the blood vessels). The resulting constriction of the bronchioles makes respiration labored and difficult. This smooth muscle action is not antagonized by atropine, because histamine acts directly on the cells of the muscles rather than on their nerve innervation.

c. **Stomach and Intestines; Uterus**. Histamine causes the stomach, intestines, and uterus to contract more powerfully. Spasm may occur.

4-26. ALLERGY AND ANAPHYLAXIS WITH HISTAMINE

Histamine has been demonstrated to have an important role in allergic reactions. Reactions produced by the injection of histamine and those seen with anaphylactic shock and allergic reaction seem identical, that is, contraction of the bronchioles, low blood pressure, increased gastrointestinal motility, increased permeability of the capillaries resulting in edema in the skin and mucous membranes, increase in lacrimal fluid, nasal discharge and fluid in the lungs. There is a nerve-ending reaction in the skin, which produces pain and itching. Since histamine is believed to cause allergic reactions, or at least many of the symptoms, antihistaminic substances are used in the control of hay fever and other allergic manifestations.

4-27. INTRODUCTION TO ANTIHISTAMINES

In 1933, it was discovered that certain compounds had the property of counteracting the effects of histamine. These antihistamine compounds directly antagonize histamine. This action is exerted directly on the peripheral effector cells, which respond to the histamine. We may think of the antihistamine compound as putting a protective coating around the susceptible cells and preventing the histamine from reaching the cells to produce its reaction.

a. **Therapeutic Uses**. The antihistamines are effective in combating conditions caused or aggravated by histamine release in the tissues. They do not cure any condition, but temporarily alleviate symptoms. There is no scientific evidence that antihistamines either prevent or alleviate the common cold. They provide good symptomatic treatment for hay fever, drug reactions, serum reactions, some cases of asthma, and other allergic reactions. Many of the antihistamine compounds are effective antiemetics, that is, agents used to treat or prevent nausea or vomiting; some are particularly effective in the prevention and treatment of motion sickness.

b. **Untoward Effects**. None of the antihistamines is particularly toxic. They have a high therapeutic index, and truly toxic manifestations are infrequent. Minor side effects do occur, such as drowsiness, depression, decreased salivation, and nausea. Drowsiness is the most common side effect. Some have lesser side effects than others do. Clients under antihistamine medication should be warned by their physician not to drive or operate heavy machinery. The sedative effect of antihistamines has been put to use in many sleeping preparations.

4-28. DIPHENHYDRAMINE HYDROCHLORIDE

a. **Uses**. Diphenhydramine (Benadryl) is highly sedative and is often used as a sedative for allergic clients. It is also a useful antiemetic in the treatment of motion sickness and other conditions producing nausea. It may be used to treat parkinsonism.

b. **Administration.** The usual oral dose is 25 to 50-mg, 3 to 4 times daily. The usual intramuscular or intravenous dose is 10 to 50-mg.

c. **Untoward Effects**. Other than sedation, the side effects may include dizziness, ringing in the ears, incoordination, fatigue, double vision, and nervousness. In addition, untoward effects involving the digestive tract may occur. These include loss of appetite, nausea, vomiting, epigastric distress, and constipation or diarrhea. The incidence of these effects can be reduced by giving the drug with food.

d. **Cautions and Contraindications**. This drug should not be administered to people such as truck drivers, aircraft pilots, and others who should stay alert. The solution of the drug for parenteral use should not be allowed to freeze.

e. **How Supplied**. Diphenhydramine hydrochloride is supplied as a powder, as 25-mg and 50-mg capsules, as an elixir, as an ingredient in an expectorant cough syrup (Benylin Expectorant), and as a solution for intravenous or intramuscular injection. The injection is supplied in 10-ml vials (10-mg per ml or 50-mg per ml) and in 1-ml ampules (50 mg each).

4-29. DIMENHYDRINATE

Dimenhydrinate (Dramamine) is a mixture of diphenhydramine (discussed above) and 8-chlorotheophylline. The latter contributes very little to the effectiveness of the mixture as an antihistamine or antiemetic. The chief use of dimenhydrinate is as an antinauseant in motion sickness. The usual dose is 50-mg, 4 times daily. It is supplied as 50-mg tablets.

4-30. MECLIZINE HYDROCHLORIDE

a. **Action and Uses.** Meclizine (Bonine, Antivert) is used to prevent or treat motion sickness, vertigo, labyrinthitis, and radiation sickness. It is long-acting (9 to 24 hours).

b. **Administration**. The usual adult dose is 25-mg daily.

c. **Contraindications**. Because of the sedative effects of this drug, it should not be used when alertness is required. It is contraindicated in pregnancy.

d. **How Supplied**. Meclizine is supplied in 12.5-mg and 25 mg tablets and as 25-mg chewable tablets.

4-31. PROMETHAZINE HYDROCHLORIDE

a. **Uses**. Promethazine (Phenergan) is a very potent phenothiazine-type antihistamine with a long duration of action. In addition to its uses as an antihistamine for allergic condition, it is also useful as an antitussive, an antiemetic, and an obstetrical, surgical, or nighttime sedative.

b. **Administration**. The usual oral or parenteral dose is 25-mg, repeated after 4 hours, if necessary.

c. **How Supplied**. Promethazine hydrochloride is supplied as an injection (25-mg per ml), 25-mg tablets, and 25-mg suppositories. It is also an ingredient in an expectorant cough syrup (Phenergan Expectorant).

4-32. CHLORPHENIRAMINE MALEATE

a. **Uses**. Chlorpheniramine maleate is an effective antihistamine with a low incidence of side effects. It is available under many trade names, including Allerest, Chlor-Trimeton, Coricidin, Extendryl, Novahistine, and Teldrin.

b. **Administration**. The usual dose is 2-4 mg, 3 or 4 times daily. The usual parenteral dose is 10-20 mg.

c. **How Supplied**. Chlorpheniramine maleate is an ingredient of numerous preparations intended for the common cold, sinusitis, and allergic rhinitis. In addition, it is available as the sole ingredient in a syrup (2-mg/5 ml), 4-mg tablets, and 8-mg timed-release tablets.

4-33. TRIPROLIDINE HYDROCHLORIDE

a. **Uses**. Triprolidine hydrochloride (Actidil) is an unusually potent antihistamine with a rapid onset of action. The maximum effect occurs in about 3 1/2 hours, and the effect lasts for about 12 hours.

b. **Administration**. The usual oral dose is 2.5-mg, 2 or 3 times daily.

c. **How Supplied**. Triprolidine hydrochloride is supplied in combination with pseudoepinephrine hydrochloride, a sympathomimetic drug included as a decongestant. Actifed is a common trade name for the mixture, available as a syrup (1.25-mg of triprolidine HC1 and 30-mg of pseudoepinephrine HC1 per 5 ml) and a tablet (2.5-mg of triprolidine HC1 and 60-mg of pseudoepinephrine HC1 per tablet).

Section VII. OTHER AGENTS

4-34. HYDROCORTISONE SODIUM SUCCINATE

a. **Action and Uses**. Except for its use in adrenal insufficiency, treatment with hydrocortisone sodium succinate (Solu-Cortef*) (HC) is only palliative. Hydrocortisone sodium succinate is used primarily for its anti-inflammatory effects. It is used in the large single dose described below for some severe life-threatening situations, including severe asthmatic or anaphylactic reactions, acute adrenal cortical insufficiency, and overwhelming infections.

b. **Administration**. This drug is given either intramuscularly or intravenously. For the treatment of emergency conditions, the usual dose is 100 mg given over a period of 60 seconds. The symptoms of stress are usually gone about 10 hours from the time of administration of the drug. However, the client may suffer a relapse if the underlying cause of his condition is severe, or if it is not treated with more definitive agents.

c. **Untoward Effects**. There are virtually no harmful effects to a single dose of this drug, nor even to the use of it for a few days. However, on prolonged use for the treatment of chronic conditions, a number of untoward reactions may occur. The principal ones include fluid and electrolyte disturbances; susceptibility to infections, including tuberculosis; failure of wounds to heal; formation of peptic ulcers, which may bleed or perforate; hyperglycemia (abnormally large amount of blood glucose) and glycosuria (sugar in the urine); a wasting or weakening of muscle tissue; osteoporosis (softening of the bone), which may result in spontaneous fractures; and psychosis. Upon the appearance of any adverse reaction, the drug should be discontinued or the dosage reduced.

d. **Cautions and Contraindications**. For immediate lifesaving therapy, there are no contraindications to the use of the drug. For the long-range treatment of chronic diseases, the drug should not be used on clients with peptic ulcers, nor on those who have a history of psychosis. The drug should be kept from freezing; also, it is subject to deterioration.

e. **Supply**. The equivalent of 100- or 250-mg of hydrocortisone base is supplied in a sterile mixing bottle. The lower section of the bottle contains the drug and the upper section contains sterile water.

4-35. MANNITOL INJECTION--AN OSMOTIC DIURETIC

a. **Action**. Diuretics are drugs, which increase the excretion of urine. An osmotic diuretic, such as Mannitol (Osmitrol), easily passes into the renal tubules, however, it is not significantly reabsorbed. It increases the osmotic pressure of the glomerular filtrate, decreases tubular reabsorption, and thus increases the volume of urine.

b. **Indications**. Mannitol injection is indicated for:

(1) Promotion of diuresis, in the prevention or treatment of the oliguric phase of acute renal failure (following hemolytic transfusion reactions) before irreversible renal failure becomes established.

(2) Reduction of intracranial pressure and treatment of cerebral edema.

(3) Reduction of elevated intraocular pressure when the pressure cannot be lowered by other means.

(4) Promoting the urinary excretion of toxic substances.

(5) Use as an irrigating solution in transurethral resection.

(6) Use as a diagnostic aid in measurement of glomerular filtration rate.

c. **Usual Dosage**. The dose of Mannitol varies with the clinical condition being treated and client response.

(1) Hemolytic transfusion reactions. Twenty-five grams are given IV over a five-minute period as soon as a reaction occurs or is suspected. Additional IV fluids should be administered to maintain urine flow at 100-ml/hr. Strict intake and output records should be maintained on the client. If urine output falls below 100-ml/hr, the initial dose of Mannitol may be repeated, but not more than 100-grams per 24 hrs.

(2) Urinary excretion of toxic substances. The passive reabsorption of toxic substances at the proximal tubule can be partially restricted by decreasing the amount of water reabsorbed at that site. An initial loading dose of 25- to 50-grams of Mannitol followed by 10 to 20 grams per hour will produce urine volumes of up to 1000 ml/hr. Fluids and electrolytes must be replaced in the client during this procedure. The effectiveness of Mannitol in increasing renal excretion of glutethimide, meprobamate, barbiturates, and salicylates has been demonstrated. It is potentially useful for all ultrafiltered poisons, which are passively reabsorbed in the proximal tubule.

(3) Test for oliguria. A test dose of 12.5-grams is administered IV over a period of 3 to 5 minutes. If urine output does not increase to 40 to 60-ml/hour over the next three hours, the condition is unresponsive to Mannitol. If a response is obtained, Mannitol should be given by IV infusion to maintain a urine output of 100-ml/hr.

d. **Cautions and Warnings**.

(1) Mannitol should be administered slowly to avoid sudden increase in plasma volume and dilutional hyponatremia.

(2) The client's fluid and electrolyte balance should be monitored and restored accordingly.

(3) Mannitol should not be mixed with blood in a transfusion set, as increased osmotic pressure may cause agglutination.

(4) The solution should be checked before administration for crystals. Directions for putting the crystals back into solution are on the bottle.

(5) Mannitol should be used with great caution in clients having congestive heart failure and renal insufficiency. It may cause increased congestion or pulmonary edema.

e. **Adverse Reactions**. Transient headache, nausea, chills, thirst, and pain in the chest may occur during administration.

f. **Supply**. Mannitol injection, 15-percent for use as a diuretic, is supplied in 150-ml bottles. Mannitol injection, 25-percent for use as a diagnostic aid, is supplied in 50-ml quantities.

Continue with Exercises

EXERCISES, LESSON 4

INSTRUCTIONS: Answer the following exercises by marking the lettered response that best answers the question or completes the incomplete statement.

After you have completed all of these exercises, turn to "Solutions to Exercises" at the end of the lesson and check your answers. For each exercise answered incorrectly, reread the material referenced with the solution.

1. The nerve endings of the parasympathetic nervous system release a substance responsible for a combination of effects referred to as cholinergic effects. What is the name of this substance?

   a. Acetylcholine.

   b. Epinephrine.

   c. Norepinephrine.

   d. Sympathin.

2. What effects should a parasympathomimetic drug produce?

   a. Adrenergic.

   b. Antiadrenergic.

   c. Cholinergic.

   d. Anticholinergic.

3. What is the basic effect of an anticholinergic drug?

   a. It enhances the action of the sympathetic nervous system.

   b. It blocks the action of the sympathetic nervous system.

   c. It enhances the action of the parasympathetic nervous system.

   d. It blocks the action of the parasympathetic nervous system.

4. What drug may be given to reduce respiratory secretions prior to the administration of ether anesthesia?

    a. Morphine.

    b. Epinephrine.

    c. Atropine.

    d. Hydrocortisone sodium succinate.

5. A drug that is extremely poisonous and the dosage of which should therefore be measured exactly is:

    a. Propantheline.

    b. Atropine.

    c. Paregoric.

    d. Diphenhydramine.

6. What is the basic effect of an adrenergic drug?

    a. It enhances the action of the sympathetic nervous system.

    b. It blocks the action of the sympathetic nervous system.

    c. It enhances the action of the parasympathetic nervous system.

    d. It blocks the action of the parasympathetic nervous system.

7. Which of the following drugs may be used to help control nosebleed?

    a. Epinephrine.

    b. Meperidine.

    c. Hydrocortisone.

    d. Diphenhydramine.

8. It is very dangerous to give a client with an open wound an overdose of a drug that will raise blood pressure because the elevated blood pressure may lead directly to:

   a. Hemorrhage.

   b. Shock.

   c. Hypersensitive reaction.

   d. Depressed respiration.

9. Which of the following sympathomimetics is effective when given orally?

   a. Ephedrine.

   b. Epinephrine.

   c. Isoproterenol.

   d. Levarterenol.

10. Which of the following properties of ephedrine makes it more suitable than epinephrine for use in the treatment of chronic asthma?

    a. Ephedrine's lesser vasoconstricting effect.

    b. Ephedrine's longer duration of action.

    c. Ephedrine's stimulating effect on the central nervous system.

    d. Ephedrine's shrinking effect on swollen nasal mucosa.

11. The subcutaneous injection of Metaraminol may result in:

    a. Sloughing of tissues.

    b. Depression of central nervous system.

    c. Overdosage effects.

    d. Rigidity of muscle tissue.

12. When Metaraminol is being administered intravenously, the client's blood pressure should be taken at which of the following time intervals.

a. 1-4 minutes.

b. 5-10 minutes.

c. 15-20 minutes.

d. 30-45 minutes.

13. The most widely used decongestant nose drops contain:

a. Epinephrine.

b. Ephedrine.

c. Levarterenol.

d. Phenylephrine.

14. A drug that acts to lower cardiac workload is:

a. Ephedrine.

b. Metaraminol.

c. Hydrocortisone.

d. Amyl nitrite.

15. Which of the following drugs is used to treat cyanide gas poisoning?

a. Nitroglycerin.

b. Amylnitrite.

c. Chloramphenicol.

d. Diphenhydramine hydrochloride.

16. Which of the following drugs is administered by inhalation?

    a. Promethazine.

    b. Diphenhydramine.

    c. Amyl nitrite.

    d. Nitroglycerin.

17. A drug that may be used to help diagnose migraine is:

    a. Caffeine.

    b. Dextroamphetamine.

    c. Hydrocortisone sodium succinate.

    d. Nitroglycerin tablets.

18. The soluble tablets of which of the following drugs are administered sublingually?

    a. Morphine.

    b. Atropine.

    c. Codeine.

    d. Nitroglycerin.

19. You attach an intravenous injection set to a bottle of 5 percent dextrose, and you do not detect a vacuum. What should you do?

    a. Select another injection set.

    b. Select another supply bottle.

    c. Milk the tubing.

    d. Continue with the preparation of the fluid.

20. When normal human serum albumin is administered to a dehydrated client, which of the following solutions should be given concurrently.

   a. Plasma; blood.

   b. Sodium chloride injection; a dextrose solution.

   c. Lactated Ringer's injection; plasma protein fraction.

   d. Sodium bicarbonate injection; potassium chloride injection.

21. Which of the following types of substances are used to reduce the intensity of allergic reactions?

   a. Antiemetics.

   b. Antihistamines.

   c. Parasympatholytics.

   d. Parasympathomimetics.

22. In addition to their use in the treatment of allergies, many antihistamines are also used for their:

   a. Analgesic and antipyretic effects.

   b. Anesthetic and antidiarrheal effects.

   c. Sedative and antiemetic effects.

   d. Stimulant and decongestant effects.

23. A drug that is useful both in the prevention of motion sickness and in the treatment of allergies is:

   a. Ephedrine.

   b. Diphenhydramine.

   c. Atropine.

   d. Epinephrine.

24. Which of the following may be used to prevent renal failure after a hemolytic transfusion reaction?

    a. Atropine.

    b. Epinephrine.

    c. Mannitol injection.

    d. Hydrocortisone sodium succinate.

25. A drug useful as an adjunct in the treatment of symptoms associated with various conditions such as anaphylactic shock is:

    a. Atropine.

    b. Ephedrine.

    c. Mannitol injection.

    d. Hydrocortisone sodium succinate.

Check Your Answers on Next Page

SOLUTIONS TO EXERCISES, LESSON 4

1. a (para 4-1)
2. c (paras 4-1, 4-2)
3. d (para 4-3)
4. c (para 4-3c)
5. b (para 4-3e)
6. a (para 4-6)
7. a (paras 4-7a(2), b)
8. a (paras 4-7e; 4-9c)
9. a (para 4-8c(1))
10. b (para 4-8c(2))
11. a (para 4-9b, d)
12. b (para 4-9d)
13. d (para 4-10)
14. d (para 4-12)
15. b (para 4-13a)
16. c (para 4-13b)
17. d (para 4-14a)
18. d (para 4-14b)
19. b (para 4-15c(4))
20. b (paras 4-16c, d; 4-18a; 4-19a)

21. b (para 4-27a)

22. c (para 4-27a, b)

23. b (para 4-28a)

24. c (paras 4-35b(1), c(1))

25. d (para 4-34a)

End of Lesson 4

LESSON ASSIGNMENT

LESSON 5	Drugs Used to Prevent and Treat Infection I.
LESSON ASSIGNMENT	Paragraphs 5-1 through 5-27.
LESSON OBJECTIVE	Upon completion of this lesson, you should be able to discuss basic concepts and terminology of microbiology; define and identify types of immunity, types of allergic reactions, and related terms; and discuss actions, uses, untoward effects, administration, cautions, and contraindications of common immunizing agents, penicillins, cephalosporins, tetracyclines, and erythromycin.
SUGGESTION	After studying the assignment, complete the exercises at the end of this lesson. These exercises will help you to achieve the lesson objectives.

LESSON 5

DRUGS USED TO PREVENT AND TREAT INFECTION I

Section I. MICROBIOLOGY

5-1. BACTERIA

Bacteria are minute, single-celled living organisms of the kingdom Protista, which exist on either living or dead hosts. While there are many hundred individual species of bacteria, only a few of them are capable of producing disease in man. Disease-producing organisms are termed pathogens; they are said to be pathogenic.

a. **Morphology**. Morphology is the study of the forms and structures of organized beings. Bacteria can be broken down into three broad groups based on their general shape. There are the spherical bacteria called cocci (coccus, singular); the rod-shaped bacteria called bacilli (bacillus, singular); and the spiral-shaped bacteria called spirochetes.

(1) Cocci. Cocci (spherical bacteria) may be arranged in pairs, chains, or clusters. Depending upon their arrangement, they are called diplococci (pairs), streptococci (chains), or staphylococci (clusters).

(2) Bacilli. The rod-shaped bacilli occur singly, in pairs, or in chains.

(3) Spirochetes. Spiral-shaped bacteria always occur singly.

b. **Locomotion (Motility)**. Since most bacteria have no special structure for locomotion, they lack the ability to move by themselves. They are carried along with the movement of food in the digestive tract or blood in the vessels. A very few of the pathogens are equipped with one or more hairlike projections called flagella. These flagella permit the organism to propel itself by whiplike motions.

c. **Capsules**. Certain bacteria can cover themselves with a gelatinous substance. This covering is called a capsule and the process is termed encapsulation. It serves to protect the organism from adverse conditions such as heat, cold, moisture, drying, or drug therapy. Encapsulated organisms are immune to the process of phagocytosis, a defensive body mechanism in which bacteria are engulfed by certain white blood cells.

d. **Size**. Bacteria are microscopic in size. Their size is usually expressed in units of microns; one micron is 1/1000 mm (1/25,400 inch). Most bacteria are from 0.5 to 2.0 microns in size.

e. **Reproduction**. Bacteria reproduce rapidly, about once every 30 minutes, through a process called binary fission. Each bacterium splits into two new organisms in this reproductive process. Under ideal conditions, a single bacterium could produce a total of 140,000,000,000,000 organisms in a period of 24 hours. Of course, conditions are never ideal. A limited food supply diminishes bacterial reproduction.

f. **Classification**. One way by which bacteria may be classified is by the manner in which they are stained by certain dyes. In this classification, most bacteria are divided into two broad groups, the gram-positive and the gram-negative bacteria. Slides are treated with a crystal violet stain followed by safranine stain. Gram-positive organisms (G+) become purple-colored because of the crystal violet. Gram-negative (G-) organisms are stained red by the safranine.

g. **Relationship to Disease**. Many diseases are wholly or partly a result of the presence of bacteria in the blood or tissues. The pathogenic effects of some of these bacteria result from the toxins they produce.

h. **Common Bacterial Diseases**. Streptococci, staphylococci, and pneumococci--all gram-positive organisms--are responsible for 80 percent to 90 percent of all clinical bacterial infections. The streptococcus is responsible for bacterial endocarditis, strep throat, and scarlet fever. The staphylococcus causes boils and other miscellaneous infections. The pneumococcus causes pneumonia. Various gram-negative bacteria are responsible for peritonitis, urinary tract infections, gonorrhea, whooping cough, plague, and wound infections.

i. **General Drug Treatment**. Most bacterial infections respond well to treatment with sulfonamides or antibiotics.

5-2. VIRUSES

The virus is an infectious agent, submicroscopic in size, that is capable of multiplication only within a living cell. Because of their extremely small size, relatively little is known about viruses.

a. **Morphology**. There is little uniformity among the viruses. They may be ovoid, spherical, rodlike, or tadpole-shaped.

b. **Locomotion (Motility)**. None of the viruses yet studied possess a mechanism for independent movement.

c. **Size**. Viruses are much smaller than bacteria. They are measured in millimicrons (1/1000th micron). An electron microscope with a magnification of 100,000 times is necessary to see an average virus. Such magnification would make a mosquito appear as large as the Empire State Building!

d. **Reproduction**. Viral nucleic acids interact with the living host cell to cause it to form the components of the progeny viruses.

e. **Classification**. In the past, viruses have been classified by the tissue in which they produce their ill effects. For example, those acting in nervous tissue were classified as neurotropic; in glandular tissue as glanulotropic; and in skin as dermatotropic. Newer classification systems are based on precise biological, chemical, and physical properties.

f. **Relationship to Disease**. Viruses produce disease symptoms by actual destruction of the cells they invade. Some produce toxins which, when absorbed by the host, add to the syndrome.

g. **Common Viral Diseases**. A few of the better known diseases caused by viruses are mumps, chicken pox, measles, influenza, yellow fever, encephalitis, polio, and parrot fever.

h. **General Drug Treatment**. In general, viral infections do not respond to specific therapeutic agents.

5-3. RICKETTSIAE

Rickettsiae are minute, obligate intracellular parasites, whose natural reservoir is the arthropods, such as ticks, lice, mites, and fleas. Once thought to be an intermediate form between viruses and bacteria, they are now known to be a specific category of true bacteria. Rickettsiae are responsible for Rocky Mountain spotted fever, typhus, trench fever, and Tsutsugamushi fever. All of these diseases are generally brought under control with the use of antibiotics.

Section II. BIOLOGICALS (IMMUNIZING AGENTS)

5-4. TERMINOLOGY

The following terms are useful in the study of immunizing agents:

a. **Immunity**--the ability to resist or overcome a specific disease or infection.

(1) Active immunity--immunity attributable to antibody formed as a result of exposure to an antigen.

(2) Passive immunity--short-term immunity acquired by the injection of antibodies that have been formed in another individual or species.

b. **Antigen**--a substance which when injected into the body stimulates production of antibodies and therefore promotes active immunity.

c. **Antibody**--substances produced by the body for its protection when pathogenic microorganisms are present in the tissues, or when an antigenic substance has been injected into the body.

d. **Toxin**--a poisonous substance produced by certain pathogenic microorganisms. Toxins stimulate the production of antibodies and thus act as antigens.

e. **Toxoid**--a suspension of a toxin, modified so that it no longer produces toxic effects in the body but still acts as an antigen.

f. **Vaccine**--a suspension of either weakened or killed bacteria or viruses, administered to create active immunity to an infectious disease.

g. **Antitoxin**--type of antibody formed in the body of an animal that has been selectively and actively immunized. Blood serum from the animal is obtained and purified; it is used to neutralize the toxins produced in certain diseases (e.g., tetanus). Thus, it is used to produce passive immunity.

h. **Immune Serum**--blood serum from either animals or humans that have been infected with the disease. Such serum contains antibodies against the particular disease-producing organisms involved; passive immunity is produced.

5-5. ALLERGIC (HYPERSENSITIVE) REACTIONS

a. **Serum Sickness**. Following injection of a drug containing animal serum, after a period of 5-14 days, there may be the sudden appearance of skin rash, fever, glandular inflammation, and joint pain. Serum sickness may last from several days to several weeks. It may require the administration of corticosteroids for its relief.

b. **Drug Fever**. In drug fever, a fever of up to 104°F appears 7-21 days after the use of a drug. Drug fever usually lasts about 2-3 days after discontinuation of the drug.

c. **Anaphylactic Reaction**. Anaphylactic reactions are unusually strong allergic reactions to the administration of a drug. Histamine is released in the body, producing urticaria (a vascular reaction characterized by reddish, pale, smooth, slightly elevated skin patches attended by severe itching), bronchial spasms, laryngeal edema, hypotension, and sometimes shock. An anaphylactic reaction may be lethal, but preparation for treatment, early recognition, and promptness of treatment reduce the possibility of death. The immediate treatment begins with the IM or IV administration of 1.0 ml of a 1:1000 solution of epinephrine. Epinephrine acts as a physiological antagonist of histamine. The most dangerous anaphylactic reactions occur very soon after the administration of the antigen. If a reaction is delayed as much as 30 minutes, it is probably less threatening and can be treated with an antihistamine.

5-6. PRECAUTIONS

A number of precautions should be taken when handling or administering immunizing drugs in order to guard against serious reactions.

a. A medical officer should be available in case serious reactions develop.

b. Epinephrine injection 1:1000 should be drawn into a syringe and placed at hand for immediate use in case the client shows signs of going into shock. A tourniquet should also be at hand.

c. The client's immunization record should be checked for evidence of previous reactions. Also, the client should be asked about previous allergic reactions.

d. Aseptic technique should be maintained. This includes using a separate needle for each injection.

e. Two or more immunizing agents should never be mixed in a vial or syringe for the purpose of giving a single, simultaneous injection. The mixing of these drugs may cause the preparations to lose their immunizing potency or to produce enhanced adverse reaction.

f. Immunizing drugs should be stored properly prior to the time they are used. Directions on the package should be followed to ensure proper storage. In general, these drugs are to be stored within a temperature range of 2°-10°C or 35°-50°F.

g. Directions on the label should be read carefully and followed exactly.

h. The expiration date on the package should be carefully checked. Outdated preparations should not be used.

i. If a person has a history of allergic reactions, an intradermal skin test should be performed, for example, using 0.1 ml of the drug to be administered. (The manufacturer's directions should always be followed for hypersensitivity tests.) Whenever serum is to be given to persons who do not report allergies to serum, it is always necessary to skin test each person before the dosage is injected to learn whether the client is sensitive to the serum. Any person who reports allergy to serum should not be skin tested and should not be given a drug suspended in serum because an allergic reaction may result.

(1) "Reading" the skin test. A positive reaction has occurred if a hivelike welt appears, or if there is redness of the skin around the site of the injection. Either of these findings indicates that the client is sensitive to the serum.

(2) Administration of serum. If the client is sensitive, the serum should not be given until he is desensitized. This is a complicated and dangerous procedure involving the injection of many small but increasingly larger doses of serum. It should be done only by a medical officer.

NOTE: In the following paragraphs we discuss individual immunizing agents. However, we do not discuss the dosage schedules for each, since they change frequently and are readily available from other sources, including AR 40-562 and information provided by the manufacturer.

5-7. SERUMS

a. **Immune Serum Globulin (Human Gamma Globulin)**. This is a solution containing antibodies derived from adult human plasma or serum. It is used for the prevention and modification of measles, infectious hepatitis, and rubella. The usual duration of protection following administration is about 4 weeks. No serious reactions occur after the use of immune serum globulin.

b. **Tetanus Immune Globulin**. Used to provide passive immunity to tetanus, tetanus immune globulin is a sterile solution of globulins from plasma of human donors who have been immunized with tetanus toxoid. Tetanus immune globulin is sometimes used for prophylaxis after injury and to treat tetanus of the newborn.

c. **Polyvalent Crotaline Antivenin**. This is a hyperimmune equine (horse) serum containing antibodies against the venoms of all members of the family of snakes called Crotalidae. Generally, the antivenin will neutralize the venoms of the rattlesnake, copperhead, and water moccasin. It is not effective against the coral snake. The manufacturer's directions must be followed closely with regard to test for hypersensitivity, dosage, and route of administration.

5-8. TOXOIDS

a. **Tetanus Toxoid**. Tetanus toxoid is a solution of growth product of the tetanus bacillus Clostridium tetani, so treated that it is no longer toxic, but still capable of inducing active immunity. The precipitated and adsorbed forms are recommended because their slower absorption produces a high degree of immunity. Severe reactions after injection of adsorbed or precipitated forms are rare. However, a nodule of insoluble suspension may remain at the site of injection for several weeks. Tetanus toxoid is most often administered in a combined preparation containing diphtheria toxoid. The primary medical approach to tetanus is immunization in childhood with tetanus toxoid, followed by the proper boosters thereafter.

b. **Adsorbed Diphtheria and Tetanus Toxoids and Pertussis Vaccine**. This product is used for active immunization against diphtheria, tetanus, and pertussis with a minimum number of injections. Protection lasts approximately 5 years. After injection some local soreness and redness may occur for 2 to 3 days. The following precautions should be observed:

(1) Adolescents and adults who have been exposed to diphtheria but have not been previously immunized should be both Schick-tested and given the Schick control test before receiving a regular injection of diphtheria toxoid. The Schick test measures an individual's immunity to diphtheria. Such testing and the use of special preparations for adults is due to the frequency of severe reactions in adults to diphtheria toxoid.

(2) Because of the pertussis component, this preparation is contraindicated in upper respiratory infection.

NOTE: A preparation called adsorbed diphtheria and tetanus toxoids, which does not contain the pertussis vaccine, is also available.

5-9. BACTERIAL VACCINES

a. **Cholera Vaccine**. Cholera vaccine is a sterile suspension of killed Vibrio comma. It is used for the protective vaccination of individuals living or traveling in areas where cholera is prevalent. Immunity lasts 4 to 6 months. As for side effects, malaise, fever, chills, and pain and swelling at the site of injection may occur.

b. **Plague Vaccine**. This is a sterile suspension of killed plague bacilli (Yersinia pestis). Partial protection persists for 4 to 6 months. The vaccine does not consistently protect against bubonic (plague) infection, but it does improve chance of recovery. Local and systemic reactions to this vaccine, which occur frequently, include malaise, headache, local swelling, and slight fever. It is not advisable to administer this vaccine to clients with an upper respiratory infection.

c. **Typhoid Vaccine**. Typhoid vaccine is a sterile suspension of killed typhoid bacilli (Salmonella typhi) for injection. This vaccine is used for prophylaxis against typhoid fever. Local reactions may include inflammation, swelling, and pain lasting for 48 hours. Systemic reactions consist of fever, malaise, headache, and nausea. The inoculated person should avoid strenuous exercise for 24 hours.

5-10. VIRAL VACCINES

a. **Live Oral Poliovirus Vaccine**. The form of poliovirus vaccine available in Army supply channels is a combination of the three types of live, attenuated polioviruses, known as type 1, type 2, and type 3. Thus, this preparation is often called trivalent live oral poliovirus vaccine. The ingested live viruses replicate in the intestine and stimulate the production of both systemic and intestinal antibodies. The result is a solid immunity to virulent polioviruses. Administration should be postponed in the presence of GI upset. This drug must never be administered parenterally. The need for a booster has not been established.

b. **Smallpox Vaccine**. Smallpox vaccine is a sterile suspension obtained from cowpox, but used to prevent smallpox. The vaccine is administered by puncturing the skin with brief stabbing movements, while the vaccine is kept in contact with the puncture sites.

(1) Primary vaccination. Within 6-8 days after a primary vaccination, there should be an area of active inflammation surrounding a central lesion. On this basis, the vaccination is recorded as successful or unsuccessful. An unsuccessful primary vaccination must be repeated until a successful lesion is obtained.

(2) Precautions and contraindications.

(a) Smallpox vaccine is not to be injected, except intradermally with jet hypodermic injection apparatus.

(b) The vaccine should not be given to anyone who has eczema or other lesions of the skin, because in such persons there is danger of systemic reaction.

(c) The site of administration should be left open to the air to aid healing. This is the reason that the arm should be used.

(d) The vaccine should be administered with utmost attention to sterile technique to prevent secondary infection of the vaccination site. A person who receives smallpox vaccine is more exposed to infection than is a person who receives a drug by injection because of the numerous punctures of the skin for smallpox vaccination.

(e) The vial, in which freeze-dried smallpox vaccine is reconstituted, and the assembly for administration contain live virus. Before these items are discarded, they should be burned, autoclaved, or boiled to prevent accidental vaccination by breakage during disposal.

(3) Supply. Smallpox vaccine is supplied as a freeze-dried powder with a colored sterile diluent to reconstitute the vaccine, in 20-, 25-, and 100-doses. It is currently available only to military service members from the Center for Disease Control (CDC) in Atlanta, Georgia. Production of the smallpox vaccine for civilian use was discontinued in May 1983.

c. **Yellow Fever Vaccine**. An attenuated strain of yellow fever virus is prepared from chick embryos and freeze-dried. It should be kept frozen for preservation. Its period of potency is 12 months. Before administration, it is reconstituted with the diluent provided. It is injected subcutaneously. It results in solid immunity for 10 years. (The vaccine should be used with caution in egg-sensitive persons. It should not be administered concomitantly with smallpox vaccine or to persons ill with other virus diseases.)

d. **Influenza Virus Vaccine**. The influenza virus vaccine is a suspension of inactivated viruses grown in chick embryos. The preparations in military supply channels are bivalent; that is, each contains two prevalent strains of influenza virus. This vaccine produces only partial immunity, and it must be injected each year, about 1 month before the beginning of the respiratory disease season (usually October in CONUS). Injection is either intramuscular or subcutaneous. Local and systemic reactions to this vaccine are common, but usually mild. However, it may cause toxic reactions in children. It is contraindicated in persons allergic to egg protein.

e. **Live Attenuated Measles**. Attenuated strains of measles virus are grown in cell culture and freeze-dried. The preparation available in military supply channels generally produces an asymptomatic infection, which results in long term immunity to measles (rubeola, not German measles, rubella). The route of administration is IM or SC. Contraindications include leukemia, age under 9 months, febrile respiratory illness or other active infection, and pregnancy. It should be deferred in children who have received immune serum globulin or a blood transfusion within the past 6 weeks.

f. **Live Mumps Virus Vaccines**. Mumps vaccine is prepared from chick embryos infected with mumps virus. The route of administration is IM. Contraindications include age under 1 year; pregnancy; allergy to eggs, chicken, or neomycin; or any active infection or other condition depressing the normal defense mechanisms. It should not be administered at the same time as other immunization. Allow 1 month to pass between elective immunizations.

g. **Live Rubella Virus Vaccine**. Attenuated strains of rubella virus, of duck cell tissue origin, are freeze-dried. The vaccine, given subcutaneously, produces a systemic infection, tolerated well by children, but sometimes causing fever and arthralgia in adults. The result is perhaps long-term immunity to rubella (German measles). The vaccine must not be given to pregnant women, or the fetus may be infected. In seronegative females, it must be assured that no pregnancy will begin within the next three months. Some physicians prefer to give the vaccine only to prepubertal girls.

NOTE: A live measles, mumps, and rubella virus vaccine is also available. It is used to produce active immunity to measles, mumps, and rubella virus and is administered subcutaneously.

h. **Rabies Vaccine**. Rabies vaccine is a dried preparation of killed rabies viruses obtained from duck embryos that have been infected with fixed rabies virus. Individuals suspected of having rabies are given daily subcutaneous injections for 14 consecutive days. Complete instructions for its use are provided by the manufacturer.

Section III. PENICILLINS AND CEPHALOSPORINS; ERYTHROMYCIN

5-11. INTRODUCTION

Antibiosis is an association between two or more organisms that is detrimental to one of them. A chemical agent responsible for this antagonistic relationship is called an antibiotic. An example of this is the relationship between certain bacteria and various plants (fungi and molds). The bacteria are unable to live and grow in the presence of these plants or their extracts. The extracts are called antibiotics. There are numerous official and nonofficial antibiotics. Their powerful antibacterial action is extremely valuable in combating diseases caused by pathogenic organisms. Antibiotics, then, are products of living microorganisms (or similar synthetic substances) that kill or inhibit the growth of other microorganisms. Penicillin is the classic example.

5-12. SPECTRUM OF ACTIVITY

The antibiotics can be classified as either "narrow" or "broad" spectrum antibiotics, depending upon the different organisms against which they are effective. Penicillin, for example, is effective against most gram-positive bacteria but against only a few gram-negative cocci. For this reason, it is called a narrow spectrum antibiotic. Tetracycline, on the other hand, is effective against the common infecting gram-positive and gram-negative organisms; it is a broad spectrum antibiotic.

5-13. PENICILLINS

The individual antibiotics can best be studied pharmacologically by first discussing penicillin and then comparing the other agents with it. Penicillin is the antibacterial substance derived from the mold <u>Penicillium notatum</u> or <u>Penicillium chrysogenum</u>. Several forms have been identified and designated as penicillin F, G, K, O, V, and X. Of these, penicillin G was found to be the best, and the manufacture of the others has been discontinued.

a. **Absorption**. When administered by intramuscular injection, potassium penicillin G is very rapidly absorbed into the circulation. Since it is also rapidly excreted by the kidneys, repeated doses must be given at frequent intervals to maintain blood levels, or a more slowly absorbed oil dispersion or sparingly soluble salt must be used.

b. **Excretion**. Penicillin is mainly excreted by the kidneys in urine. Most of a therapeutic intramuscular dose of potassium penicillin G is excreted in 5 hours, but lessening amounts are detected for as long as 7 to 12 hours.

c. **Mechanism of Action**. The mode of action of penicillin has long been in dispute. The present concept, arrived at after long study by several researchers, is that penicillin's antibacterial activity is due to an inhibition of vital metabolic functions within the cell wall of the bacteria concerned. Briefly, this inhibition prevents conversion of muramic acid in the cell wall to new cell wall material. The organism thus cannot survive or grow.

d. **Solubility and Stability**. Penicillin is a high-molecular- weight organic acid, and as such is not soluble in water. Its salts, however, are soluble. The potassium salt is most frequently used. These solutions are stable at a pH of 5 through 8 for about 2 weeks. They must be buffered to maintain their pH. Potassium penicillin G is stable at room temperature, but its solution should be kept refrigerated.

e. **Adverse Reactions**. Possible reactions include urticarial reactions, serum sickness, dermatitis, and anaphylactic shock. Topical applications may produce sensitivity; therefore, it should not be used indiscriminately. The few cases of anaphylactic shock that occur are so severe that sensitivity tests should be performed before administering this agent. Other than allergic reactions, penicillin produces few adverse effects.

f. **Standardization**. The potency of penicillin is expressed in terms of international units. One unit is equivalent to 0.6 mcg of crystalline sodium penicillin G. There are 1,667 units in 1 mg.

g. **Acquired Resistance to Penicillin**. The massive use of penicillin in the past has promoted the development of strains resistant to penicillin. One of the chief bacterial means of resisting penicillin is to produce an enzyme called <u>penicillinase</u>, which destroys penicillin. As a consequence, semisynthetic penicillins not so susceptible to penicillinase have been developed. These should be used only when the other penicillins--penicillin G, penicillin V, and ampicillin--are not effective in treating a particular malady.

5-14. POTASSIUM PENICILLIN G FOR INJECTION

Potassium penicillin G is also known as aqueous penicillin G or crystalline penicillin G.

a. **Indications**. This is the penicillin of choice for intravenous administration. It is effective against most gram-positive cocci and bacilli, some gram-negative cocci, and some spirochetes. (In addition, some species of gram-negative bacilli are sensitive to high concentrations of the drug obtained with intravenous therapy. These include most strains of <u>E. coli</u>, all strains of <u>Proteus mirabilis</u>, <u>Salmonella</u> and <u>Shigella</u>, and some strains of <u>Aerobacter aerogenes</u> and <u>Alcaligenes faecalis</u>.) Potassium penicillin G for injection is indicated in the therapy of severe infections caused by penicillin G-sensitive microorganisms when rapid and high penicillin blood levels are required. Therapy should be guided by culture and sensitivity studies and by clinical response. The following infections will usually respond to adequate doses of potassium penicillin G for injection.

(1) Streptococcal infections. Potassium penicillin G for injection is the penicillin dosage form of choice for bacteremia, empyema, severe pneumonia, pericarditis, endocarditis, meningitis, and other severe infections caused by sensitive strains of this organism.

(2) Pneumococcal infections.

(3) Staphylococcal infections (penicillin-G sensitive).

(4) Anthrax.

(5) Actinomycosis.

(6) Clostridial infections (to include tetanus).

(7) Diphtheria (to prevent carrier state).

(8) Erysipeloid endocarditis.

(9) Fusospirochetal infections.

(10) Gram-negative bacillary infections (bacteremias).

(11) Listeria infections.

(12) Pasteurella infections.

(13) Bacteremia and meningitis.

(14) Rat-bite fever.

(15) Gonorrheal endocarditis.

(16) Syphilis.

(17) Prophylaxis against bacterial endocarditis in clients with rheumatic or congenital heart disease when undergoing dental or upper respiratory tract surgery or instrumentation, surgery of the lower intestinal tract, childbirth, and instrumentation of the genitourinary tract.

b. **Usual Dosage**. Potassium penicillin G for injection has a short duration of effect (approximately 60 percent of a total dose is excreted in the urine within a 5-hour period). Thus, high and frequent doses are required to maintain the elevated serum levels necessary to treat certain severe infections in individuals with normal kidney function.

(1) Severe infections due to susceptible strains of streptococci, pneumococci, and staphylococci--a minimum of 5 million units daily.

(2) Gonorrheal endocarditis--a minimum of 5 million units daily.

(3) Meningococcal meningitis--1 to 2 million units IM every 2 hours or continuous IV drip of 20 to 30 million units daily.

(4) Actinomycosis--up to 20 million units/day.

(5) Rat-bite fever--12 to 15 million units/day.

(6) Erysipeloid endocarditis--2 to 20 million units/day.

(7) Gram-negative bacillary infections (E. coli, A. aerogenes, A. faecalis, Salmonella, Shigella, and Proteus mirabilis)--bacteremia--20 to 80 million units/day.

(8) Diphtheria (carrier state)--300,000 to 400,000 units/day in divided doses for 10 to 20 days.

(9) Anthrax--a minimum of 5 million units of penicillin/day in divided doses until cure is achieved.

c. **Cautions and Warnings**.

(1) A history of a previous allergic reaction to any of the penicillins is a contraindication.

(2) Anaphylaxis and other serious hypersensitivity reactions are more frequent following injection of penicillin. These reactions are more likely to occur in clients with a history of sensitivity to multiple allergens or asthma.

(3) Continue therapy for a minimum of 10 days for streptococcal infections.

(4) Frequent evaluation of electrolyte balance, renal, and hematopoietic function is recommended during therapy when high doses of intravenous potassium penicillin G are used.

(5) Prolonged use of antibiotics may promote a superinfection of nonsusceptible organisms.

d. **Adverse Reactions**.

(1) The following allergic reactions have been reported: skin rashes, urticaria, and reactions resembling serum sickness including chills, fever, edema, arthralgia, and prostration. Severe and occasionally fatal anaphylaxis has occurred.

(2) Hemolytic anemia, leukopenia, thrombocytopenia, nephropathy, and neuropathy are rarely observed and usually associated with high intravenous dosage.

(3) Severe or even fatal potassium poisoning can occur, especially if renal insufficiency is present in clients given continuous intravenous therapy with potassium penicillin G in high dosage (10 to 100 million units/day).

(4) The Jarisch-Herxheimer reaction (increase in syphilitic symptoms) has been reported in clients treated for syphilis.

e. **Supply**. This preparation, in dry powder form, must be reconstituted. It is available in bottles of 1 and 5 million units for IM or IV use. It is also supplied as a 20 million unit vial for reconstitution and intravenous infusion only.

5-15. PROCAINE PENICILLIN G

a. **Indications**. Procaine penicillin G is a natural penicillin composed of procaine and penicillin G administered intramuscularly as a suspension. Plateau-type blood levels occur about 4 hours after injection and fall slowly over a period of the next 15 to 20 hours. Procaine penicillin G is indicated in the treatment of moderately severe infections due to penicillin G-sensitive microorganisms that are sensitive to the low and persistent serum levels common to this dosage form. The following infections will usually respond to adequate doses of intramuscular procaine penicillin G.

(1) Pneumococcal infections.

(2) Staphylococcal infections except penicillinase-resistant strains.

(3) Streptococcal infections Group A (without bacteremia). Group D (enterococcus) are resistant.

(4) Fusospirochetosis (Vincent's gingivitis and pharyngitis).

(5) <u>Treponema pallidum</u> (syphilis); all stages.

(6) <u>Neisseria gonorrhoea</u> (acute and chronic stages of gonorrhea).

(7) Yaws, bejel, pinta.

(8) <u>Corynebacterium diphtheriae</u>--procaine penicillin G as an adjunct to antitoxin for prevention of the carrier state of diphtheria.

(9) Anthrax.

(10) Erysipeloid.

(11) Prophylaxis against bacterial endocarditis.

NOTE: In the above infections when high sustained serum levels are required, potassium penicillin G for injection should be used.

b. **Usual Dosage**. This preparation is given IM only. The usual recommended dose is 600,000 to 2,400,000 units daily according to the susceptibility of the organism and the severity of the infection. For the treatment of gonorrhea, the usual doses are as follows:

(1) Males--2.4 million to 4.8 million units in one-day treatment.

(2) Females--4.8 million units in one-day treatment.

(3) Probenecid (1 gram orally) should be used to potentiate the action of procaine penicillin G in gonorrhea.

c. **Cautions and Warnings**.

(1) A previous hypersensitivity reaction to any penicillin is a contraindication.

(2) Avoid accidental intravenous administration.

(3) Use with caution in individuals with histories of significant allergies or asthma.

(4) In suspected staphylococcal infections, proper laboratory studies, including sensitivity tests, should be performed.

(5) The use of antibiotics may result in overgrowth of nonsusceptible organisms.

(6) Periodic evaluation of renal and hematopoietic systems are recommended in prolonged therapy with penicillin, particularly with high dosage schedules.

(7) Monthly serological tests should be made for at least four months when treating gonococcal infections in which primary or secondary syphilis may be suspected.

d. **Adverse Reactions**.

(1) Hypersensitivity reactions to penicillin are common and include: skin rashes, urticaria, and serum sickness-like reactions. Severe and often fatal anaphylaxis have been reported.

(2) The Jarisch-Herxheimer reaction (increase in syphilis symptoms) has been reported with the treatment for syphilis.

e. **Supply**.'

(1) Procaine penicillin for aqueous injection in dry powder form, 300,000 units and 1,500,000 units.

(2) Sterile procaine penicillin G suspension with cartridge- needle units:

(a) 600,000 units, 1-ml size.

(b) 1,200,000 units, 2-ml size.

(c) 2,400,000 units 4-ml size.

5-16. BENZATHINE PENICILLIN G

Benzathine penicillin G (Bicillin) is always given IM. It is absorbed into the bloodstream much more slowly than are the other penicillins and is, therefore, longer acting. Depending upon the size of the dose, a single intramuscular injection produces an effective blood level for 1 to 4 weeks. The drug may be used when prolonged action at low blood levels is desirable. For example, it is the preferred drug for preventing recurrence of rheumatic fever in those who have had previous attacks. The usual dose is 1,200,000 units, once a month. The usual dose range is 600,000 to 3,000,000 units, from three times a week to once a month. Preparations containing benzathine penicillin G are given below.

a. **Sterile Benzathine Penicillin G Suspension**. This preparation is supplied in cartridge-needle units with one plastic cartridge syringe. The available sizes are 1 ml (600,000 units) and 2 ml (1,200,000 units).

b. **Sterile Benzathine Penicillin G and Procaine Penicillin G Suspension**. This preparation is also supplied in cartridge-needle units with one plastic cartridge syringe. The 1-ml size contains 300,000 units of each penicillin, and the 2-ml size contains 600,000 units of each penicillin.

c. **Benzathine Penicillin G, Procaine Penicillin G, and Potassium Penicillin G for Injection**. This is a dry powder form that must be reconstituted. It contains 600,000 units of benzathine penicillin G, 300,000 units of potassium penicillin G, and 300,000 units of procaine penicillin G.

5-17. POTASSIUM PHENOXYMETHYL PENICILLIN (PENICILLIN V)

a. **Indications**.

(1) Penicillin V is the phenoxymethyl analog of penicillin G. It has the same basic activity as penicillin G and is intended for oral use only. Penicillin V is not active against the penicillinase-producing bacteria. Penicillin V has the distinct advantage over penicillin G in resistance to inactivation by gastric acid and that it may be given with meals.

(2) Penicillin V is indicated for the treatment of mild to moderately severe infections due to penicillin G-sensitive microorganisms that are sensitive to the low serum levels common to this particular dosage form.

NOTE: Therapy should be guided by bacteriological studies and by clinical response. Severe pneumonia, empyema, bacteremia, pericarditis, meningitis, and arthritis should not be treated with penicillin V during the acute stage.

b. **Usual Dosage**.

(1) The dosage of penicillin V should be determined according to the sensitivity of the causative microorganism, the severity of the infection, and adjusted to the client's clinical response.

(2) The usual dose range for adults and children who are 12 years of age and older is 200,000 to 500,000 units every 6 to 8 hours.

c. **Cautions and Warnings**.

(1) A previous hypersensitivity reaction to any penicillin is a contraindication.

(2) Hypersensitivity reactions are more likely to occur in clients with a history of sensitivity to multiple allergens or asthma.

(3) The oral route of administration should not be relied on in clients with severe illness or with nausea, vomiting, gastric dilatation, cardiospasm or intestinal hypermotility.

(4) Therapy must be maintained for at least 10 days in streptococcal infections to completely eliminate the organism.

(5) Prolonged use of an antibiotic may promote a superinfection due to nonsusceptible organisms including fungi.

d. **Adverse Reactions**.

(1) All degrees of hypersensitivity to include fatal anaphylaxis have been reported with oral penicillin. The incidence is much less frequent than with injected forms.

(2) Other common reactions reported include nausea, vomiting, epigastric distress, diarrhea, and black hairy tongue.

e. **Supply**.

(1) Potassium phenoxymethyl penicillin for oral solution. This is in the form of granules or powder and is reconstituted to make an oral solution containing 400,000 units/5 ml.

(2) Potassium phenoxymethyl penicillin tablets. Tablets are available in 400,000- and 800,000-unit sizes.

5-18. AMPICILLIN

a. **Indications**. Ampicillin (Omnipen) is a broad-spectrum, semi- synthetic derivative of penicillin. A special feature of ampicillin is its effectiveness against many gram-negative bacteria, as well as against most of the gram-positive bacteria affected by penicillin G and penicillin V. It can be used in conditions caused by the following organisms:

(1) Shigella.

(2) Salmonella (including S. typhi).

(3) Haemophilus influenzae.

(4) E. coli.

(5) Proteus mirabilis.

(6) Neisseria meningitidis.

(7) Streptococci.

(8) Diplococcus pneumoniae.

(9) Nonpenicillinase-producing staphylococci.

(10) Bacillus anthracis.

(11) Clostridia.

(12) Most strains of enterococci.

b. **Usual Dosage**. Adult--250 to 500 mg, 4 times daily orally, or 250 to 500 mg, every 6 hours IM or IV.

c. **Cautions and Warnings: Adverse Reactions**. The cautions and warnings for ampicillin, as well as possible adverse reactions, are the same as with penicillin V.

d. **Supply**. Ampicillin is supplied as 250-mg and 500-mg capsules and as a flavored dry mix for oral suspension (3.75 gm to be reconstituted to 150 ml of 125 mg/5 ml suspension, 5 gm to be reconstituted to 100 ml of 250 mg/5 ml suspension, 7.5 gm to be reconstituted to 150 ml of 250 mg/5 ml suspension).

5-19. PENICILLINS RESISTANT TO PENICILLINASE

The following semisynthetic penicillins, which are resistant to penicillinase, should be used only to treat infections caused by strains of bacteria, particularly staphylococci, which have developed a resistance to penicillin. This limited use helps discourage the further development of strains resistant to these drugs also. The precautions and contraindications for these drugs are similar to those for the other penicillins.

a. **Sodium Methicillin (Staphcillin)**. Methicillin is given IM or IV.

b. **Sodium Oxacillin (Prostaphlin)**. Sodium oxacillin may be given orally 1 or 2 hours before meals. Since absorption by the oral route is unreliable, it should not be used for the most serious infections. Preparations for IM or IV administration are also available.

c. **Sodium Dicloxacillin (Dynapen)**. Sodium dicloxacillin should be given orally 1-2 hours before meals. May be used to initiate therapy in any client in whom a staphylococcal infection is suspected.

d. **Sodium Nafcillin (Unipen)**. Serum levels of nafcillin after oral administration are low and unpredictable. Use parenteral therapy initially in severe infections and change to oral therapy as the condition warrants.

5-20. CEPHALOSPORINS

The cephalosporins are a family of antibiotics resembling the penicillins. They are bactericidal agents, active against both gram-positive and gram-negative bacteria. The cephaloporins resist the action of penicillinase. They are divided into first, second, and third generation agents. In general, progression from first to third generation reveals greater gram-negative spectrum, loss of efficacy against gram-positive organisms, greater efficacy against resistant organisms, and increased costs.

a. **Indications**. These agents are most useful in:

(1) The treatment of serious gram-negative bacterial infections due to susceptible organisms that do not respond to agents of first choice.

(2) The treatment of urinary tract or respiratory tract infections due to susceptible organisms.

(3) The treatment of infections with penicillinase-producing staphylococci. In addition, a cephalosporin may be occasionally used as a substitute in known penicillin-allergic clients. CAUTION: Some cross-hypersensitivity exists.

b. **Usual Dosage**.

(1) Cephalothin (Keflin). Cephalothin, a first generation agent, is for parenteral use only; it may be given intravenously or by deep intramuscular injection. The usual adult dose range is 500 mg to 1 gram every 4 to 6 hours. In life-threatening infections, doses up to 2 grams every 4 hours may be required.

(2) Cephapirin (Cefadyl). Cephapirin, a first generation agent, is for parenteral use only and has a spectrum of activity similar to cephalothin.

(3) Cephalexin (Keflex). Cephalexin, another first generation agent, is for oral administration only; the usual adult dose is 250 mg qid, with a maximum of 4 grams daily for more severe infections. The daily dose for children is 25 to 50 mg per kg of body weight, divided into four doses.

(4) Cefoxitin (Mefoxin). Cefoxitin, a second generation agent, is for parenteral use only. It has greater activity against gram negative organisms than first generation agents.

(5) Cefaclor (Ceclor). Cefaclor is a second generation agent for oral use only. It is employed primarily for otitis media and respiratory tract infections.

(6) Ceftriaxone (Rocephin). Ceftriaxone, a third generation cephalosporin, is for parenteral use only. It is administered once daily either IM or IV.

c. **Cautions and Warnings**.

(1) All cephalosporins are contraindicated in clients who have shown hypersensitivity to any one cephalosporin.

(2) In penicillin-sensitive clients, the cephalosporin derivatives should be used with great caution. It has been estimated that about 10 percent of penicillin-hypersensitive clients are also allergic to the cephalosporins.

(3) The addition of 10 to 25 mg of hydrocortisone to intravenous solutions containing 4 to 6 grams of cephalothin may reduce the incidence of thrombophlebitis.

(4) Prolonged use of the cephalosporins may result in the overgrowth of nonsusceptible organisms (superinfection).

(5) The cephalosporins will produce a false-positive reaction for glucose in the urine with Benedict's solutions and Clinitest tablets but not with Tes-Tape.

(6) Safety of the cephalosporins for use in pregnancy has not been established.

d. **Adverse Reactions**.

(1) Injectable forms can produce severe pain after intramuscular injection, while repeated intravenous injection may result in thrombophlebitis.

(2) Anaphylaxis, urticaria, skin rashes, fever, eosinophilia, granulocytopenia, and hemolytic anemia may occur.

(3) Renal toxicity has occurred with cephaloridine but not with cephalothin.

(4) Oral cephalosporins have produced diarrhea, nausea, and vomiting.

e. **Supply**.

(1) Sterile sodium cephalothin (Keflin). Cephalothin is a semisynthetic cephalosporin antibiotic for parenteral use only. Its use has not been associated with renal toxicity. It is supplied in 1-gram, 2-gram, and 4-gram vials for reconstitution. It may be refrigerated for 48 hours after reconstitution without loss of potency.

(2) Cephapirin for injection (Cefadyl). Cephapirin can be administered IM or IV. Adults receive 500 mg to 1 gram every 4 to 6 hours. For serious infections up to 12 grams daily may be administered. The IV route must be used when higher doses are required. Cephapirin is supplied in 500 mg, 1 gm, 2 gm, 4 gm, and 20 gm vials for reconstitution.

(3) Cephalexin monohydrate (Keflex). Cephalexin is a semi- synthetic cephalosporin intended for oral use only. It is included in the Battalion Aid Station Medical Equipment Set. The main indications for this drug are as a follow-up antibiotic for clients switching from a parenteral cephalosporin and for the treatment of urinary tract infections resistant to antibiotics of first choice (that is, sulfonamides, ampicillin,

and so forth). It is supplied as a 250-mg capsule; quantities of 2.5 grams are available to be reconstituted to 100 ml of oral suspension (125 mg/5 ml).

(4) Cefoxitin for injection (Mefoxin). The adult dose of cefoxitin is 1 to 2 grams every 6 to 8 hours. IM doses need to be injected well within a large muscle. It is supplied in 1 gram, 2 gram, and 10 gram vials.

(5) Cefaclor (Ceclor). Cefaclor is commonly used to treat respiratory tract infections and otitis media. The usual dose is 250 mg every eight hours. In more severe infections, 500 mg every eight hours may be administered. It is supplied in 250 mg and 500 mg capsules and as powder for suspension 125 mg per 5 ml and 250 mg per 5 ml. The suspension must be refrigerated after reconstitution.

(6) Ceftriaxone (Rocephin). Ceftriaxone can be administered IM or IV. The adult dose is 1 to 2 gm once daily. A total daily dose of 4 gm should not be exceeded. IM doses should be injected well within the body of a large muscle. Ceftriaxone is supplied in 250 mg, 500 mg, 1 gram, 2 gram, and 10-gram vials.

5-21. ERYTHROMYCIN

Erythromycin (Erythrocin) is often used to treat clients who are hypersensitive to penicillin. Its antibacterial activity is similar to that of penicillin. Erythromycin is effective against gram-positive organisms, especially pneumococci, streptococci, staphylococci, and corynebacteria. It is also effective against neisseriae, Haemophilus, and Mycoplasma.

a. **Indications**.

(1) Upper and lower respiratory tract, skin, and soft-tissue infections due to beta-hemolytic streptococcus.

(2) Short-term prophylaxis against bacterial endocarditis prior to dental procedures in clients with a history of rheumatic fever or congenital heart disease and who are allergic to penicillin.

(3) Acute infections of the skin or soft tissue due to Staphylococcus aureus.

(4) Upper and lower respiratory tract infections due to Diplococcus pneumoniae.

(5) Treatment of primary atypical pneumonia due to Mycoplasma pneumoniae.

(6) Treatment of primary syphilis in penicillin-allergic clients.

(7) Treatment of gonorrhea in clients allergic to penicillin.

b. **Adverse Effects**.

(1) The most frequent side effect of oral administration is abdominal cramping and other GI discomfort. Nausea, vomiting, and diarrhea do occur in some clients.

(2) Allergic reactions ranging from simple skin rash to anaphylaxis have been reported.

(3) Superinfections may occur during long-term therapy.

c. **Cautions and Warnings**.

(1) The safety of this drug in pregnancy has not been established.

(2) The administration of erythromycin estolate has been associated with cholestatic hepatitis.

(3) This drug should be used cautiously in clients with impaired hepatic function.

(4) Intramuscular injection is not recommended in small children, since small children do not have the large muscle mass needed for deep placement of the injection.

(5) Intramuscular injections may cause severe pain, sterile abscess formation, and necrosis.

d. **Usual Dosage**. Dosage varies with the sensitivity of the organism and severity of the infection.

(1) Adult: 250 mg every 6 hours.

(2) Child: 30-50 mg/kg/day, in divided doses.

e. **Supply**.

(1) Erythromycin stearate or base capsules, 250 mg each.

(2) Erythromycin estolate capsules, 250 mg each.

(3) Erythromycin estolate for oral suspension, 125 mg/5 ml when mixed with water.

(4) Erythromycin ethylsuccinate for oral suspension, 200 mg/5 ml. when reconstituted.

(5) Erythromycin ethylsuccinate tablets, 200 mg each, chewable.

(6) Erythromycin lactobionate for injection, powder in 1-gram vials for reconstitution.

(7) Erythromycin stearate or base tablets, 250 mg each.

Section IV. TETRACYCLINES

5-22. INTRODUCTION

The tetracyclines are a group of closely related, broad-spectrum antibiotics that are effective against the same range of microbes. The ones we discuss here are tetracycline (Achromycin), chlortetracycline (Aureomycin), and oxytetracycline (Terramycin).

5-23. INDICATIONS

The tetracyclines are bacteriostatic antibiotics effective against a wide range of gram-positive and gram-negative bacteria.

a. Tetracyclines are considered agents of first choice in:

(1) Infections caused by Mycoplasma pneumoniae (PPLO, Eaton agent). (Erythromycin is considered equally effective.)

(2) Infections caused by rickettsiae.

(3) Infections caused by agents of psittacosis, lymphogranuloma venereum (LGV), granuloma inguinale, Chlamydia trachomatis, and the virus of inclusion conjunctivitis.

(4) Infections caused by Vibrio comma (cholera) and Borrelia recurrentis (relapsing fever).

(5) Infections caused by Haemophilus ducreyi (chancroid), Brucella organisms (with or without streptomycin), and gastrointestinal forms of Bacteroides.

b. In addition, tectracyclines may be considered in the following situations:

(1) Acute amebiasis--adjunctive therapy with other amebicides.

(2) When penicillin is contraindicated, tetracyclines are alternative drugs in treatment of gonorrhea, syphilis, yaws, actinomycosis, and infections caused by gram-positive bacilli (anthrax, gas gangrene, and tetanus).

(3) Oral forms of tetracycline may be a useful adjunct to the chronic management of severe acne.

(4) Other infections caused by gram-negative and gram-positive organisms when bacteriologic testing indicates appropriate susceptibility. However, other antibiotics are usually considered agents of first choice.

5-24. USUAL DOSAGE

The doses for tetracycline hydrochloride and oxytetracycline are given below:

a. **Intramuscular**. Intramuscular administration is not recommended since IM injections are painful and tetracycline is poorly absorbed from the muscles. The usual daily dose of tetracycline or oxytetracycline is 250 mg IM once every 24 hours or 300 mg given in divided doses at 8- to 12-hour intervals.

b. **Intravenous**. Intravenous administration should be considered only if rapid, high blood levels are needed especially in an acutely ill client. Oral therapy should be instituted as soon as possible, as IV therapy given over prolonged periods of time may result in thrombophlebitis. The usual adult dose of tetracycline or oxytetracycline is 250 to 500 mg IV every 12 hours, not to exceed 500 mg every 6 hours or 2 grams per day.

c. **Oral**. Oral forms of tetracyclines should be given one hour before or two hours after meals. The usual adult daily dose of tetracycline is 1 to 2 grams orally per day, divided in 2 to 4 equal doses depending on the severity of the infection. In the treatment of acne, an initial dose of 0.5 to 1.0 gram daily is used for a few weeks, then decreased to 250 mg per day for maintenance.

NOTE: The absorption of oral tetracyclines is impaired when they are taken with antacids containing aluminum, calcium, or magnesium. Food and some dairy products (milk) also interfere with absorption. Recent evidence also suggests that iron compounds interfere with absorption.

5-25. ADVERSE REACTIONS

a. **Gastrointestinal**--anorexia, nausea, vomiting, diarrhea, glossitis, and lesions with Candida overgrowth in the anogenital region. These are the most common reasons for discontinuing tetracycline therapy.

b. **Dermatological**--rashes, photosensitivity, especially with demeclocycline.

c. **Renal**--rise in BUN (blood urea nitrogen) reported which is dose- related.

d. **Hypersensitivity reactions**--urticaria, angioedema, anaphylaxis, etc.

e. **Bulging Fontanels**--reported in young infants following full therapeutic dosage.

f. **Hematological**--blood dyscrasias only rarely reported.

g. **Bone Lesions and Staining and Deformity of Teeth**--in children up to 8 years old and in the newborn when given to pregnant women after fourth month of pregnancy.

h. **Liver Damage**--parenteral doses may cause serious liver damage, especially in pregnant women and clients with renal disease receiving 1 gram or more daily.

5-26. CAUTIONS AND WARNINGS

a. The tetracyclines are contraindicated in clients who have shown hypersensitivity to these antibiotics.

b. Tetracycline drugs should not be used during tooth development (last half of pregnancy, infancy, and childhood to 8 years of age) unless other drugs are contraindicated or are likely to be ineffective. The use of the tetracyclines in this age group may cause permanent discoloration of the teeth (yellow, gray, brown). Enamel hypoplasia has been reported also.

c. Reduce oral and parenteral doses of tetracyclines if renal impairment exists.

d. Photosensitivity reactions may develop as an exaggerated sunburn; thus, clients who will be exposed to direct sunlight or ultraviolet light should be warned.

e. In pregnant women, tetracyclines cross the placenta and can have direct toxic effects (usually related to retardation of skeletal development) on the developing fetus.

f. Tetracyclines will occur in the milk of lactating women.

g. Since bacteriostatic drugs may interfere with the bactericidal action of the penicillins, avoid the use of a tetracycline in conjunction with a penicillin.

h. Superinfections may result due to overgrowth of nonsusceptible organisms including fungi.

i. Using outdated and deteriorated tetracyclines may cause renal damage.

5-27. SUPPLY

Since the tetracyclines are essentially the same therapeutically, the choice of one may be based on duration of action and relative cost.

a. **Tetracycline Hydrochloride (Achromycin)**. Tetracycline hydro-chloride is the most frequently used member of this group, the least expensive, and associated with the lowest incidence of side effects. It is supplied as a tablet, capsule, oral syrup, and injection. The usual dose is 250 mg, four times daily (see discussion above).

b. **Chlortetracycline Hydrochloride (Aureomycin)**. Chlortetracycline hydrochloride is supplied in 1% and 3% ointments. Chlortetracycline is valuable in the treatment of trachoma and inclusion conjunctivitis. Oral sulfonamides such as sulfisoxazole (Gantrisin) are often used concurrently.

c. **Oxytetracycline (Terramycin)**. Oxytetracycline has the same actions, usage, and dosage as tetracycline. It is supplied in oral and parenteral dosage forms. It is also available in an ophthalmic ointment, which contains polymyxin B sulfate, another antibiotic.

Continue with Exercises

EXERCISES, LESSON 5

INSTRUCTIONS: Answer the following exercises by marking the lettered response that best answers the question or completes the incomplete statement.

After you have completed all of these exercises, turn to "Solutions to Exercises" at the end of the lesson and check your answers. For each exercise answered incorrectly, reread the material referenced with the solution.

1. Resistance to a certain infection or disease is called:

   a. Antigen.

   b. Antitoxin.

   c. Immunity.

   d. Antibody.

2. If a substance is injected into the body to stimulate the production of antibodies, the resulting immunity is called:

   a. Active.

   b. Latent.

   c. Passive.

   d. Refractory.

3. Immunity that affords short-term protection to a person exposed to an infectious disease is called:

   a. Active immunity.

   b. Passive immunity.

   c. Natural immunity.

   d. Antigenic immunity.

4. Passive immunity results from the injection of a substance containing:

   a. Antibodies.

   b. Antigens.

   c. Toxins.

   d. Vaccine.

5. When a vaccine is administered, the body should produce which of the following substances?

   a. Antibodies.

   b. Antigens.

   c. Toxins.

   d. Toxoids.

6. An antitoxin is a type of:

   a. Antibiotic.

   b. Antibody.

   c. Antihistamine.

   d. Antipruritic.

7. A client who received an injection of an immunizing drug two minutes ago is now breathing with difficulty and is scratching himself. What kind of reaction is the client exhibiting?

   a. Serum sickness.

   b. Anaphylactic reaction.

   c. Immune reaction.

   d. Normal reaction.

8. What is the proper procedure concerning the administration of serum to a person who reports that he is allergic to serum?

   a. Skin test with 0.1 ml of the drug.

   b. Apply a tourniquet and give the drug.

   c. Give one-third of the full dose.

   d. Do not give any of the drug.

9. The primary medical approach to the problem of tetanus is:

   a. The administration of penicillin.

   b. The administration of tetanus antitoxin.

   c. The administration of tetanus immune globulin.

   d. Childhood immunization with tetanus toxoid followed by necessary boosters.

10. Severe reactions to diphtheria toxoid are particularly common in which of the following groups?

   a. Children.

   b. Adults.

   c. Females.

   d. Males.

11. By what method should live poliovirus vaccine be administered?

   a. Oral.

   b. Sublingual.

   c. Rectal.

   d. Parenteral.

12. To have immunity against poliomyelitis, a person must be immune to which of the following strains of the virus?

    a. All of the below.

    b. Type 1.

    c. Type 2.

    d. Type 3.

13. A smallpox vaccine is actually obtained from:

    a. Rubella.

    b. Rubeola.

    c. Smallpox.

    d. Cowpox.

14. By what method should smallpox vaccine be administered?

    a. Oral.

    b. Subcutaneous.

    c. Intramuscular.

    d. None of the above.

15. If the reaction obtained following primary administration of smallpox vaccine is read as "unsuccessful," what should be done?

    a. Skin test the client.

    b. Put tape over vaccination site.

    c. Revaccinate.

    d. Assume immunity.

16. Following the use of smallpox vaccine, the empty vials should be burned, boiled, or autoclaved before they are disposed of in order to avoid accidental:

    a. Breakage.

    b. Dispersion.

    c. Vaccination.

    d. Cross-contaminations.

17. What is the main adverse effect of penicillin?

    a. CNS depression.

    b. Postural hypotension.

    c. Allergic reactions.

    d. Respiratory depression.

18. A primary mechanism used by bacteria to develop resistance to penicillin is the production of an enzyme called:

    a. Methicillin.

    b. Oxacillin.

    c. Cholinesterase.

    d. Penicillinase.

19. The penicillin referred to as crystalline penicillin G is actually which of the following products?

    a. Benzathine penicillin G.

    b. Procaine penicillin G.

    c. Potassium penicillin G.

    d. Penicillin V.

20. Penicillin G is generally least effective against which of the following?

    a. Gram-negative bacilli.

    b. Gonococci (cause of gonorrhea).

    c. Pneumococci.

    d. Streptococci.

21. The penicillin best suited for use in the long-term prophylaxis of rheumatic fever is:

    a. Benzathine penicillin G.

    b. Procaine penicillin G suspension.

    c. Potassium penicillin G.

    d. Penicillin V.

22. An advantage of ampicillin is its:

    a. Natural derivation.

    b. Long duration of action.

    c. Resistance to penicillinase.

    d. Effectiveness against many gram-negative bacteria.

23. An advantage of methicillin and oxacillin is their:

    a. Natural derivation.

    b. Long duration of action.

    c. Resistance of penicillinase.

    d. Effectiveness against many gram-negative bacteria.

24. What is the preferred cephalosporin for parenteral use, especially when renal function is impaired?

    a. Cephalothin.

    b. Cefaclor.

    c. Cephalexin.

25. What drug is indicated in the treatment of primary atypical pneumonia due to Mycoplasma pneumoniae?

    a. Erythromycin or a tetracycline.

    b. Erythromycin or a cephalosporin.

    c. Potassium penicillin G or a tetracycline.

    d. Potassium penicillin G or a cephalosporin.

26. What is the most frequent side effect to the oral use of erythromycin?

    a. Liver damage.

    b. Blood dyscrasias.

    c. Renal toxicity.

    d. Gastrointestinal discomfort.

27. Which of the following is bacteriostatic, not bactericidal?

    a. Penicillin.

    b. Ampicillin.

    c. Tetracyclines.

    d. Cephalosporins.

28. What is the most common reason for discontinuing treatment with tetracyclines?

  a. Liver damage.

  b. Skin disorders.

  c. Kidney dysfunction.

  d. Gastrointestinal disorders.

Check Your Answers on Next Page

SOLUTIONS TO EXERCISES, LESSON 5

1. c (para 5-4a)
2. a (para 5-4a(1), b)
3. b (para 5-4a(2))
4. a (para 5-4a(2), h)
5. a (para 5-4a(1), c, f)
6. b (para 5-4g)
7. b (para 5-5c)
8. d (para 5-6i)
9. d (para 5-8a)
10. b (para 5-8b(1))
11. a (para 5-10a)
12. a (para 5-10a)
13. d (para 5-10b)
14. d (para 5-10b)
15. c (para 5-10b(1))
16. c (para 5-10b(2)(e))
17. c (para 5-13e)
18. d (para 5-13g)
19. c (para 5-14)
20. a (paras 5-14a, 5-15a)
21. a (para 5-16)

22. d (para 5-18a)

23. c (para 5-19)

24. a (para 5-20b(1), d(3))

25. a (paras 5-21a(5), 5-23a(1))

26. d (para 5-21b(1))

27. c (para 5-23)

28. d (para 5-25a)

End of Lesson 5

LESSON ASSIGNMENT

LESSON 6	Drugs Used to Prevent and Treat Infection II
LESSON ASSIGNMENT	Paragraphs 6-1 through 6-38
LESSON OBJECTIVE	Upon completion of this lesson, you should be able to discuss actions, uses, untoward effects, administration, cautions, and contraindications of common aminoglycosides, sulfonamides, antifungals, anti-malarials, and anthelmintics, as well as metronidazole and gamma benzene hexachloride.
SUGGESTION	After studying the assignment, complete the exercises at the end of this lesson. These exercises will help you to achieve the lesson objectives.

LESSON 6

DRUGS USED TO PREVENT AND TREAT INFECTION II

Section I. AMINOGLYCOSIDES

6-1. INTRODUCTION

The aminoglycosides, a group of antibiotics including streptomycin, neomycin, gentamicin, and kanamycin, are similar in mode of antimicrobial action, toxic effects, pharmacology, and chemistry.

6-2. STREPTOMYCIN SULFATE

a. **Indications**. Streptomycin is a narrow-spectrum antibiotic used for the following organisms:

(1) Mycobacterium tuberculosis.

(2) Yersinis pestis (bubonic plague).

(3) Francisella tularensis (tularemia).

(4) Other organisms of known sensitivity.

b. **Usual Dosage**.

(1) For tuberculosis--1 gram, given once daily, usually in combination with other drugs.

(2) For tularemia--1 to 2 grams daily in divided doses for 7 to 10 days.

(3) For plague--2 to 4 grams daily in divided doses.

(4) For severe fulminating infections caused by known sensitive organisms, usually in combination with other antibiotics.

(a) Adult--2 to 4 grams daily, given in divided doses every 6 to 12 hours.

(b) Child--20 to 40 mg/kg of body weight, in divided doses every 6 to 12 hours.

NOTE: This drug is given intramuscularly only.

c. **Cautions and Warnings**.

(1) This drug should be used cautiously in pregnant women because of the fact that it can cross the placenta and cause ototoxicity (see d (1) below) in the fetus.

(2) Baseline audiometric tests should be run initially prior to therapy and then frequently during therapy to guard against ototoxicity.

d. **Adverse Reactions**.

(1) Ototoxicity. Ototoxicity is toxicity to the eighth nerve possibly resulting in damage to hearing and the sense of balance. Initial signs may include vestibular damage causing nausea, vomiting, and vertigo. Other symptoms include tinnitis, roaring noises, or a sense of fullness in the ears. Hearing loss, often permanent, may develop. The frequency and severity of ototoxicity are proportionate to the age of the client, the dosage level, and the duration of administration.

(2) Other Reactions. Other common adverse reactions include parathesia (abnormal sensation) of the face, rash, fever, urticaria, angio-neurotic edema, and eosinophilia. Allergic reactions occur most frequently with prolonged contact, either in clients with a long course of therapy or in medical personnel administering the drug; personnel preparing streptomycin solutions should wear gloves.

(3) Superinfection. Superinfection may occur.

e. **Supply**. Streptomycin sulfate is supplied in 1-gram quantities of powder, which must be reconstituted before injection. Streptomycin sulfate injection, 0.4 gram/ml, is supplied in 2.5-ml cartridge-needle units.

6-3. KANAMYCIN SULFATE INJECTION

a. **Indications**. Kanamycin (Kantrex) is a broad-spectrum bactericidal antibiotic. Because of its potential for toxic side effects, its use is limited mainly to certain serious gram-negative infections. It should not be used when less toxic anti-infective agents are available. It is effective in the treatment of E. coli, Proteus species, Enterobacter aerogenes, Klebsiella pneumoniae, Serratia marcescens, and Mima-Herrelea. Although kanamycin is not the drug of choice for staphylococcal infections, it may be indicated under certain conditions for the treatment of known or suspected staphylococcal disease. These situations include:

(1) The initial therapy of severe infections where the organism is thought to be either a gram-negative bacterium or a staphylococcus.

(2) Infections due to susceptible strains of staphylococci in clients allergic to other less toxic antibiotics.

(3) Mixed staphylococcal and gram-negative infections.

b. **Administration**. The usual dose is 7.5 mg/kg of body weight, IM every 12 hours. The average daily adult dose is 1.0 gram.

(1) Uncomplicated infections of sensitive organisms should respond in 24 to 48 hours. Should no improvement be seen in 3 to 5 days, therapy should be stopped and bacterial sensitivity rechecked.

(2) Partially used vials should be discarded after 48 hours, and kanamycin should not be physically mixed with other anti-infective agents.

c. **Cautions and Warnings**.

(1) Prior to and during therapy, audiograms should be obtained on clients with kidney dysfunction if therapy is to last more than 5 days.

(2) Kanamycin therapy should be stopped if client complains of tinnitus or hearing loss.

(3) Clients should be well hydrated to prevent chemical irritation to the renal tubules. Concurrent use of kanamycin and potent diuretics, such as furosemide and ethacrynic acid, should be avoided.

(4) Concurrent administration of kanamycin and other potentially nephrotoxic and ototoxic drugs should be avoided.

(5) Safety in pregnancy has not been established.

(6) Renal function should be checked prior to and during therapy. If azotemia or oliguria occurs, therapy should be discontinued.

(7) Bacterial or mycotic superinfections may occur with therapy.

(8) Allow for complete recovery from anesthesia and muscle relaxants before intraperitoneal instillation to avoid neuromuscular paralysis with respiratory depression.

d. **Adverse Reactions**.

(1) Pain or irritation may occur at the site of injection.

(2) Eighth cranial nerve damage, affecting mainly hearing, may be irreversible. In some clients, this hearing loss may not be detected until after therapy has been discontinued. Nerve damage is more likely to occur in clients with renal impairment.

(3) Renal function impairment with nitrogen retention and proteinuria can occur during kanamycin therapy, especially in clients with pre-existing kidney damage.

(4) Neuromuscular paralysis with respiratory depression has been reported following parenteral or intraperitoneal administration.

e. **Supply**. Kanamycin sulfate injection, 37.5-mg/ml for pediatric use, is supplied in 2-ml units. The preparation for adult use, 333-mg/ml, is supplied in 3-ml units.

6-4. GENTAMICIN SULFATE

a. Gentamicin sulfate (Garamicin) has the same general uses and warnings as kanamycin (above). It is effective against most strains of staphylococci, E. coli, Klebsiella, Enterobacter, and Pseudomonas aeruginosa, and many strains of Proteus and Serratia.

b. The concomitant use of carbenicillin (a penicillin) with gentamicin may result in synergistic activity against some strains of Pseudomonas and may allow for lower doses of gentamicin to be used.

c. Gentamicin is not considered the drug of choice for treating gram-negative sepsis because of susceptible organisms.

d. It is available as gentamicin sulfate cream (1-mg of gentamicin per gram) and as gentamicin sulfate injection (40-mg/ml) in a 2-ml bottle for intramuscular use.

6-5. NEOMYCIN SULFATE

Neomycin is very similar to kanamycin, as discussed above, but it is usually restricted to topical applications and to oral use for reduction of microbes in the gut before surgery. It has a wide range of activity; it is effective against both gram-negative and gram- positive bacteria. It is useful in many local infections, including burns, wounds, ulcers, and other sites of infection. However, Pseudomonas species and streptococci tend to be resistant.

NOTE: Neomycin is often combined with the narrow-spectrum antibiotic bacitracin. Bacitracin (not an aminoglycoside) is especially effective against gram-positive organisms. It too is usually confined to topical use. It is often effective in the treatment of infections associated with wounds, carbuncles, superficial and deep abscesses, and infected ulcers. It is available alone in bacitracin ointment and bacitracin ophthalmic ointment.

a. **Neomycin Sulfate**. Neomycin sulfate is available alone in a powder and in 350-mg tablets.

b. **Bacitracin and Neomycin Sulfate Ointment**. Bacitracin and neomycin sulfate (Bacimycin) ointment contains 500-units of bacitracin and 3.5-mg of neomycin sulfate in each gram. This ointment must not be used in the eyes, deep or puncture wounds, or severe burns. Prolonged use may result in superinfection; if this occurs, use of the ointment should cease and other treatment used.

c. **Neomycin Sulfate and Dexamethasone Sodium Phosphate Ophthalmic Ointment**. This ophthalmic ointment (NeoDecadron) is included in a chemical agents casualty treatment set. An ophthalmic solution of the same drugs is also available. It is indicated for severe conditions such as corneal burns and ocular infections in which vision is threatened by acute, severe uveitis and stromal edema. (More extensive information should be consulted prior to its use.) Dexamethasone, a synthetic drug similar to hydrocortisone, is included for its anti-inflammatory and anti-allergic effects, but it may also reduce tissue resistance to infection. Neomycin generally helps to control infections which may result from suppression of the inflammatory response or which may be secondary to the original irritation.

d. **Neomycin Sulfate, Hydrocortisone, and Polymyxin B Sulfate Suspension**. These eardrops (Cortisporin Otic Drops) may be used to treat otitis external (inflammation of the external ear) caused by organisms susceptible to neomycin or polymyxin B (also an antibiotic). Hydrocortisone is included for its anti-inflammatory effects; however, it may also reduce tissue resistance to infection. An ophthalmic suspension of the same drugs is also available.

e. **Neomycin Sulfate, Gramicidin, and Polymyxin B Sulfate**. These three antibiotics are available both in a cream and in an ophthalmic solution.

Section II. SULFONAMIDES

6-6. INTRODUCTION

In the 1930's, chemists in Germany developed a substance, prontosil, which was effective against hemolytic streptococci. Later, researchers in France added hydrogen to a portion of the prontosil molecule and thus created the basic sulfonamide, which had a therapeutic efficacy no less than that of prontosil. These were the first chemical agents to be successfully employed systemically for the prevention and cure of bacterial infections. In the following years, many more alterations were made in the sulfonamide molecules, creating a large number of antibacterial drugs. Even with the advent of antibiotics, the sulfonamides are still drugs of choice for some types of infection. In fact, because of their low cost and their usefulness in some common infections, they are still among the most widely used antibacterial agents.

6-7. EFFECTIVENESS

a. The sulfonamides are bacteriostats. They stop bacterial growth by interfering with the production of folic acid in the bacteria cells. They do not interfere with human utilization of folic acid.

b. The ranges of effectiveness of the various sulfonamides are very similar to each other. However, some sulfonamides may be more potent against specific types of infection than others. The sulfonamides are effective against gram-positive and gram-negative bacteria, as well as several other types of microorganisms.

6-8. SULFISOXAZOLE

a. **Indications**. Sulfisoxazole (Gantrisin) is rapidly absorbed and rapidly excreted. It is useful in:

(1) Acute, recurrent, or chronic urinary tract infections (primarily cystitis, pyelitis, pyelonephritis) because of susceptible organisms (usually E. coli, Klebsiella-Aerobacter, Staphylococcus, Staphylococcus aureus, Proteus mirabilis).

(2) Meningococcal meningitis because of susceptible organisms.

(3) Haemophilus influenzae meningitis when used with parenteral streptomycin; acute otitis media because of H. influenzae when used with adequate penicillin.

(4) Trachoma.

(5) Inclusion conjunctivitis.

(6) Nocardiosis.

(7) Chancroid.

b. **Usual Dosage**.

(1) Child. The initial dose for children is one-half of the 24-hour dose. The maintenance dose is 150 mg/kg/24 hours or 4 grams/m^2 is 6 grams.

NOTE: Systemic sulfonamides are contraindicated for infants under two months of age.

(2) Adult. The initial adult dose is 2 to 4 grams. The maintenance dose is 4 to 8 grams daily, divided into 4 to 6 doses.

c. **Cautions and Warnings**.

(1) This product should be used very cautiously in pregnant women and nursing mothers, because this drug passes the placenta and is excreted in the milk and may cause kernicterus (condition of severe neural symptoms, with high blood levels of bilirubin).

(2) Adequate fluid intake must be maintained in order to prevent crystalluria (crystals in the urine) and stone formation.

(3) Sulfonamides should be given cautiously in clients with impaired renal or hepatic function and to those with severe allergy or bronchial asthma.

(4) Use this drug cautiously in clients with glucose-6-phosphate dehydrogenase (G6PD) deficiency.

(5) Complete blood counts should be done frequently to guard against severe blood dyscrasias.

d. **Adverse Reactions**.

(1) Allergic reactions including rashes, pruritis, and fever are the most common adverse effects.

(2) Nausea, vomiting, headache, lassitude, dizziness, mental depression, abdominal pain, arthralgia, leukopenia, and photosensitivity may occur.

(3) Less common reactions include crystalluria, hepatotoxicity, jaundice, and serious blood dyscrasias.

(4) Clients with G6PD deficiency may develop hemolytic anemia.

e. **Supply**. Sulfisoxazole tablets, 0.5 gram each, are available.

6-9. SODIUM SULFACETAMIDE

a. **Indications**. Sodium sulfacetamide (Sodium Sulamyd) is used topically:

(1) For the treatment of conjunctivitis, corneal ulcer, and other superficial ocular infections.

(2) As adjunctive treatment in systemic therapy of trachoma.

b. **Usual Dosage**.

(1) Ophthalmic solution, 15 percent. For conjunctivitis or corneal ulcer, instill one or two drops into the lower conjunctival sac every two or three hours during the day, but use less at night. For trachoma, use four drops every two hours with concomitant systemic therapy with sulfonamides or tetracycline.

(2) Ophthalmic ointment, 30 percent. Apply a small amount four times daily and at bedtime. The ointment may be used adjunctively with the solution. The ointment is not sterile.

c. **Cautions and Warnings**.

(1) Sulfacetamide is contraindicated in individuals who are hypersensitive to sulfonamide preparations.

(2) Solutions are incompatible with silver preparations.

(3) Ophthalmic ointments may retard corneal healing.

(4) Nonsusceptible organisms, including fungi, may proliferate with use of these preparations.

(5) Sulfonamides are inactivated by para-aminobenzoic acid present in purulent exudates.

(6) Use with caution in clients who are deficient in glucose-6-phosphate dehydrogenase.

(7) Keep in a cool place.

d. **Adverse Reactions**. Common side effects are fever, skin rashes, urticaria, photosensitivity, and conjunctivitis.

e. **Supply**. Sodium sulfacetamide is supplied as a 15 percent ophthalmic solution and as a 10 percent ophthalmic ointment. It is also available in combinations called sodium sulfacetamide, phenylephrine hydrochloride, and prednisolone acetate ophthalmic suspension and sodium sulfacetamide and prednisolone acetate ophthalmic suspension.

Section III. ANTIFUNGAL AGENTS

6-10. INTRODUCTION

A dermatophyte is a fungus parasite upon the skin. For convenience, fungal infections are classified as deep (systemic) mycoses and superficial mycoses (dermatophytoses; fungal infections of the skin, hair, or nails).

a. **Superficial Mycoses**. Superficial infections of the skin are often chronic and resistant to treatment, but the general health of the client is rarely affected. The drugs discussed in this section are useful only for superficial mycoses. The names of some common dermatophytoses are provided below with the affected area of the body indicated after the dash.

(1) Tinea axillaris--armpit.

(2) Tinea palmaris--palm of the hand.

(3) Tinea pedis (athlete's foot)--foot.

(4) Tinea corporis (ringworm)--nonhairy skin.

(5) Tinea capitis (ringworm)--scalp.

(6) Tinea cruris ("jock itch")--upper surface of the thighs.

(7) Tinea versicolor--brownish-red scaling patches on the neck, arms, and trunk.

b. **Candidiasis**. Candidiasis (moniliasis) is an infection caused by Candida (the pathogenic species in man is Candida albicans). This yeast-like fungus is normally present on the mucous membranes of the gastrointestinal, respiratory, and female genital tracts, but when the body defense mechanisms are weakened or when other microbes have been destroyed by antimicrobial therapy, Candida albicans can establish dominance in these and other areas. Candidiasis of the throat is called thrush.

c. **Deep Mycoses**. Deep mycoses are often accompanied by systemic involvement, can be fatal, and are exceedingly difficult to treat. Fortunately, they are not common.

6-11. GRISEOFULVIN TABLETS

a. **Indications**. Griseofulvin (Fulvicin U/F) tablets are indicated for the treatment of dermatophytosis, including ringworm.

b. **Usual Dosage**. The usual oral dose is 0.5- to 1.0-gram daily, given in a single dose or divided doses after meals. Administration after a fatty meal increases its absorption. Treatment must be continued 3 to 6 weeks for skin infections, and up to 6 months if hair or nails are involved.

c. **Adverse Reactions**. Griseofulvin is a relatively safe drug although some allergic type reactions (rashes, serum sickness) have been reported. Photosensitivity, headache, and mental and neurologic problems have been seen in some clients.

d. **Cautions and Warnings**.

(1) Griseofulvin is ineffective in treating Candida, tinea versicolor, and bacterial infections. If a mixed infection is present, a second agent must also be employed.

(2) This drug should not be used unless laboratory findings indicate a sensitive organism.

(3) In severe cases, concomitant administration of a topical antifungal (tolnaftate) may be needed.

(4) Griseofulvin may increase the rate of metabolism of oral anticoagulants.

(5) Contraindicated in clients with acute porphyria or with a history of the disease.

e. **Supply**. The drug is available as 0.5-gram tablets, compressed from microsized powder to allow maximum absorption.

6-12. TOLNAFTATE SOLUTION

a. **Indications**. Tolnaftate (Tinactin) is a topical antifungal useful in athlete's foot, ringworm, and other fungal infections. However, if the scalp, nails, palms, or soles are infected, an oral preparation such as griseofulvin is indicated.

b. **Usual Dosage**.

(1) One to 2 drops of solution are rubbed into the lesion twice a day for 2 to 3 weeks.

(2) Tinea versicolor: Rub in sufficient amount of solution to cover the area, twice a day.

c. **Cautions and Warnings**.

(1) A diagnosis of a fungal infection should be supported by laboratory findings.

(2) Tolnaftate is of no use in Candida or bacterial infections.

(3) It should not be applied to areas, which are acutely inflamed or infected.

(4) It may be of limited use in nail infections in conjunction with oral antifungals. Nails should be trimmed to facilitate use of solution and prevent spread of infection.

(5) It is less effective with hyperkeratotic lesions. Treat areas alternately with 10 percent salicylic acid ointment and tolnaftate.

(6) It is useful in tinea versicolor, although relapses are common with all types of therapy.

d. **Adverse Effects**. Adverse effects are relatively rare, although local irritation characterized by erythema, pruritis, and a burning sensation may occur. In such cases, the drug should be discontinued.

e. **Supply**. Tolnaftate solution is a nonaqueous 1 percent solution for dermatological use only.

6-13. NYSTATIN

a. **Indications**.

(1) Nystatin (Mycostatin; Nilstat) is indicated in the treatment of Candida albicans (candidiasis, moniliasis, and thrush) infections of the skin, mucous membranes, vagina, and gastrointestinal tract. This is often associated with prolonged therapy with broad-spectrum antibiotics.

(2) Nystatin may be given with other antibiotics and may be indicated with prolonged broad-spectrum antibiotics or steroid therapy to prevent superinfections.

b. **Usual Dosage**.

(1) Oral.

(a) Tablets--500,000 units to 1,000,000 units tid.

(b) Suspension--5 ml (500,000 units) swished in mouth and swallowed qid.

(2) Topical. Ointment or cream--applied locally 3 to 4 times daily.

(3) Vaginally. 100,000 to 200,000-units daily for 2 weeks.

c. **Cautions and Warnings**.

(1) Nystatin is not absorbed from the GI tract and is not suitable for systemic fungal infections.

(2) Drug should be discontinued if client develops local irritation following topical administration.

d. **Adverse Reactions**. Adverse reactions are relatively rare, although local irritation may occur following topical application. Diarrhea may be associated with large oral doses.

e. **Supply**. Nystatin is supplied as nystatin oral suspension (100,000 units/ml), nystatin tablets (oral 500,000-unit tablets and vaginal 100,000-unit tablets), nystatin ointment (100,000-units/grams), nystatin topical powder (100,000-units/grams), and nystatin cream (100,000-units/grams). It is also available in a topical combination of nystatin and triamcinolone acetonide cream.

6-14. IODOCHLORHYDROXYQUIN AND HYDROCORTISONE

a. **Indications**. Iodochlorhydroxyquin and hydrocortisone (Vioform-HC) is possibly effective in the control of acute and chronic inflammatory skin diseases, particularly when complicated by bacterial, protozoal, and the following fungal conditions: tinea palmaris, t. pedis, t. cruris, t. corporis, t. axillaris, and candidiasis.

b. **Usual Dosage**. Apply a small amount to affected areas 3 or 4 times daily.

c. **Cautions and Warnings**.

(1) This preparation should not be used in the eye or topically in the presence of tuberculosis, vaccinia, varicella, or other viral skin conditions.

(2) The client should be warned that this preparation may stain the skin, hair, and clothing yellow.

(3) Prolonged use of this combination product can lead to the toxicities associated with hydrocortisone. Because of this fact, the client should be switched to plain iodochlorhydroxyquin, if available, when inflammation is no longer present.

d. **Adverse Reactions**.

(1) Local burning, irritation, and itching have been noted.

(2) This product may cause staining of the skin, hair, and clothing.

e. **Supply**.

(1) Cream: Three percent iodochlorhydroxyquin with 0.5 percent or 1 percent hydrocortisone, 28.35 grams (1 oz).

(2) Ointment: Three percent iodochlorhydroxyquin with 1 percent hydrocortisone, 5 grams.

NOTE: The cream has a slightly drying effect, which is useful for moist, weeping lesions. The ointment is especially indicated for dry lesions accompanied by thickening and scaling of the skin.

6-15. SELENIUM SULFIDE LOTION

a. **Indications**. Selenium sulfide lotion (Selsun) is indicated for the treatment of:

(1) Common dandruff.

(2) Mild to moderately severe seborrheic dermatitis.

(3) Tinea versicolor.

b. **Usual Dosage**.

(1) Dandruff or seborrheic dermatitis:

(a) Lather 1 to 2 teaspoonfuls into wet scalp.

(b) Allow to remain 2 to 5 minutes.

(c) Rinse thoroughly.

(d) Repeat procedure.

(e) After treatment, wash hands.

(f) Make two applications each week for 2 weeks, then decrease frequency to maintain control.

(2) Tinea versicolor:

(a) Apply sufficient amounts to cover affected areas of body (except face). Allow to remain 5 minutes and rinse thoroughly.

(b) Lather face and allow suspension to remain 10 minutes; then rinse thoroughly.

(c) After treatment, wash hands.

(d) This procedure should be done once daily for 3 successive days. For persistent or recurring cases, the procedure may be repeated.

c. **Cautions and Warnings**.

(1) Toxic if taken orally, but little toxic effect topically.

(2) Irritating to mucous membranes.

(3) Do not allow contact with eyes or genital region.

(4) Unpleasant odor and taste.

(5) Should be a 4-day lapse prior to use following tinting, dyeing, or waving hair.

(6) May cause excessive oiliness of hair.

(7) May tint gray hair orange because of incomplete rinsing.

d. **Adverse Effects**.

(1) Discontinue use if skin sensitivity occurs.

(2) Chemical conjunctivitis can occur if allowed to enter the eye.

(3) Application to acutely inflamed scalp may result in cutaneous absorption with possible systemic toxic effects, which include nervousness, drowsiness, convulsions, death from vasomotor and respiratory depression.

e. **Supply**. Selenium sulfide lotion is supplied as a 2.5-percent suspension in a 4-fl oz container.

6-16. UNDECYLENIC ACID

a. Undecylenic acid (Desenex) is a fungistat, which is used to treat athlete's foot and ringworm of the body. Since it is only fungistatic and not fungicidal, attention must be directed to other hygiene, especially where there are raw lesions. Fungicidal foot powder and undecylenic acid ointment both contain, in addition, the astringent zinc undecylate to help reduce rawness and irritation. Response of athlete's foot to the drug is often dramatic, but the infection sometimes persists despite treatment.

b. Undecylenic acid is available as a 10 percent solution in 59-ml bottles; as an ointment in 1-ounce (28.35-gram) containers; and as a 1 percent foot powder in 1-ounce (28.35-gram) containers.

Section IV. ANTIMALARIAL DRUGS

6-17. MALARIA

a. **Cause and Transmission**. Malaria is caused by a microbe called the plasmodium. There are four principal species of malaria-producing plasmodia--P. falciparum, which caused about 84 percent of the cases of malaria contracted by Americans in Vietnam; P. vivax, a more benign plasmodium which caused about 85 percent of the cases of malaria contracted in the United States in 1971; P. malariae, which causes the form of malaria called quartan malaria; and P. ovale, a plasmodium rarely seen except in certain parts of South America and East and West Africa. These parasites are generally transmitted by the Anopheles mosquito, of which there are many species. (An important method of defense against malaria, in addition to control of the mosquito and its environment, is personal measures taken to avoid mosquito bites.) In addition to transmission by mosquitos, malaria may also be transmitted in a blood transfusion or in a contaminated needle used for an injection.

b. **Progression of Malaria in Man**. After a person has been infected with malaria by a mosquito, there is a latent period called the tissue stage, when the parasites, or schizonts, are multiplying in liver cells. This stage without overt effects generally lasts from 10 days to 6 weeks, depending on the type of malaria, but may last as long as several months. Eventually, however, the parasites, now called merozoites, enter the red blood cells, where they develop into small, ring-shaped forms called trophozoites. The trophozoites grow rapidly and fill the cells, and some of them develop into still other forms, sexual forms called gametocytes. During this stage, called the erythrocytic stage, many of the red blood cells burst and the typical symptoms of malaria--a chill followed by a fever, profuse sweating, headache, and backache--ensue. Meanwhile, some of the schizonts may remain in the liver, and, if not destroyed, cause a relapse of the disease even when the parasites in the blood have been destroyed by drugs. The details of the life cycle of the Plasmodium are illustrated in Figure 6-1.

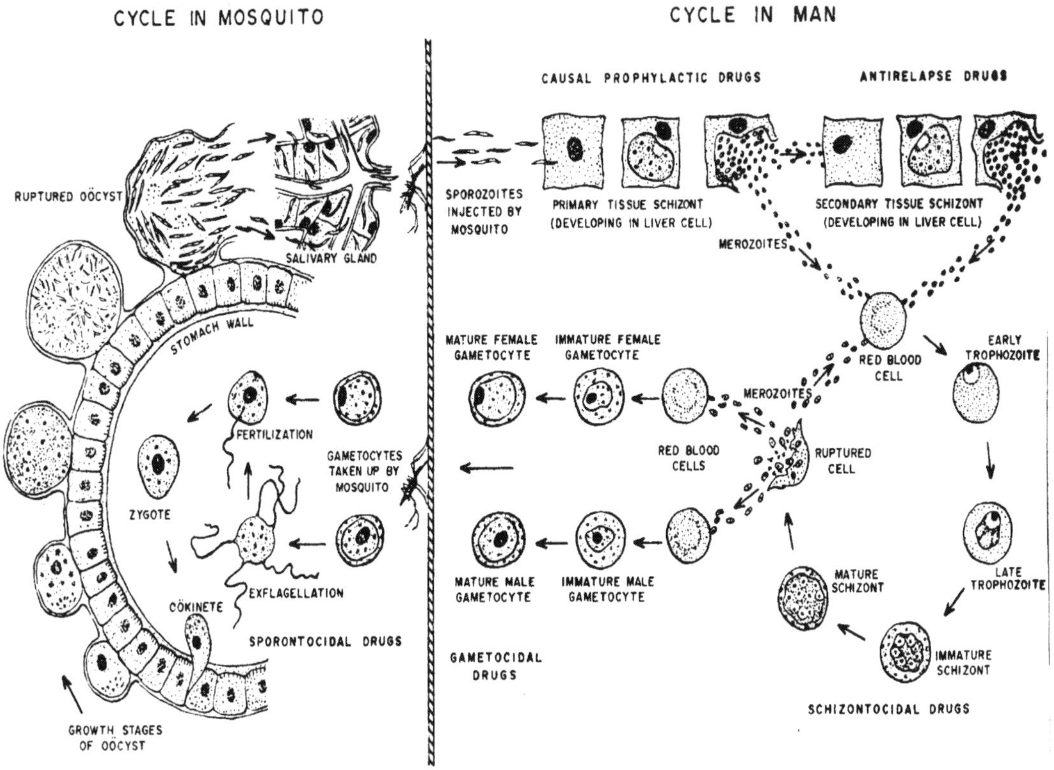

Figure 6-1. Life cycle of Plasmodium, the malaria parasite.

6-18. CLASSIFICATION OF ANTIMALARIAL DRUGS

Antimalarial drugs are often classified according to the stage in the life cycle of the Plasmodium against which they are capable of acting. The categories are the primary tissue schizonticides, the secondary tissue schizonticides, the blood schizonticides, the gametocides, and the sporontocides.

a. **Antimalarial Drugs Beneficial in the Treatment of Clinical Malaria.**

(1) Primary tissue schizonticides. These drugs destroy the primary tissue schizonts in the liver soon after infection by the mosquito. An example is primaquine.

(2) Secondary tissue schizonticides. These drugs destroy the secondary tissue schizonts in the liver and thus prevent the relapsing fevers characteristic of P. vivax, P. malariae, and P. ovale (but not characteristic of P. falciparum, the most lethal form of malaria). Primaquine serves this purpose also.

(3) Blood schizonticides. These drugs destroy the schizonts and merozoites in the red blood cells and thus relieve the symptoms of malarial infection. They include quinine, quinacrine, and chloroquine. These drugs are often capable of curing malaria because of P. falciparum.

b. **Drugs Useful in the Prevention of Transmission of Malaria**. The following two categories of drugs do not necessarily help the immediate client, but they do help prevent transmission to other people by way of mosquitoes.

(1) Gametocides. These drugs (primaquine is an example of this category too) prevent mosquitoes from acquiring the infection from a client by destroying the gametocytes in the client's blood.

(2) Sporontocides. The sporontocidal drugs (for example, pyrimethamine) act inside the mosquito after it has ingested the client's blood. There they prevent the reproduction of the zygote, the formation of sporozoites.

6-19. CHLOROQUINE AND PRIMAQUINE PHOSPHATE TABLETS

a. **Action and Uses**. The standard chloroquine-primaquine (CP) tablet is used for malaria prophylaxis in all geographic areas where malaria is endemic. Each tablet contains 500-mg of chloroquine phosphate (equivalent to 300-mg of chloroquine base), which is a blood schizonticide for all four types of malaria mentioned above. It is thus used to prevent the appearance of symptoms of malaria. The 79-mg of primaquine phosphate (equivalent to 45 mg of primaquine base) in each tablet acts to destroy the primary tissue schizonts of P. falciparum or P. vivax and the secondary tissue schizonts of the malarias characterized by relapses, that is, P. vivax, P. malariae, and P. ovale. (Thus, primaquine can be used to cure malaria as well as to prevent it or treat its symptoms. However, CP tablets should NOT be used for therapy of acute attacks of malaria. The toxic effects of taking more than one CP tablet in 1 day are severe.)

b. **Usual Dosage**.

(1) Adults and children over 100 pounds: One tablet weekly on the same day of each week, starting at least 1 day before entering the area. After leaving the area, continue this schedule (one tablet weekly) for 8 weeks.

(2) Younger children: Make a suspension of two CP tablets in 75-ml of water so that each 5-ml equals 40-mg of chloroquine base and 6-mg of primaquine base.

Children's weekly dose:	10-15 pounds	=	1/2 tsp
	16-25 pounds	=	1 tsp
	26-35 pounds	=	1 1/2 tsp
	36-45 pounds	=	2 tsp
	46-55 pounds	=	2 1/2 tsp
	56-100 pounds	=	1/2 tablet

c. **Adverse Effects**. Occasionally, CP tablets produce intestinal cramps and loose stools. Serious hematologic effects have been reported with G6PD deficiency. Diarrhea can be handled by breaking up tablets, taking with meals or cheese, or combating with Lomotil if other measures fail.

d. **Cautions and Warnings**.

(1) The CP tablet should not be used in the treatment of malaria.

(2) Some individuals may respond to the primaquine in the CP tablet with a hemolytic reaction. If this happens and is severe enough, plain chloroquine tablets at the same dosage may be substituted for prophylaxis.

(3) Concurrent use of quinacrine with primaquine may cause agranulocytosis.

(4) Dapsone, 25-mg daily, may be used as an adjunct to the CP tablet in resistant falciparum areas.

6-20. CHLOROQUINE

a. **Indications**. Chloroquine (Aralen) is a blood schizonticide indicated in the:

(1) Treatment of uncomplicated attacks of malaria except resistant P. falciparum.

(2) Parenteral treatment of severe malaria illness except resistant P. falciparum.

(3) Prophylaxis and suppression of malaria while in an endemic area.

NOTE: This drug is also indicated for treatment of discoid lupus erythematosis, rheumatoid arthritis, and extraintestinal amebiasis.

b. **Usage Dosage**. Oral administration is preferred whenever possible.

(1) Prophylaxis of malaria: 500-mg (300-mg base) once weekly, beginning 2 weeks before exposure and continuing for 8 weeks after last exposure in endemic area.

(2) Oral administration for treatment of malaria: One gram (2 tablets) to start, followed by one tablet (0.5 -gram) in 6 hours. One tablet is then given daily for the next two days. Total dosage is four doses over a 3-day period for a total of 2.5-grams of chloroquine phosphate (1.5-grams of chloroquine base).

(3) Parenteral administration in critically ill malaria clients: One 5-ml ampule equivalent to 200--mg of base is given intramuscularly. This may be repeated in 6 hours, but total parenteral dosage in first 24 hours should not exceed 4 ampules or 800-mg of chloroquine base.

(4) For blackwater fever in areas where drug resistance has not been encountered: 200-mg base diluted with 40--ml of normal saline given slowly intravenously.

c. **Adverse Effects**.

(1) Mild transient headaches, pruritis, anorexia, blurring of the vision, vertigo, diarrhea, malaise, and urticaria have been infrequently reported.

(2) Signs of acute chloroquine intoxication include myocardial depression, disturbances in cardiac conduction, arrhythmias, hypotension, CNS stimulation with convulsion, and eventual paralysis of vital brain centers.

d. **Cautions and Warnings**.

(1) Chloroquine is extremely toxic for young children. The toxic dose for children is 20 mg/kg and the lethal dose is 100-mg/kg.

(2) Prolonged use of large doses of chloroquine has commonly produced retinal changes or visual impairment after several months or years of treatment.

(3) Chloroquine accumulates in the liver and should be used with caution in clients with liver disease.

(4) It is contraindicated in clients with psoriasis.

(5) Avoid its use in pregnancy unless there is an overwhelming need for it.

(6) Chloroquine may color urine rusty yellow or brown.

e. **Supply**.

(1) Chloroquine phosphate tablets, 0.5-gram (each contains 300-mg of base).

(2) Chloroquine hydrochloride injection, 5-ml ampules containing equivalent of 200-mg of base.

6-21. PRIMAQUINE

a. **Uses**. Since primaquine, a tissue schizonticide, is not effective against blood schizonts, it will not provide immediate relief to acute symptoms of malaria such as fever. However, it is capable of preventing infection because of P. falciparum if it is administered soon after the mosquito bite. It is used along with blood schizonticides in radical (complete) cures of the relapsing malarias, that is, those due to P. vivax, P. malariae, and P. ovale. Unfortunately, there are some strains of P. vivax, which are partially resistant to primaquine. Since primaquine inhibits gametocytes, it is effective in preventing the transmission of malaria to other persons by way of mosquitoes.

b. **Toxicity**.

(1) Primaquine sensitivity. Some people have an inherited sensitivity to primaquine because of a deficiency of a substance called G6PD, which is important to metabolism in the red blood cells. They may react to large doses of primaquine with chills, malaise, and weakness, resulting from hemolysis. The incidence of this deficiency is much greater among people whose ancestors have lived in areas where malaria due to P. falciparum is common. These people include blacks, Greeks, Iranians, Sardinians, and Sephardic Jews. The prophylactic dose, such as that found in the CP tablet, seldom causes any intense reaction. However, when these groups are treated with primaquine for preexisting malarial infections, that is, when the doses are greater, the clients should be observed closely for hemolysis. Each such client receiving primaquine should be told to report signs of hemolysis, such as red or dark coloration of the urine.

(2) Side effects. The side effects of primaquine may include difficulty in focusing, itching, nausea, headache, and abdominal cramps (which antacids relieve). Some blood disorders may occur.

c. **Contraindications**. Primaquine should not be given to clients with a tendency toward active rheumatoid arthritis, granulocytopenia, lupus erythematosus, or any very serious systemic disease. Primaquine should not be given concurrently with quinacrine or any drug, which depresses the bone marrow. Large doses of primaquine should usually be avoided.

d. **Dosage**. Primaquine is given orally. The usual dose is one tablet daily for 14 days.

e. **Supply**. Each 26.3-mg tablet contains the equivalent of 15-mg of primaquine base.

6-22. DAPSONE

a. **Indications**. Dapsone (Avolsulfon) is indicated:

(1) In all forms of leprosy.

(2) In combination with other antimalarial agents for the treatment of resistant Plasmodium falciparum.

b. **Usual Dosage**.

(1) Leprosy--initiate small oral doses during the first few weeks until a maintenance dose of 50-mg/day is achieved. Clients should be hospitalized for the first few weeks of therapy and should be treated by a specialist.

(2) Malaria--25-mg daily for 21 to 28 days in combination with other antimalarials (quinine and pyrimethamine).

c. **Cautions and Warnings**.

(1) It is not rapidly effective in terminating acute attacks of malaria.

(2) It is not effective against P. falciparum gametocytes, P.vivax, or primary tissue forms of P. falciparum.

(3) If used alone in treatment of malaria, parasites rapidly develop resistance to the drug.

(4) Periodic blood checks should be performed during entire period of therapy. If anemia develops, the drug should be stopped and anemia treated.

(5) Use with caution in persons with a G6PD deficiency, as dapsone can precipitate a hemolytic reaction.

d. **Adverse Reactions**. Dapsone can produce a wide range of adverse reactions affecting the GI tract, the blood, skin, central nervous system, and the liver:

(1) Nausea, vomiting, headache, psychosis.

(2) Liver enlargement and damage.

(3) Skin rashes.

(4) Hemolysis and methemoglobinemia.

e. **Supply**. Dapsone tablets each contain 25-mg of dapsone.

6-23. QUININE

a. **Uses**. Quinine is used to treat acute attacks of malaria because of strains of P. falciparum resistant to chloroquine. It can also suppress the symptoms of an acute attack of the other three types of malaria (P. vivax, P.malariae, and P. ovale), but since it does not kill the tissue schizonts, it is incapable of curing these three relapsing malarias. When quinine is used to treat chloroquine- resistant strains of P. falciparum, it is more effective when combined with pyrimethamine or dapsone and pyrimethamine.

b. **Administration as an Antimalarial**.

(1) Oral dosage. Two quinine sulfate tablets (324-mg per tablet) are given three times daily after meals for 14 days. Care must be exercised not to use old tablets of quinine, which may have hardened, since such tablets will fail to be absorbed in the bowel.

(2) Intravenous administration. One 2-ml ampule of quinine dihydrochloride injection (containing 300-mg per ml) is diluted in 300-ml of normal saline, dextrose-saline, plasma, or other intravenous fluid appropriate to the client's condition, and given slowly (not less than 30 minutes), since low blood pressure may occur if it is infused too rapidly. The blood pressure and pulse should be monitored constantly while the infusion is running to detect a fall in blood pressure or the appearance of an abnormal rhythm of the pulse. This dosage may be repeated every 6 to 8 hours, as necessary, but not more than three such doses (a total of 2-gm of quinine dihydrochloride) should be administered during a 24-hour period. Oral administration should be substituted or resumed as soon as possible. If falciparum malaria recurs a few days after treatment with quinine, re-administration as described above may be required for a duration of 10 to 21 days.

c. **Toxicity**.

(1) If too much quinine is used, an effect called cinchonism results. Cinchonism may include headache, ringing of the ears, symptoms of cerebral congestion, flushing, sweating, nausea, diarrhea, and blurred vision. When it is severe, there may be deafness, skin rashes, drowsiness, damage to vision, cardiac arrhythmia, and abdominal pain.

(2) Administration of quinine can cause effects such as GI discomfort when given orally, painful noninfected abscesses when given IM, and damage to the lining of the blood vessels and even clotting when given IV.

(3) Some authorities believe that quinine is responsible for the condition called blackwater fever, found among people where malaria is endemic. It is

characterized by black or red-colored urine. This is due to hemolysis, which in turn leads to sludging in the kidney tubules. From 25 percent to 50 percent of the victims of black-water fever die.

(4) Quinine causes hemolysis in about 1 in every 2000 people. Quinine can also cause other blood disorders.

(5) Massive hemolysis followed by kidney failure has occurred in pregnant women after large doses of quinine. Pregnant women, nearing the time to give birth, who have shown a sensitivity to quinine or who have ever had tinnitus (characterized by false sounds in the ears), a hemolytic episode, atrial fibrillation, or optic neuritis should be warned to stay out of areas where there are strains of P. falciparum treatable only with quinine. No pregnant woman should ever take quinine.

(6) The lethal dose of quinine is about 8 gm.

d. **Supply**. The drug is available as 324-mg quinine sulfate tablets and as 2-ml ampules of quinine dihydrochloride injection (300-mg per ml).

6-24. PYRIMETHAMINE

a. **Uses**. Pyrimethamine (Daraprim), if administered for at least 10 weeks, can produce a suppressive cure of an infection with one of the relapsing malarias. However, it acts too slowly to be useful in relieving acute attacks. It can be used weekly for suppressive prophylaxis against malaria and for its sporonticidal effects, which deter the transmission of the infection from a person who already has malaria. Given concurrently with quinine sulfate or dapsone or both, it can quickly terminate acute attacks of chloroquine-resistant falciparum malaria in nonimmune clients and also make a relapse less likely. Pyrimethamine is also sometimes used in combination with oral sulfonamides to treat toxoplasmosis (infection with organisms of the genus Toxoplasma, one of which causes enlargement of the spleen and progressive anemia).

b. **Usual Dosage**.

(1) For malarial prophylaxis, one 25-mg tablet is given orally each week to adults.

(2) For the treatment of resistant Plasmodium falciparum, the drug is administered orally in a dosage of 25-mg twice daily for three days in combination with quinine or dapsone.

(3) For the treatment of toxoplasmosis in the adult, the starting dose is 50 to 75-mg daily combined with 1 to 4-grams of a sulfonamide drug (that is, sulfadiazine). This dosage is continued for 1 to 3 weeks. The dosage may then be reduced to about one-half that previously given for each drug and continued for an additional 4 to 5 weeks.

c. **Cautions and Warnings**.

(1) Do not administer to pregnant women, clients with oliguria, liver disease, heart disease, or allergy to pyrimethamine.

(2) Overdosage may cause hypotension, arrhythmias of the heart, and shock.

(3) Because this is a folic acid antagonist, it tends to cause bone marrow depression when given at high doses. Periodic blood counts should be run. If signs appear, then the drug dosage should be reduced.

d. **Adverse Reactions**. Anorexia, vomiting, megaloblastic anemia, and bone marrow depression with leukopenia and thrombocytopenia have been observed.

e. **Supply**. Pyrimethamine is supplied in 25-mg tablets.

6-25. SULFADOXINE AND PYRIMETHAMINE

a. **Uses**. Sulfadoxine and pyrimethamine (Fansidar) is used in the treatment of plasmodium falciparum malaria in clients in whom chloroquine resistance is suspected and for the prophylaxis of malaria for travelers to areas where chloroquine-resistant plasmodium falciparum malaria is endemic.

b. **Usual Dosage**.

(1) For treatment of malaria, adults take 2 or 3 tablets in a single dose alone or in sequence with quinine regimen.

(2) For prophylaxis of malaria for travelers in endemic areas, adults take one tablet one or two days before departure and then take one tablet weekly during the stay and for 4 to 6 weeks after return.

c. **Cautions and Warnings**.

(1) Fatalities have been associated with sulfadoxine/pyrimethamine use. Discontinue use if skin rash appears, if the count of any formed blood elements is reduced significantly, or if active bacterial or fungal infections occur.

(2) Clients must maintain adequate fluid intake to prevent crystalluria and stone formation.

(3) Take contraceptive measures to avoid pregnancy during therapy.

(4) Avoid breastfeeding during therapy.

d. **Adverse Reactions**. Agranulocytosis, aplastic anemia, stomatitis, nausea, emesis, abdominal pains, headache, peripheral neuritis, erythema multiforme, Stevens-Johnson syndrome, generalized skin eruptions, drug fever, and chills have been observed.

e. **Supply**. Sulfadoxine and pyrimethamine (Fansidar) are supplied as scored tablets containing 500 mg sulfadoxine and 25-mg pyrimethamine.

Section V. ANTHELMINTIC DRUGS

6-26. INTRODUCTION

An anthelmintic is a drug used to counteract infections with worms or helminths. There are two phyla (categories) of helminths--the nemathelminths (roundworms) and the platyhelminths (flatworms, a phylum composed of flukes and tapeworms). Roundworms are also called nematodes. Flukes are called trematodes. Tapeworms are called cestodes.

6-27. DRUGS OF CHOICE FOR SPECIFIC INFECTIONS

Below is a list of different types of helminthic infections, followed in parentheses by the common name of the infection, followed (after a dash) by the names of the drugs of choice for treating that particular infection. Names of alternate drugs for treating an infection are placed in parentheses.

a. **Infections with Roundworms**.

(1) Ascaris lumbricoides (giant intestinal roundworm)--paperazine, mebendazole (or pyrantel pamoate).

(2) Ancylostoma duodenale (hookworm, Old World type)--mebendazole (or pyrantel pamoate).

(3) Necator americanus (hookworm, tropical type)--mebendazole.

(4) Strongyloides stercoralis (threadworm)--thiabendazole (or perhaps pyrvinium pamoate).

(5) Enterobius vermicularis (pinworm)--pyrantel pamoate (or mebendazole).

(6) Trichuris trichiura (whipworm)--mebendazole.

(7) Trichinella spiralis (trichinosis)--ACTH, corticosteroids, or thiabendazole. The effectiveness of thiabendazole against trichinosis is not established.

(8) Wuchereria bancrofti (filariasis) or W. (Brugia) malayi--diethylcarbamazine.

(9) Onchocerca volvulus (onchocerciasis)--suramin plus diethylcarbamazine. Suramin is available for investigational use only.

b. **Infections with Tapeworms**.

(1) Taenia saginata (beef tapeworm)--niclosamide.

(2) Taenia solium (pork tapeworm)--niclosamide.

(3) Diphyllobothrium latum (fish tapeworm)--niclosamide.

(4) Hymenolepis nana (dwarf tapeworm), H. diminuta (rat tapeworm), and Dipylidium caninum--niclosamide.

c. **Infections with Flukes**. THE RECOMMENDATION OF DRUGS FOR INFECTION WITH FLUKES, AS GIVEN BELOW, IS IN SOME CASES ONLY TENTATIVE. Stibocaptate bithionol is available for investigational use only.

(1) Schistosoma mansoni--praziquantel.

(2) Schistosoma japonicum--praziquantel.

(3) Schistosoma haematobium--praziquantel.

NOTE: Infection with one of the three flukes above is called schistosomiasis.

(4) Fasciolopsis buski (large intestinal fluke) praziquantel or niclosamide.

(5) Heterophyes heterophyes--praziquantel or tetrachloroethylene.

(6) Metagonimus yokogaway--praziquantel or tetrachloroethylene.

(7) Clonorchis sinensis (liver fluke)--praziquantel.

(8) Opisthorchis felineus--praziquantel.

(9) Paragonimus westermani (lung fluke)--praziquantel (or bithionol).

(10) Fasciola hepatica (sheep liver fluke)--praziquantel (or bithionol).

6-28. MEBENDAZOLE

a. **Indications**. Mebendazole (Vermox) is the drug of choice for the treatment of whipworm, pinworm, roundworm, and hookworm in single or fixed infections.

b. **Usual Dosage**. The same dosage schedule applies to both adults and children. The tablets may be chewed, swallowed, or crushed and mixed with food. No special procedures, such as fasting or purging are required. If the client is not cured 3 weeks after treatment, a second treatment course is advised.

(1) Hookworm infection: One tablet morning and evening on three consecutive days.

(2) Pinworm infection: A single tablet given once.

c. **Cautions and Warnings**.

(1) Mebendazole is not recommended for use in pregnant women. During pregnancy, especially during the first trimester, use only if the potential benefit justifies the potential risk to the fetus.

(2) Safety and efficacy for use in children under 2 years of age have not been established.

d. **Adverse Reactions**.

(1) Transient abdominal pain and diarrhea have been observed in massive infection and expulsion of worms.

(2) Fever, a possible response to drug-induced necrosis, has been reported.

e. **Supply**. Mebendazole (Vermox) is supplied as 100-mg tablets.

6-29. DIETHYLCARBAMAZINE CITRATE

a. **Indications**. Diethylcarbamazine citrate (Hetrazan) is orally effective in the treatment of filariasis caused by Wuchereria bancrofti, W. (Grugia) malayi or Loa loa. Diethylcarbamazine also has limited usefulness in Onchocerca vulvulus infection ("river blindness").

b. **Usual Dosage**.

(1) W. bancrofti, W. malayi, and Loa loa--2-mg/kg of body weight three times a day after meals for 3 to 4 weeks. The microfilariae in the blood are rapidly killed, but repeated courses of therapy may be required to destroy adult worms. Three to 4 weeks should be allowed between each course of therapy.

c. **Adverse Effects**. Diethylcarbamazine citrate is a relatively safe drug. The major problem is allergic reactions because of the foreign protein from the dying microfilarial worms. The intensity of these reactions can be lessened by the concomitant administration of antihistamines during the first 5 days of therapy.

d. **Cautions and Warnings**. If a client is suspected of having malaria, he should be treated with chloroquine prior to the administration of diethylcarbamazine. This drug may provoke a relapse of nonsymptomatic malaria.

e. **Supply**. Diethylcarbamazine citrate is supplied as 50-mg tablets.

6-30. PYRANTEL PAMOATE

a. **Indications**. Pyrantel pamoate (Antiminth) is a depolarizing neuromuscular blocking agent, resulting in spastic paralysis of the worm. It is active against Enterobius vermicularis (pinworm) and Ascaris lumbricoides (roundworm).

b. **Dosage**. A single dose of 11-mg/kg (maximum total dose of 1 gram) which corresponds to a simplified dosage regimen of 1-ml/10-lb. Pyrantel may be administered without regard to meals or time of day. Purging is not necessary. It may be taken with milk or fruit juices.

c. **Cautions and Warnings**.

(1) Safety and efficacy for use in children under 2 years of age have not been established.

(2) Safety in pregnant women has not been established.

d. **Adverse Effects**. Anorexia, nausea, vomiting, abdominal cramps, diarrhea, headache, dizziness, and skin rash have been observed with the administration of this medication.

e. **Supply**. Pyrantel pamoate (Antiminth) is supplied as an oral suspension containing 50-mg pyrantel per ml.

6-31. PIPERAZINE CITRATE

a. **Indications**. Piperazine citrate (Antepar) is an alternate drug of choice for roundworms (Ascaris lumbricoides) and pinworms (Enterobius vermicularis). Piperazine blocks the response of acetylcholine in the worm causing flaccid paralysis of the worm. The worm is then dislodged and expelled by peristalsis.

b. **Usual Dosage**. Piperazine is best taken on an empty stomach. The surface contact between drug and parasite is diminished in the presence of food.

(1) Roundworms can be treated with 75-mg/kg daily for two consecutive days (maximum daily dose = 3.5-grams).

(2) Pinworms can be treated with 65 mg/kg daily for 7-8 consecutive days (maximum daily dose = 2.5-grams).

c. **Cautions and Warnings**.

(1) It has been reported that clients with a predisposition to grand mal or petit mal have been reported to have an exacerbation of seizures following administration of piperazine.

(2) Piperazine may be used during the third trimester of pregnancy.

d. **Adverse Reactions**. Mild adverse reactions include nausea, vomiting, mild diarrhea, abdominal pain, and headache.

e. **Supply**. Each 5-ml of piperazine citrate syrup, as available in supply channels, contains the equivalent of 0.5-gram of piperazine hexahydrate.

6-32. NICLOSAMIDE

a. **Indications**. Niclosamide inhibits oxidative phosphorylation in cestodes. The scolex and segments are killed on contact with the drug. It is effective in the treatment of Taenia saginata (beef tapeworm), Diphyllobothrium latum (fish tapeworm), and Hymenolepis nana (dwarf tapeworm).

b. **Usual dosage**. Tablets should be thoroughly chewed, then swallowed with a small amount of water. No special dietary restrictions are required although niclosamide should be taken after a light meal. Segments of the ova may be present in the stool for up to 3 days following treatment. A second course of therapy should be administered if ova are still present after 7 days following therapy. A client is not cured unless the stool has been negative for a minimum of 3 months.

T. saginata and D. latum (beef and fish tapeworm)		
Adults	4 tablets (2 grams) in a single dose	
Children	>75-lbs	3 tablets in a single dose
	25 to < 75-lbs	2 tablets in a single dose
Hymenolepis nana (dwarf tapeworm)		
Adults	4 tablets as a single daily dose for 7 days	
Children	>75-lbs	3 tablets on 1st day, then 2 tablets daily for the next 6 days
	25 to 75-lbs	2 tablets on 1st day followed by 1 tablet daily for the next 6 days.

c. **Cautions and Warnings**.

(1) Safety for use during pregnancy has not been established.

(2) Safety and efficacy for use in children under 2 years of age have not been established.

d. **Adverse Reactions**. Nausea and vomiting, abdominal discomfort, loss of appetite, drowsiness, dizziness, and skin rash have been observed.

e. **Supply**. Niclosamide (Niclocide) is supplied as 500-mg chewable tablets.

6-33. QUINACRINE

a. **Indications**. Quinacrine (Atabrine), once used extensively in the suppression and treatment of malaria, is an alternate agent used to treat infections of Taenia saginata (beef tapeworm), T. solium (pork tapeworm), and Diphyllobothrium latum (fish tapeworm). It is also an alternate drug for the treatment of Hymenolepis nana (dwarf tapeworm), H. diminuta (rat tapeworm), and Dipylidium caninum.

b. **Administration for Treatment** of Taenia saginata, T. solium, and Diphyllobothrium latum. The client is placed on a semisolid, bland, nonfat diet for 1 day prior to administration. The client must fast at least from suppertime the evening before because the gastrointestinal tract should be as empty as possible. A saline laxative should be given about an hour before therapy is begun. Four doses of 200-mg each should be administered orally 10 minutes apart. Sodium bicarbonate, 600-mg in about 75 ml of water, should be given with each dose to reduce the tendency to nausea and vomiting. Enough saline laxative should be given 1 to 2 hours after the last dose to produce a copious evacuation, removing the worm, alive and stained yellow, from the GI tract within 4 to 10 hours. Since only one worm is usually present in Taenia infections, the discovery of the scolex (head and neck) in the stool usually indicates that the client is cured.

c. **Administration for Treatment** of H. nana, H. diminuta, and D. caninum. The initial treatment of these tapeworms is the same as for Taenia infections above. However, on the following three days after the initial treatment, 100-mg (adult dose) of quinacrine, three times daily, must be administered. It may be necessary to repeat the entire course of treatment 2 weeks later.

d. **Adverse Effects**. The use of quinacrine may result in toxic reactions such as gastrointestinal upset, skin eruptions, and mental disorders. These effects are reversible when administration of the drug is stopped. The client's skin and his urine may become stained yellow, although these effects are not toxic.

e. **Cautions and Warnings**. The drug should not be given to clients with a history of psychosis or to people with psoriasis. It is also contraindicated in clients who are receiving primaquine. It should not be given to pregnant women because this drug readily reaches the fetus.

f. **Supply**. Quinacrine (Atabrine) is available as 100-mg quinacrine hydrochloride tablets.

6-34. TETRACHLOROETHYLENE

a. **Indications**. Tetrachloroethylene (perchloroethylene) is an alternate drug of choice for treating Heterophyes heterophyes (intestinal fluke).

b. **Usual Dosage**. A single dose of 0.12-ml/kg of body weight up to a maximum of 5-ml is given in capsule form. The client should be kept on bed rest for 4 hours following therapy. A purge should not be given as it may increase side effects and reduce effectiveness of the drug. The client must avoid alcohol and fatty foods 24 hours prior to and also after therapy. Food should be withheld during the day of therapy. Two or more treatments at 4- to 7-day intervals may be necessary to effect a complete cure.

c. **Adverse Effects**. This drug is relatively free of side effects if administered correctly. Nausea, vomiting, abdominal cramping, dizziness, and drowsiness may occur. Fainting and hypotensive episodes have been reported in severely anemic clients.

d. **Cautions and Warnings**.

(1) It should not be taken with fatty foods or alcohol as they will increase the systemic absorption of tetrachloroethylene and side effects.

(2) It should not be used in the treatment of small, severely ill children.

(3) It is contraindicated in pregnancy, hepatic disease, gastroenteritis, alcoholism, and clients undergoing heavy metal therapy.

(4) It should be stored in a cool dark place; broken capsules should not be used.

(5) Stool specimens should be checked at the end of a week to determine effectiveness of therapy.

e. **Supply**. Tetrachloroethylene is supplied in 1-ml capsules.

6-35. THIABENDAZOLE

a. **Indications**. Thiabendazole (Mintezol) is the drug of choice for the treatment of Strongyloides stercoralis (threadworm) and cutaneous larva migrans (creeping eruption, a type of nematode also), and it may be effective in the treatment of trichinosis and visceral larva migrans.

b. **Usual Dosage**. For the treatment of threadworm and cutaneous larva migrans, the usual dose is 25-mg/kg twice daily for 2 days. The maximum single dose is 1.5-grams, and the maximum total daily dose is 3.0-grams. If necessary, the course of treatment may be repeated 1 week later. For the treatment of trichinosis, the current dosage is the same as for threadworm, but the drug may be continued as long as 4 days.

c. **Adverse Reactions**. Common side effects include dizziness, anorexia, nausea, and vomiting. Less common side effects are diarrhea, abdominal cramping pains, headache, lethargy, drowsiness, and pruritus. Bradycardia, hypotension, visual disturbances, perianal rashes, tinnitus, and paresthesias occur rarely. Occasionally, the client's urine has an unaccustomed odor during treatment and 24 hours thereafter. Leukopenia, crystalluria, and hematuria have been occasionally reported, but all subsided when treatment with thiabendazole was discontinued.

d. **Contraindications and Cautions**. Experience is very limited in the effects of thiabendazole upon children weighing less than 15-kg. Alternate drugs may be indicated when there is hepatic dysfunction. Thiabendazole must be used with caution when drug-induced vomiting may be dangerous. If ascarids are present, they may become hypermotile and appear at the nose or mouth. Thiabendazole should not be used when complete mental alertness is required.

e. **Supply**. Thiabendazole is supplied as an oral suspension containing 500 mg in each 5-ml.

6-36. PRAZIQUANTEL

a. **Indications**. Praziquantel increases cell membrane permeability in worms, resulting in a loss of intracellular calcium, massive contractions, and paralysis of the worm's musculature. It is indicated in the treatment of infections caused by <u>Schistosoma mekongi</u>, <u>S. japonicum</u>, <u>S. mansoni</u>, and <u>S. hematobium</u> (blood flukes).

b. **Usual dosage**. Praziquantel tablets should be swallowed with some liquid during meals. Tablets should not be chewed. Three doses should be administered as a 1-day treatment in doses of 20-mg/kg. The interval between doses should not be less than 4 hours and not more than 6 hours. Dosage for children under 4 years of age has not been established.

c. **Cautions and Warnings**.

(1) Safety in pregnancy has not been established.

(2) Praziquantel appears in breast milk. Women should not nurse on the day of treatment and during the subsequent 72 hours.

(3) Safety and efficacy in children under 4 years of age have not been established.

d. **Adverse Reactions**. Praziquantel is well tolerated and side effects are usually mild. The most frequently reported side effects are malaise, headache, dizziness, and abdominal discomfort.

e. **Supply**. Praziquantel (Biltricide) is supplied as 600 mg film-coated tablets.

Section VI. OTHER AGENTS

6-37. METRONIDAZOLE

a. **Indications**. Metronidazole (Flagyl) is indicated in protozoal infections caused by the following organisms:

(1) Trichomonas vaginalis in both males and females.

(2) Giardia lamblia.

(3) Entamoeba histolytica (a species of amebas).

b. **Usual Dosage**.

(1) Trichomoniasis--concurrent treatment of sexual partners:

(a) Female--one tablet three times a day for 10 days.

(b) Male--one tablet twice a day for 10 days.

(2) Giardiasis--two courses of metronidazole therapy: 500-mg daily for 5 days, repeated after a 15-day interval.

(3) Amebiasis (infection with amebas, especially E. histolytica, both intestinal infections and hepatic abscesses: 750-mg three times a day for 5 to 10 days.

c. **Adverse Reactions**. There is a low incidence of untoward effects. Nausea, vomiting, a metallic taste, and a darkening of the urine are the most commonly reported side effects.

d. **Cautions and Warnings**.

(1) Metronidazole is inactive against Candida albicans infections.

(2) A total decrease in leukocytes has been reported with therapy. Total and differential white blood cell counts should be made, especially if the client needs to undergo a second course of therapy.

(3) Clients should be warned not to consume alcohol while receiving metronidazole; it may lead to a reaction characterized by flushing, nausea and vomiting, and a feeling of impending doom.

(4) It is well tolerated in pregnancy, but should be used with caution during the first trimester.

e. **Supply**. Metronidazole is supplied as 250-mg tablets.

6-38. GAMMA BENZENE HEXACHLORIDE (LINDANE)

Gamma benzene hexachloride (Kwell, lindane) is very effective in the treatment of both scabies ("itch" mite) and pediculosis (lice and "crabs"). When used to treat scabies, a thin layer of the cream is rubbed into the skin from the neck to the soles of the feet (15- to 25-grams for an adult). The cream is to be left on the client for a full 24 hours before being removed. No water is to be used on the client during this time. After this 24-hour period, the client should bathe and put on clean clothing. Pruritis (itching) is usually relieved after 24 hours, and there is rarely a need for a second application. However, if necessary, a second and third application may be made at weekly intervals. Gamma benzene hexachloride is both effective and safe to use where there is secondary infection of the skin. However, subsequent treatment with a bactericide may be needed to clear up the infection. When used in the treatment of pediculosis, the cream is applied to the area that is infected with the lice (head, body, or pubic region) and is washed off the following day. A single application is usually sufficient. The drug is supplied as a 1 percent cream packaged in 60-gram containers.

Continue with Exercises

EXERCISES, LESSON 6

INSTRUCTIONS: Answer the following exercises by marking the lettered response that best answers the exercise or completes the incomplete statement.

After you have completed all of these exercises, turn to "Solutions to Exercises" at the end of the lesson and check your answers. For each exercise answered incorrectly, reread the material referenced with the solution.

1. For systematic effect, streptomycin is given by which of the following routes?

   a. Any of the below

   b. Orally

   c. Rectally

   d. Intramuscularly

2. Which of the following untoward effects may occur with the use of streptomycin?

   a. Deafness

   b. Blindness

   c. Loss of speech

   d. Loss of sense of touch

3. Personnel preparing streptomycin solutions should wear rubber gloves to protect themselves from:

   a. Resistant organisms

   b. Allergic reactions

   c. Systemic absorption of the drug

   d. Discoloration of their hands

4. Which of the following factors is likely to produce toxic effects when streptomycin is being administered?

   a. Giving it without food or milk

   b. Giving it at mealtime

   c. Giving it over a prolonged time

   d. Giving it with another antibiotic

5. Which of the following drugs exhibits ototoxic effects?

   a. All of the below

   b. Streptomycin

   c. Kanamycin

   d. Gentamicin

   e. Neomycin

6. Bacitracin is most frequently administered in which of the following ways?

   a. IM

   b. IV

   c. Orally

   d. Topically

7. Bacitracin is effective primarily against:

   a. Gram-negative bacteria

   b. Gram-positive bacteria

   c. Rickettsiae

   d. Viruses

8. A sulfonamide commonly used for treatment of infections of the genitourinary tract is:

   a. Nystatin

   b. Griseofulvin

   c. Sulfisoxazole

   d. Sulfacetamide

9. Crystalluria may be a complication of treatment with which of the following drugs?

   a. Kanamycin

   b. Primaquine

   c. Sulfisoxazole

   d. Streptomycin

10. How is griseofulvin administered?

    a. Orally

    b. Rectally

    c. Topically

    d. Parenterally

11. Tolnaftate is used topically in the treatment of athlete's foot, ringworm, and other fungal infections. However, if the scalp, nails, palms, or soles are infected, which of the following oral preparation is indicated.

    a. Nystatin

    b. Griseofulvin

    c. Sulfisoxazole

    d. Iodochlorhydroxyquin and hydrocortisone

12. Which of the following drugs is indicated in the treatment of candidiasis?

    a. Tolnaftate

    b. Nystatin

    c. Griseofulvin

    d. Selenium sulfide

13. Which of the following is indicated in the treatment of common dandruff, seborrheic dermatitis, and tinea versicolor?

    a. Nystatin

    b. Selenium sulfide

    c. Undecylenic acid

    d. Iodochlorhydroxyquin and hydrocortisone

14. At the time that an infected <u>Anopheles</u> mosquito bites a person, the malaria parasite introduced into the person is called a:

    a. Merozoite

    b. Gametocyte

    c. Schizont

    d. Sporozoite

    e. Zygote

15. The clinical symptoms of malaria occur during the part of the life cycle of the malaria parasite when it is called:

   a. A merozoite

   b. An ookinete

   c. A gametocyte

   d. A schizont

   e. A sporozoite

16. A particular antimalarial drug, which falls into only one of the categories below, will relieve symptoms of malaria, but it will not cure or prevent an infection with one of the relapsing malarias. It is a:

   a. Primary tissue schizonticide

   b. Secondary tissue schizonticide

   c. Blood schizonticide

   d. Gametocide

   e. Sporonticide

17. A CP tablet is taken once every:

   a. Hour

   b. Day

   c. Week

   d. Month

18. What is the preferred method for the administration of chloroquine?

a. Oral

b. Subcutaneous

c. Intramuscular

d. Intravenous

19. When chloroquine is given orally to treat malaria, a course of treatment consists of:

a. 4 doses

b. 8 doses

c. 16 doses

d. 24 doses

20. According to some authorities, which drug is responsible for blackwater fever?

a. Quinine

b. Quinacrine

c. Primaquine

d. Chloroquine

21. Which of the following dose regimens of chloroquine phosphate would ordinarily be sufficient to produce a significant danger of eye damage?

a. A weekly dose of 500 mg given for long-term prophylaxis

b. A total of 2.5 gm given in divided doses over a period of 3 days

c. Large doses given in short-term treatment

d. Large doses given chronically

22. A drug that is effective in preventing transmission of malaria because it kills the sexual form of the parasite is:

    a. Chloroquine

    b. Quinine

    c. Quinacrine

    d. Primaquine

23. What drug is used for the treatment of leprosy and, in combination with quinine and pyrimethamine, for chloroquine-resistant falciparum malaria?

    a. Chloroquine

    b. Primaquine

    c. Quinacrine

    d. Dapsone

24. The blood schizonticide quinine is used to treat acute attacks of malaria resistant to which drug?

    a. Chloroquine

    b. Dapsone

    c. Primaquine

    d. Quinacrine

25. What is the drug of choice for treating the giant intestinal roundworm?

    a. Niclosamide

    b. Mebendazole

    c. Quinacrine

    d. Thiabendazole

26. Which of the following drugs should not be given concurrently with quinacrine?

a. Quinine

b. Chloroquine

c. Primaquine

d. Metronidazole

27. A drug that stains tapeworms yellow is:

a. Quinacrine

b. Quinine

c. Piperazine citrate

d. Pyrantel pamoate

28. The disease that results from infection with E. histolytica is:

a. Amebiasis

b. Typhoid fever

c. Rocky Mountain spotted fever

d. Typhus fever

29. When gamma benzene hexachloride is applied to treat scabies, the person should not bathe until after:

a. 4 hours

b. 12 hours

c. 24 hours

d. 3 days

Check Your Answers on Next Page

SOLUTIONS TO EXERCISES, LESSON 6

1. d (para 6-2b)
2. a (para 6-2d(1))
3. b (para 6-2d(2))
4. c (para 6-2d(1), (2))
5. a (paras 6-1; 6-2d(1); 6-3d(2); 6-4a; 6-5)
6. d (para 6-5)
7. b (para 6-5)
8. c (para 6-8a(1))
9. c (para 6-8c(2), d(3))
10. a (para 6-11b)
11. b (para 6-12a)
12. b (para 6-13a)
13. b (para 6-15a)
14. d (fig. 6-1)
15. a (para 6-17b, fig. 6-1)
16. c (para 6-18a(3))
17. c (para 6-19b(1))
18. a (para 6-20b)
19. a (para 6-20b(2))
20. a (para 6-23c(3))
21. d (para 6-20d(2))

22. d (paras 6-17b; 6-18b(1); 6-21a)

23. d (paras 6-22a; 6-23a; 6-24a)

24. a (para 6-23a)

25. b (paras 6-27a(1), 6-31a)

26. c (paras 6-33e, 6-21c)

27. a (para 6-33b)

28. a (para 6-37b(3))

29. c (para 6-38)

END OF LESSON 6